Basic Sciences for
Dental Students

Basic Sciences for Dental Students

Edited by Simon A. Whawell and Daniel W. Lambert

School of Clinical Dentistry,
University of Sheffield,
Sheffield, UK

WILEY Blackwell

Registered Office(s)
John Wiley & Sons, Inc., 111 River Street, Hoboken, NJ 07030, USA
John Wiley & Sons Ltd, The Atrium, Southern Gate, Chichester, West Sussex, PO19 8SQ, UK

Editorial Office
The Atrium, Southern Gate, Chichester, West Sussex, PO19 8SQ, UK

For details of our global editorial offices, customer services, and more information about Wiley products visit us at www.wiley.com.

Wiley also publishes its books in a variety of electronic formats and by print-on-demand. Some content that appears in standard print versions of this book may not be available in other formats.

Library of Congress Cataloging-in-Publication Data

Names: Whawell, Simon A., 1965– editor. | Lambert, Daniel W., 1976– editor.
Title: Basic sciences for dental students / edited by Simon A. Whawell, Daniel W. Lambert.
Description: First edition. | Hoboken, NJ : Wiley, 2018. | Includes bibliographical references and index. |
Identifiers: LCCN 2017033954 (print) | LCCN 2017035293 (ebook) | ISBN 9781118906095 (pdf) |
    ISBN 9781118906088 (epub) | ISBN 9781118905579 (pbk.)
Subjects: | MESH: Dentistry–methods | Biological Science Disciplines | Dental Care
Classification: LCC RK76 (ebook) | LCC RK76 (print) | NLM WU 100 | DDC 617.60071/1–dc23
LC record available at https://lccn.loc.gov/2017033954

Cover Design: Wiley
Cover Image: Courtesy of Heather Wallis

Set in 10/12pt Warnock by SPi Global, Pondicherry, India
Printed and bound in Singapore by Markono Print Media Pte Ltd

10 9 8 7 6 5 4 3 2 1

Contents

List of Contributors

Fiona M. Boissonade
School of Clinical Dentistry,
University of Sheffield,
Sheffield, UK

Aileen Crawford
School of Clinical Dentistry,
University of Sheffield,
Sheffield, UK

Paula M. Farthing
School of Clinical Dentistry,
University of Sheffield,
Sheffield, UK

Paul V. Hatton
School of Clinical Dentistry,
University of Sheffield,
Sheffield, UK

Stuart Hunt
School of Clinical Dentistry,
University of Sheffield,
Sheffield, UK

Peter P. Jones
Otago School of Medical Sciences,
University of Otago,
Dunedin, New Zealand

Daniel W. Lambert
School of Clinical Dentistry,
University of Sheffield,
Sheffield, UK

Cheryl A. Miller
School of Clinical Dentistry,
University of Sheffield,
Sheffield, UK

Angela H. Nobbs
Bristol Dental School,
University of Bristol,
Bristol, UK

Gordon B. Proctor
King's College London Dental Institute,
London, UK

Alistair J. Sloan
School of Dentistry,
University of Cardiff,
Cardiff, UK

John J. Taylor
School of Dental Sciences,
Newcastle University,
Newcastle upon Tyne, UK

Abigail S. Tucker
Department of Craniofacial
Development and Stem Cell Biology,
King's College London,
London, UK

Simon A. Whawell
School of Clinical Dentistry,
University of Sheffield,
Sheffield, UK

About the Companion Website

Don't forget to visit the companion website for this book:

www.wiley.com/go/whawell/basic_sciences_for_dental_students

There you will find valuable material designed to enhance your learning, including:

1) Figures from the book available for download
2) MCQs to test your knowledge

Scan this QR code to visit the companion website:

1

Biomolecules

Daniel W. Lambert and Simon A. Whawell

School of Clinical Dentistry, University of Sheffield, Sheffield, UK

Learning Objectives

- To understand the basis of molecular structure and bonding.
- To outline the basic structure and function of proteins, carbohydrates, lipids and nucleic acids.
- To be able to describe the biological role of enzymes and explain how their activity is regulated.
- To understand basic energy-yielding pathways and how they are controlled.

Clinical Relevance

An understanding of basic biomolecule structure and function provides a foundation for all normal cell and tissue structure and physiology. The structure of biomolecules present in the human body closely relates to their function, as is the case for cells and tissues. In disease, drugs can be used that target specific biochemical pathways, so an appreciation of biochemistry underlies patient care as well as the diagnosis, prognosis and treatment of disease.

Introduction

As complex as the human body is, it is heavily dependent on just four atoms for its composition: carbon, hydrogen, nitrogen and oxygen. These atoms form structurally diverse groups of biologically important molecules, their structure always relating to their function in the same way that the cells and tissues of the body are adapted. Biomolecules commonly take part in relatively simple reactions which are subject to complex control to finely tune the essential processes that they mediate. Biomolecules are often large polymers made up from smaller molecular monomers and even though there are thousands of molecules in a cell there are relatively few major biomolecule classes. Fatty acids, monosaccharides, amino acids and nucleotides form di- and triglycerides, polysaccharides, proteins and nucleic acids respectively. Small molecules are also important to biology, as we will see; adenosine triphosphate (ATP), for example,

Basic Sciences for Dental Students, First Edition. Edited by Simon A. Whawell and Daniel W. Lambert.
© 2018 John Wiley & Sons Ltd. Published 2018 by John Wiley & Sons Ltd.
Companion website: www.wiley.com/go/whawell/basic_sciences_for_dental_students

stores energy for catabolic and anabolic process and nicotinamide adenine dinucleotide (NADH) is the principle electron donor in the respiratory electron transport chain.

Biological Bonding

Molecular bonds are dependent on the arrangement of electrons in the outermost shell of each atom, being most stable when this is full. This can be achieved by transferring electrons, which takes place in ionic bonding (e.g. NaCl) or by sharing electrons in a covalent bond. Biological systems are also crucially dependent on **non-covalent bonds**, namely hydrogen bonds (or H bonds), electrostatic interactions and van der Waals' forces. While these 'bonds' are associated with at least an order of magnitude lower energy than covalent bonds they are collectively strong and can have significant influence on biological reactions. Non-covalent bonds differ in their geometry, strength and specificity. Hydrogen bonds are the strongest and form when hydrogen that is covalently linked to an electronegative atom such as oxygen or nitrogen has an attractive interaction with another electronegative atom. They are highly directional and are strongest when the atoms involved are co-linear. Hydrogen bonds are important in the stabilization of biomolecules such as DNA and in the secondary structure of proteins. Charged groups within biomolecules can be electrostatically attracted to each other. Amino acids, as we will discuss later, can be charged and such electrostatic interactions are important in enzyme–substrate interactions. The presence of competing charged ions such as those in salt would weaken such interactions. Finally, the weakest of the non-covalent interactions is the non-specific attraction called the van der Waals' force. This results from transient asymmetry of charge distribution around a molecule which, by encouraging such asymmetry in surrounding molecules, results in an attractive interaction. Such forces only come into play when molecules are in close proximity and although weak can be of significance when a number of them form simultaneously.

Water, Water Everywhere

The human body is of course comprised mostly of water but it is worth mentioning the profound effects that water has on biological interactions. Two properties of water are particularly important in this regard, namely its **polar nature** and **cohesion**. A water molecule has a triangular shape and the polarity comes from the partial positive charge exhibited by the hydrogen atom and the partial negative charge of the oxygen. The cohesive properties of water are due to the presence of hydrogen bonding (Figure 1.1). Water is an excellent solvent for polar molecules and does this by weakening/competing for hydrogen bonds and electrostatic interactions. In biology, water-free microenvironments must be created for polar interactions to have maximum strength.

Amino Acids and Proteins

Proteins are **polymers of amino acids** and are the most **abundant** and **structurally and functionally diverse** group of biomolecules. They form structural elements within the cell and extracellular matrix, act as transport and signalling molecules, interact to enable muscles to contract and form the biological catalysts (enzymes) without which most cell functions would cease. Amino acids consist of a tetrahedral alpha C atom (Cα) attached to a hydrogen atom, amine and carboxyl groups and a substituted side group (R) (Figure 1.2a), which can be anything from

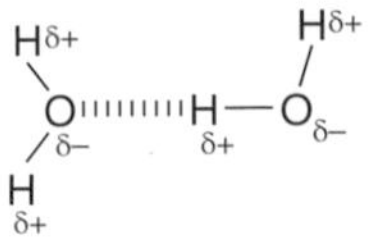

Figure 1.1 The chemical structure of water.

(a)

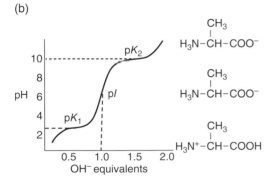

(b)

Figure 1.2 (a) Peptide bond and (b) amino acid ionization.

a hydrogen atom to a more complicated structure. Amino acids are chiral and in biology all are the left-handed (L) isomers. Many possible amino acid structures exist but only 20 occur naturally and are used for protein synthesis. Some of these are synthesized in the body from other precursors and some amino acids have to come from our diet (called essential amino acids). Amino acids can be broken down to form glucose as an energy source and can also act as precursors for other molecules such as neurotransmitters.

Urea Cycle

Amino acids cannot be stored or secreted directly so must be broken down prior to their removal from the body. Their carbon skeletons may be converted to glucose (**glucogenic** amino acids) or acetyl-CoA or acetoacetate (**ketogenic**), which can be fed into the tricarboxylic acid (TCA) cycle, generating energy. The **nitrogen** is then removed in three steps starting with transfer of the amino group (transamination) to glutamate which is then converted to ammonia by glutamate dehydrogenase in the liver. Finally **ammonia** enters the urea cycle, a series of

five main biochemical reactions that results in the formation of urea, which is excreted in urine. The urea cycle is a good example of a disposal system where 'feed-forward' regulation through allosteric activation of the enzymes involved results in a higher rate of urea production if there is a higher rate of ammonia production (see Allosterism later in this chapter). This is important given that ammonia is toxic and also explains why a high-protein diet and fasting, which results in protein breakdown, induce urea cycle enzymes.

Amino Acid Ionization

The amide and carboxyl groups and some side chains of amino acids are **ionizable** and their state is dependent on the pH (Figure 1.2b). If you were to titrate an amino acid, at low pH all groups are protonated, the amino group carries a positive charge and the carboxyl group is uncharged. As the pH increases the proton dissociates from the carboxyl group, half being in this form at the first pK value of around pH 2 (pK_1 on Figure 1.2b). As the pH increases further the amino acid is zwitterionic with both positive and negatively charged groups. As the net charge is zero this is the **isolectric point** of an amino acid (pI on Figure 1.2b). At the second pK of pH 9 (pK_2 on Figure 1.2b) half of the amine groups carry charge and the overall charge is negative. Titration curves for amino acids are not linear around the pK values as there is resistance to changes in pH as the amino acids act as weak buffers. If there is an ionizable side chain present there would be a third pK value; acidic amino acids lose a proton at pH 4 and thus have a negative charge at neutral pH. For basic amino acids this occurs around pH 10 and thus such amino acids are positively charged at neutral pH.

Classification of Amino Acids

As the only difference between amino acids is the nature of the substituted side chain this determines the characteristics of the

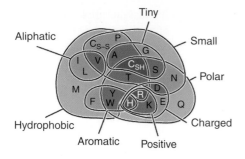

Figure 1.3 Classification of amino acids. Note that amino acids can be referred to using one- or three-letter codes. This figure uses the former; so C represents cysteine, which in the three-letter code would be Cys. SH is the thiol group of cysteine that can react to form a disulphide bridge (represented elsewhere by S–S) with another cysteine residue.

amino acid, such as the **shape, size, charge, chemical reactivity** and **hydrogen bonding** capability. This ultimately determines the structure and function of the protein polymer that the amino acids form. Amino acids can be classified according to their structure or chemical nature; the latter is summarized in Figure 1.3. Polar amino acids have uneven charge distribution even though they have no overall charge. The hydroxyl and amide groups are capable of hydrogen bonding with water or each other and thus these amino acids are hydrophilic and often found on the surface of water-soluble globular proteins. Cysteine is often included in this group and is very important in protein structure as it can from covalent disulphide bonds with other amino acids in the protein polymer. Tyrosine is an aromatic amino acid containing a six-carbon phenyl ring but as this contains a hydroxyl group capable of hydrogen bonding it is polar. Non-polar amino acids have side chains with evenly distributed electrons and therefore do not form hydrogen bonds. They tend to form hydrophobic cores within proteins. Phenylalanine and tryptophan are aromatic and methionine contains sulphur. Aspartate and glutamate have carboxylic groups that carry a negative charge at neutral pH, which is why they are referred to as '-ate' and not acid. Their presence in a protein would impart a negative charge that would allow electrostatic interactions to take place. Three amino acids carry a positive charge at neutral pH and these are highly hydrophilic. Lysine and arginine are always charged at biological pH, but histidine has a pK close to neutral pH and thus its charge is dependent on the local environment. It is this feature that gives this amino acid an important role in the active site of enzymes.

Peptide Bonding

Amino acids form protein polymers through a condensation reaction resulting in the formation of a **peptide bond** between the carboxyl group of one amino acid and the amine group of another (Figure 1.2a). The sequence of amino acids in the resultant protein is determined by the genetic code of the messenger RNA (mRNA) with the average protein having approximately 300 amino acids. The peptide bond is rigid and the atoms are in the same geometric plane; there is, however, considerable flexibility around the bond which has a significant effect on protein structure. Peptide bonds are very stable and are only physiologically broken by proteolytic enzymes.

Protein Structure

Whether they are globular, fibrous or span the cell membrane, proteins take part in highly specific interactions the nature of which is intimately associated with the **conformation** and **shape** of the protein. The structure provides binding sites for these specific interactions and determines the flexibility, solubility and stability of the protein (Feature box 1.1). Protein structure is influenced by the amino acid sequence and character of the side chains in particular. Cysteine, as we have mentioned previously, carries out a special role in the formation of disulphide linkages and hydrogen bonding is very important in protein structure. Water influences shape as proteins will naturally fold with hydrophilic residues exposed to the aqueous environment and hydrophobic residues hidden away inside the protein. **Chaperones** are barrel-shaped proteins that also assist in the folding of some proteins and by overcoming kinetic barriers to folding and providing a water-free micro-environment and template. The structure of proteins is often divided into the following levels: the **primary** structure refers to the linear sequence of amino acids, the **secondary** structure relates to how this sequence is formed into regular structures such as helices or sheets and the **tertiary** structure is how the secondary structure is folded in three dimensions (Figure 1.4). Finally some proteins have a **quaternary** structure which is the spatial arrangement of individual polypeptide subunits.

Posttranslational Modifications

Additions are commonly made to amino acids after they have been formed into proteins which can significantly change their properties. **Glycosylation** is the addition of carbohydrate and acts as a 'tag'. **Phosphorylation** is the addition of phosphate to serine, tyrosine and threonine which by adding a significant negative charge changes the local structure of the protein allowing it to be recognized by other molecules. Intracellular signalling pathways are often cascades of phosphorylation reactions controlled by kinase enzymes that add phosphate and phosphatase enzymes that remove it. (See Other Regulatory Mechanisms later in this chapter.)

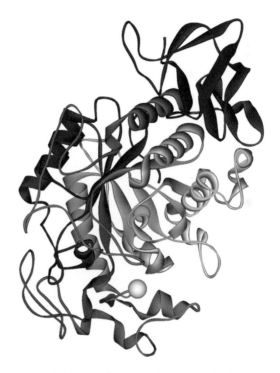

Figure 1.4 Three-dimensional structure of salivary amylase.

Enzymes

Enzymes are proteins that **catalyse** biological reactions; that is, they speed them up without themselves being permanently altered. They also regulate many of the biochemical pathways in which they play a role (see Control of Metabolism in this chapter). Enzymes bind **substrates** in their active sites and convert them into **products**. The substrates are bound to specific regions in the **active site**: these are the **functional groups** (in basic terms this means bits of the molecules which can have electrostatic interactions with the substrate) of the amino acids making up the substrate-binding site, or those of coenzymes and metal ions. This specificity of binding makes enzymes extremely selective for their substrates. In the course of any reaction, a transition-state complex is formed. This is an intermediate with the highest energy of any component of the reaction: the energy needed to overcome this to form the products is called the **activation energy**. Enzymes reduce the activation energy by stabilizing the complex, and thereby increase the rate of the reaction (Figure 1.5). This specificity can be exploited by drugs and toxins which potently and selectively inhibit enzymes. These can be covalent inhibitors, which form covalent bonds with functional groups in the active site, or transition-state analogues, which mimic the transition-state complex (Feature box 1.2).

Regulation of Enzyme Activity

pH and Temperature

The binding of substrate to the active site is determined by **electrostatic interactions**. Changes in pH alter the properties of functional groups within the active site and therefore change the interactions. Enzymes are hence very sensitive to pH, with different enzymes having different optimum pH values according to their function. As they are proteins with complex tertiary structures, enzymes are also sensitive to temperature. Basic thermodynamic principles dictate that

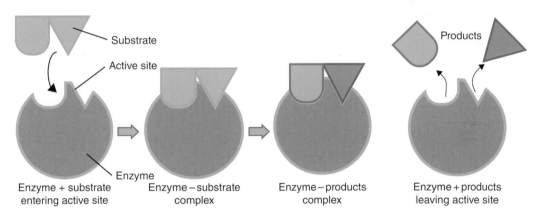

Enzyme + substrate entering active site — Substrate — Active site — Enzyme

Enzyme–substrate complex

Enzyme–products complex

Enzyme + products leaving active site — Products

Figure 1.5 Enzyme–substrate complexes and the transition state.

Feature box 1.2 Penicillin, a transition-state analogue

Penicillin is a widely used antibiotic, derived from the fungus *Penicillum*. The discovery of penicillin's antimicrobial properties is widely credited to the observation in 1925 by Alexander Fleming that contamination by *Penicillum* of culture plates on which a bacterium, *Staphylococcus*, was being grown, inhited the growth of the bacteria. Penicillin was subsequently isolated from the fungus and has been used to treat a wide range of infections for decades, although bacterial resistance to the drug is now widespread. Penicillin is effective as it inhibits a transpeptidase enzyme required to form bacterial cell walls, causing the bacteria to 'burst'. Penicillin inhibits the enzyme as it tightly binds to the transition-state complex formed during the transpeptidase-catalysed reaction, preventing the formation of products.

In the 1960s scientists were investigating whether bacteria could survive at high temperatures, in environments such as hot springs. They identified a species, *Thermus aquaticus*, which was found thriving at temperatures of 70°C in the geysers of Yellowstone National Park. The researchers quickly realized that to survive at this temperature the bacterium must have evolved enzymes that could function at temperatures that would denature most proteins. Later, the DNA polymerase enzyme catalysing replication of the bacterial DNA was isolated and developed for use in the polymerase chain reaction (PCR), a method now used in thousands of laboratories worldwide to amplify short sections of DNA.

the speed of the reactions will increase with temperature owing to increased substrate energy and probability of collisions, but in an enzyme-catalysed reaction this only occurs up to the point at which the temperature begins to break bonds within the enzyme; even small changes in the shape of the enzyme can interfere with substrate binding. Most enzymes function best below 40°C; however, some organisms living in deep-sea vents have enzymes that function at 95°C! (See Feature box 1.3.)

Substrate

The rate of all enzyme reactions is dependent on substrate concentration; they show saturation kinetics, with rate of reaction increasing with increasing substrate concentration (or [S]) until saturation, when maximum velocity (V_{max}) is reached. The relationship between substrate concentration and reaction velocity is described by the **Michaelis–Menton equation**:

$$v = V_{max}[S] / K_m + [S]$$

This equation is useful because the Michaelis constant (K_m) is a measure of the affinity an enzyme has for its substrate, and together with V_{max} can be used to determine the nature of a particular inhibitor, which may act in a competitive, non-competitive or uncompetitive manner (Figure 1.6).

Allosterism

Many enzymes are **allosteric**; that is, they are inhibited or activated by molecules binding to them at a site other than the active site (Figure 1.7). This binding alters the shape of the active site by changing the overall shape of the enzyme. Allosteric inhibitors can be either homotrophic (the substrate itself binds to the enzyme somewhere other than its active site) or heterotrophic (a molecule other than the substrate binds to the enzyme away from its active site). Allosteric regulation is particularly important in the regulation of metabolic pathways, which are often regulated by the rate of one key enzyme. In many pathways, this enzyme is regulated (often allosterically) by the end product of the pathway (see Control of Metabolism).

Other Regulatory Mechanisms

Enzymes can also be regulated in a variety of other ways. One of these is **covalent modification**, probably best illustrated by the addition of a phosphate group to an amino acid residue in the enzyme, which alters the shape of the active site. This **phosphorylation** is carried out by another enzyme called a kinase, and can be reversed by another type of enzyme, termed a phosphatase. It may sound a trifle unexciting but this is a big deal: virtually all cellular signalling processes are carried out by cascades of enzymes phosphorylating and dephosphorylating each other and defects in this are responsible for many diseases, particularly cancer. A closely related regulatory mechanism is through **protein–protein interactions**, which as you might surmise is alteration of enzymic activity caused by the binding of another protein.

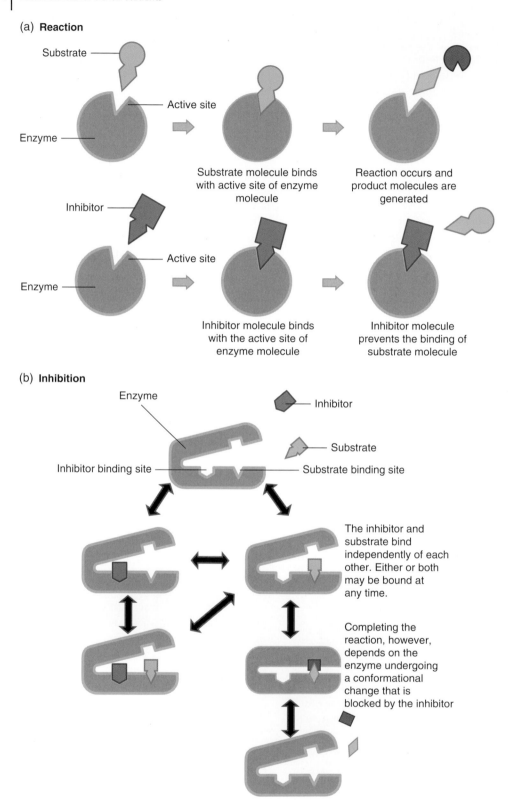

Figure 1.6 Mechanisms of enzyme inhibition. (a) Competitive inhibition. (b) Non-competitive inhibition.

(a) **Reaction**

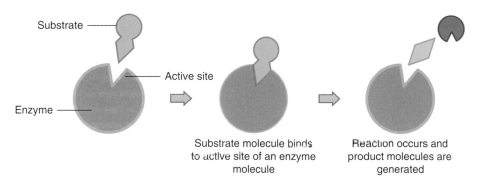

Substrate molecule binds
to active site of an enzyme
molecule

Reaction occurs and
product molecules are
generated

(b) **Inhibition**

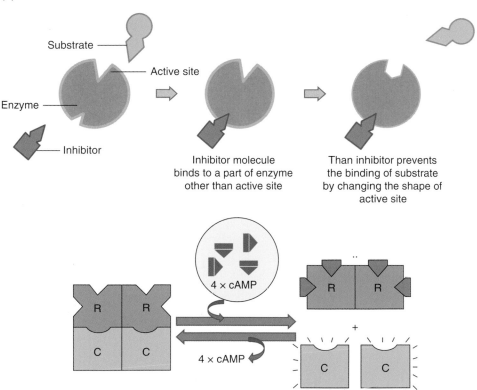

Inhibitor molecule
binds to a part of enzyme
other than active site

Than inhibitor prevents
the binding of substrate
by changing the shape of
active site

Figure 1.7 Allosteric regulation of protein kinase A.

A calcium-binding protein, calmodulin, is one of the proteins that do this and its importance is illustrated by the fact that it is present in large quantities in every type of cell and that it is evolutionarily ancient, being identical in nearly every species. Some enzymes are also regulated by being synthesized as an inactive 'zymogen', only becoming active when cut by another enzyme. This is often the case with proteases which would otherwise damage the cell in which they are synthesized.

Nucleic Acids

Deoxyribonucleic acid (**DNA**) contains all the information required to produce and maintain all the components of a cell. It comprises four bases – adenine (A), guanine (G), cytosine (C) and thymine (T) – each of which is bonded to a **deoxyribose**: each of these is termed a **nucleoside**. A nucleoside bound to a phosphate is termed a **nucleotide**, and nucleotides form a linear string along a **phosphate backbone** (Figure 1.8). It is the sequence of these four nucleotides that determines the sequence of every protein in the cell, which determines the function of the cell, which determines, ultimately, you. Two strands of nucleotides line up opposite each other, with each string going in the opposite direction; that is, one going 5′–3′ and one going 3′–5′ (termed antiparallel chains; Figure 1.9). The structure of the bases preferentially places adenine opposite thymine, and guanine opposite cytosine on the antiparallel chains; this allows the greatest

number of bonds to form (other combinations are possible, but this is generally undesirable). The two strands are coiled into a helix (called a **double helix** as there are two strands). The majority of the DNA in a human cell is contained within the nucleus; this is covered in more detail in Chapter 2.

The other major form in which nucleic acids are found in the cell is **ribonucleic acid** (**RNA**). RNA is also made up of chains of nucleosides, but in this case the base thymine is replaced by uracil. RNA does not form double-stranded helices but is instead a single-stranded molecule that can fold up on itself to form a wide array of structures. The sequence of RNA is copied from DNA by **transcription** (covered in more detail in Chapter 2), a process traditionally considered to produce three major types of RNA molecule – ribosomal RNA (rRNA), messenger RNA (mRNA) and transfer RNA (tRNA) – all of which play important roles in protein synthesis. In recent years, it has become apparent that many other forms of RNA exist, many of which have functions unrelated to protein synthesis (Feature box 1.4).

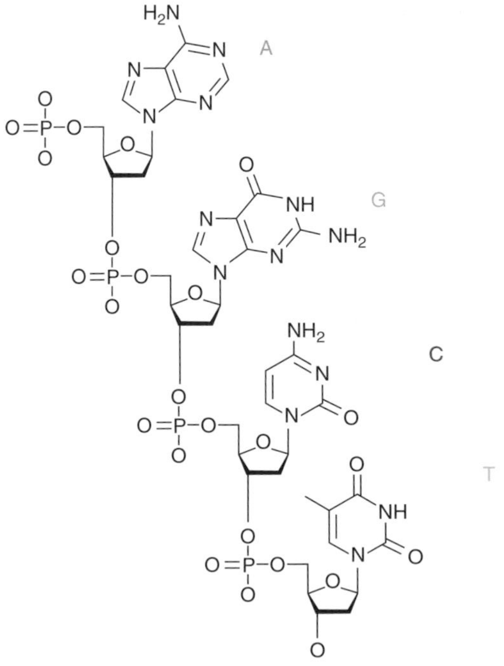

Figure 1.8 The structure of the four nucleotides of DNA.

Carbohydrates

The Structure of Carbohydrates

Carbohydrates are essential components of all living organisms and are the most abundant class of biological molecule. The basic carbohydrate unit is a **monosaccharide**. Monosaccharides are classified according to the chemical nature of their **carbonyl group** (the carbon in the aldehyde (aldoses) or ketone (ketoses) group) and the number of carbon atoms (e.g. hexose, 6C; heptose, 7C). The carbons in sugars with a ring structure are numbered in a clockwise manner, with the carbonyl carbon designated 1 (Figure 1.10). Monosaccharides form **disaccharides** by forming glycosidic linkages with other monosaccharides. Further linkages can be formed to form oligosaccharides and polysaccharides.

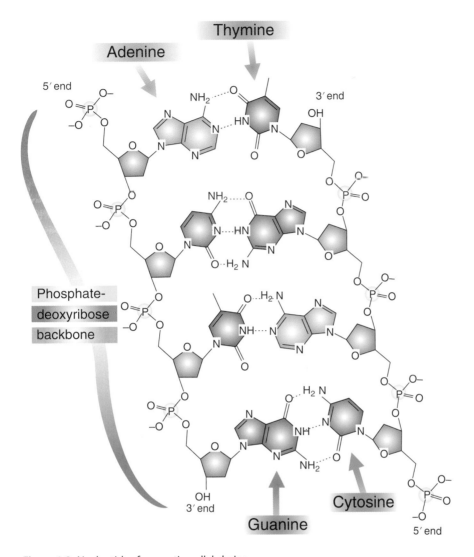

Figure 1.9 Nucleotides form antiparallel chains.

Feature box 1.4 Non-coding RNA, the dark matter of the cell

Scientists have long been puzzled that a large proportion of the human genome, perhaps as much as 95%, does not encode known proteins. In recent years it has become apparent that much of this DNA is transcribed into various types of non-coding RNA; collectively this is sometimes termed the 'dark matter' of the cell, as its function was until very recently largely unknown. Advances in RNA sequencing technology have now revealed that much of this RNA does appear to have an important functional role, and can be divided into many different classes of RNA, including lncRNA, miRNA and snoRNA. One of these lncRNAs, Xist, is critical in determining the sex of a developing embryo, and mutations in others have been found to occur in a number of diseases, but much is still not known of this uncharted RNA world.

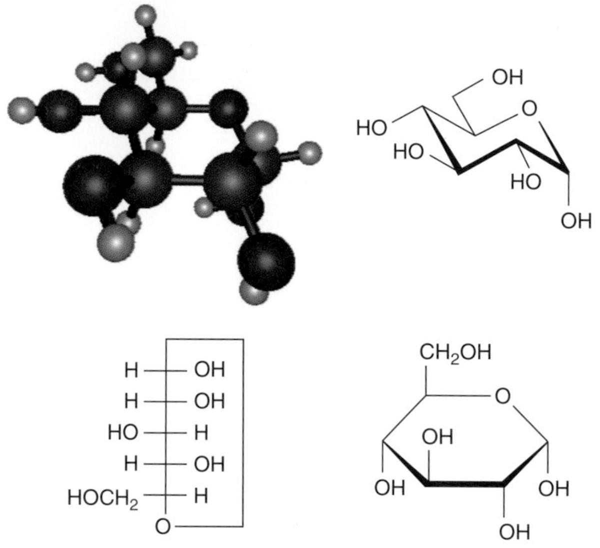

Figure 1.10 The structure of glucose.

Oligosaccharides and Polysaccharides

Monosaccharides are metabolized to provide energy (see sections Carbohydrates as a Fuel and The TCA Cycle for more on this) or, as just outlined, act as building blocks to form polysaccharides. Polysaccharides perform a wide variety of roles in the cell. They can be made up of either one type of monosaccharide (homopolysaccharide) or either more than one (heteropolysaccharide) and can form either linear or branched chains. A good example of a linear polysaccharide is cellulose, which is the main structural component of plant cell walls. The long chains of monosaccharides are heavily hydrogen-bonded to neighbouring chains and, in the plant cell wall, are embedded in a matrix of other polysaccharides, making it very strong and insoluble. A closely related polysaccharide, chitin, forms the exoskeleton of insects and crustaceans and has similar properties. As well as having structural roles, polysaccharides are also very important storage molecules. Starch, the storage molecule of plants, is made up of two polysaccharides: amylose and amylopectin. Amylose is a coiled string of glucose molecules whereas amylopectin is a heavily branched molecule.

Starch is partially digested by a salivary enzyme, amylase (see Figure 1.4), which hydrolyses the glycosidic bonds. In animals, carbohydrate storage is accomplished by glycogen, a heavily branched polysaccharide (much like amylopectin) that is hydrolysed by glycogen phosphorylase. Polysaccharides also occur as glycosaminoglycans. These are elastic, flexible molecules that are a component of cartilage, skin and tendons.

When biochemists were first purifying proteins they were often confounded by their preparations being contaminated with carbohydrates, causing problems when trying to solve their structure. This was the case until the 1960s when it was realized that the carbohydrate was not a contaminant but actually covalently linked to the protein. It has since become clear that most proteins (particularly intramembrane and secreted ones) are 'glycosylated'; that is, they are bound to carbohydrate molecules. The nature of these carbohydrate molecules tends to be quite variable (Figure 1.11). The glycoproteins perform diverse roles, from structural roles in connective tissue to modulating interactions with bacteria and intracellular signalling. Glycoproteins are also an important feature of bacterial cell walls.

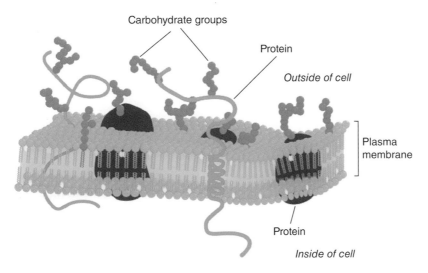

Figure 1.11 Protein glycosylation.

Carbohydrates as a Fuel

Every human cell is able to generate adenosine triphosphate (**ATP**) from **glycolysis**, even in anaerobic conditions. Glycolysis occurs in the cytoplasm and utilizes glucose; this is particularly important in the brain, which relies on glucose as its main source of fuel. The first step is the phosphorylation of glucose to glucose 6-phosphate by an enzyme, hexokinase. Each glucose 6-phosphate is oxidized by a series of reactions to two pyruvate molecules, generating two molecules of nicotinamide adenine dinucleotide (**NADH**) and two molecules of ATP (Figure 1.12). The ATP is generated by direct transfer of phosphate groups (**substrate-level phosphorylation**) rather than via oxidative phosphorylation (covered in the next section). In aerobic conditions, the pyruvate is then oxidized to produce CO_2 and ATP via the **tricarboxylic acid (TCA) cycle** and **oxidative phosphorylation** (this is explained in more detail below). In anaerobic conditions (for example, during intense exercise), cells have to resort to anaerobic glycolysis. This is necessary to regenerate the NAD required earlier in the glycolysis pathway, and involves reducing pyruvate to lactate. While necessary, this pathway is inefficient and will eventually produce enough lactate to cause **lactic acidaemia** (it makes your muscles burn a bit too). In certain situations, such as in a growing tumour, cells may preferentially undergo anaerobic respiration (Feature box 1.5).

The TCA Cycle

In the presence of oxygen, the pyruvate generated by glycolysis is first converted into **acetyl-CoA**. The pathways for oxidation of other fuels, including fatty acids, amino acids and ketone bodies, also produce acetyl-CoA, which then enters the tricarboxylic acid (TCA) cycle (sometimes known as the Krebs' cycle or the citric acid cycle). The TCA cycle accounts for the majority of ATP generated from fuel by oxidizing acetyl-CoA to the electron donors NADH and **FADH$_2$**, which enter the **electron transport chain**. The intermediates in the TCA cycle are shown in Figure 1.13, some of which are utilized for other biosynthetic reactions such as the production of amino acids and fatty acids. Overall, the TCA cycle is remarkably efficient: over 90% of the available energy from the oxidation of acetyl-CoA is conserved.

Adenosine Triphosphate (ATP)

ATP is the molecule used to drive most processes in the cell because of its high-energy

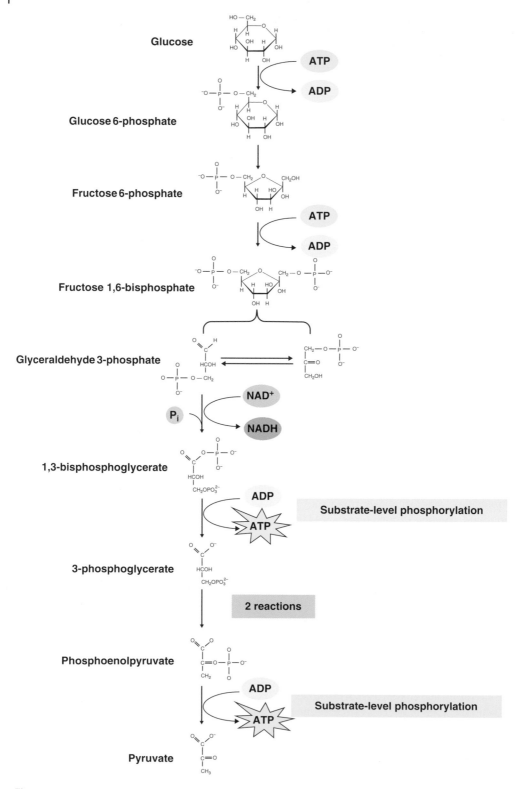

Figure 1.12 Glycolysis.

Feature box 1.5 The Warburg effect: glycolytic metabolism in cancer

Most cells predominantly generate ATP via oxidative phosphorylation under normal conditions, when oxygen is plentiful. Cancer cells, however, frequently utilize glycolysis to generate ATP, even in aerobic conditions, a phenomenon termed the Warburg effect, after Otto Warburg, who first proposed the hypothesis that this is a feature of cancer cells. Although the mechanisms underlying the effect are not fully understood, the high level of glycolysis in cancer cells is detected by positron emission tomography (PET), an imaging technique used to detect and monitor tumours.

---

phosphoanhydride bonds between the phosphate groups. Phosphate groups are negatively charged and repel each other; it requires a lot of energy to keep them together and this is released when one of the phosphate groups is released. The release of a phosphate group converts ATP to adenosine diphosphate (**ADP**) and drives most energy-dependent processes in the cell (Figure 1.14). ADP can then be converted back into ATP by **ATP synthase**, using reduced coenzymes formed during glycolysis and the TCA cycle, in the electron transport chain. This process is known as oxidative phosphorylation.

Oxidative Phosphorylation

As already seen, most of the energy generated in the TCA cycle is in the form of the reduced electron-accepting/-donating coenzymes NADH and FADH$_2$. In oxidative phosphorylation the electron transport chain oxidizes NADH and FADH$_2$ and donates the electron to O$_2$, which is reduced to H$_2$O. This is why it can only occur in aerobic conditions. The energy generated by this reduction is used to phosphorylate ADP. The net yield of all of this is approximately 2.5 moles of ATP per mole of NADH and 1.5 moles of ATP per mole FADH$_2$.

So how is the energy from the reduction of O$_2$ actually used to generate ATP? Well, this is rather clever. The electron transport chain contains proteins which span the inner membrane of the mitochondria (**protein complexes I**, **III** and **IV**). Electrons pass through these proteins via a series of oxidation–reduction reactions, simultaneously pumping **protons** (hydrogen ions) across the inner mitochondrial membrane (from matrix towards outside). This creates an electrochemical gradient, down which the protons return to the matrix, passing through a pore in ATP synthase, the enzyme responsible for synthesizing ATP. It is the change in conformation of ATP synthase caused by the passage of the protons which causes it to synthesize and release ATP. This process is also known as the **chemiosmotic model** of ATP synthesis (Figure 1.15). Uncoupling of proton movement from ATP generation, by allowing protons to leak back across the inner mitochondrial membrane into the matrix, generates heat and occurs in the brown fat cells of young babies and animals during hibernation for warmth.

Control of Metabolism

Metabolic pathways must be dynamic, able to respond to the changing energy needs of the cell and fuel availability. Cells must therefore be able to respond to changing environments, not just in isolation but as part of a particular tissue and the body as a whole. Cells therefore employ a remarkably complex array of regulatory systems to ensure everything runs smoothly. The most fundamental level of regulation of metabolic pathways is achieved by tight control of the activity of enzymes catalysing certain reactions within those pathways. The most tightly regulated enzymes are those involved in **irreversible reactions** that are effectively a point of no return; that is, to convert the product of the reaction back into the reactants is either impossible or inefficient for the cell to do. Perhaps the best example of this is found in glycolysis, in which the

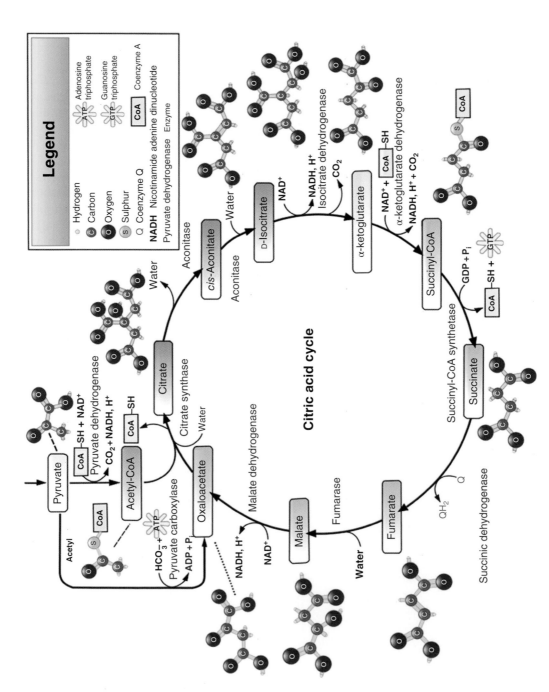

Figure 1.13 The TCA cycle.

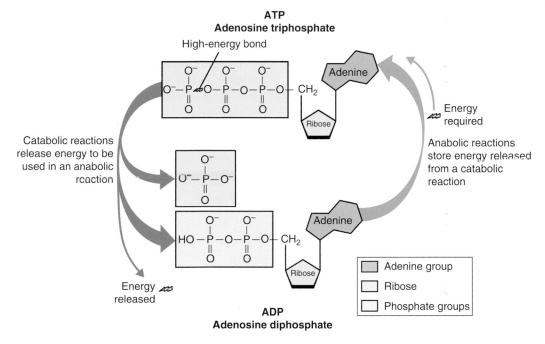

Figure 1.14 ATP structure and function.

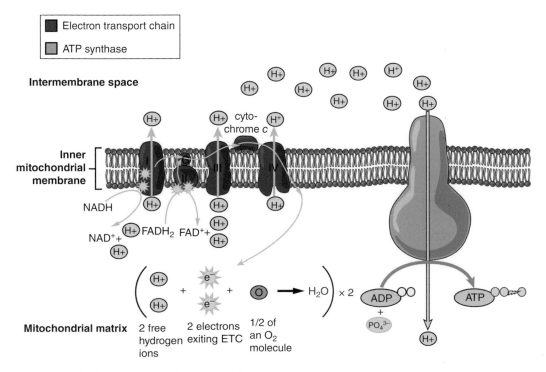

Figure 1.15 Oxidative phosphorylation and ATP synthesis.

enzyme phosphofructokinase-1 is subject to an array of allosteric regulation which either speeds up its activity (feed-forward allosteric activation), or slows it down (feedback allosteric inhibition). This is a classic example of an enzyme's activity being regulated according to the availability of substrate or product, and is summarized in (Figure 1.16). Other enzymes within the glycolysis pathway and the TCA cycle are regulated in a similar manner, or by covalent modification by phosphorylation (for example pyruvate dehydrogenase) or changes in the amount of a metabolic enzyme synthesized by a cell.

Lipids

The major remaining class of biomolecules to be considered is fats, more accurately known as lipids. Lipids are a diverse group of

molecules which share the property of being insoluble in water due to their **hydrophobic** nature. The most commonly encountered lipids are **fatty acids**, which may be of varying lengths, saturated or unsaturated, and are often found linked by ester bonds to **glycerol**, forming **triacylglycerols** (Figure 1.17). The major role of triacylglycerols is for storage; the body has essentially unlimited capacity to store triacylglycerols that can subsequently be used to release energy (see Metabolism in the Fed and Fasting States) as required. Fatty acids are also found linked to glycerol along with a phosphate group; this class of lipids, the **phospholipids**, are the main components of the membranes which surround cells and intracellular organelles (see Chapter 2). **Cholesterol** is another important lipid, playing a role in the structure of cell membranes (see Chapter 2) and circulating lipoproteins

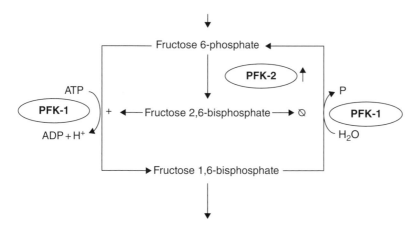

Figure 1.16 Regulation of phosphofructokinase.

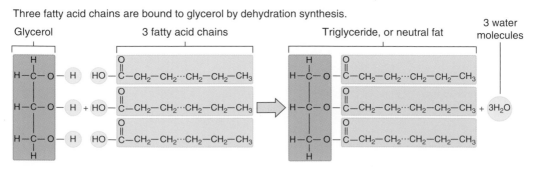

Figure 1.17 Structure of fatty acids and triacylglycerols.

(see Sources of Lipids), as well as being a precursor for the formation of bile salts, steroid hormones and vitamin D.

Sources of Lipids

Lipids may be obtained from the diet or synthesized from other biomolecules. Dietary lipids, largely in the form of triacylglycerols, are **emulsified** by bile salts secreted from the gall bladder, and digested by **lipases** released by the pancreas to form micelles of fatty acids and 2-monoacylglycerol, which can be absorbed by the cells lining the gut. Once absorbed, the triacylglycerols are reformed and packaged with proteins (apolipoproteins, or Apo), phospholipids and cholesterol to form chylomicrons, which are subsequently released into lymph vessels and ultimately the bloodstream (Figure 1.18).

Once circulating in the bloodstream, the lipids contained in chylomicrons are digested by **lipoprotein lipase** (LPL) present on the surface of cells such as adipose and muscle cells and activated by the lipoproteins present in the chylomicrons, and the triacylglycerols absorbed. The remnant components of the chylomicrons are recycled to the liver. Cholesterol may also be obtained from the diet by diffusion into the cells lining the gut or may be synthesized from **acetyl-CoA** (see Carbohydrates as a Fuel). The first step in

this sequence of reactions has become an important target of drugs to reduce circulating levels of cholesterol, which have been associated with heart disease. Triacylglycerols may also be synthesized in the liver from glucose, a key link between carbohydrate and lipid metabolism (see Metabolism in the Fed and Fasting States). Once synthesized, fatty acids are combined with apolipoproteins (derived from high-density lipoprotein, HDL), cholesterol and phospholipids to form very-low-density lipoprotein (VLDL), which is secreted from the liver into the bloodstream and digested by lipoprotein lipase on the surface of cells such as adipose cells and muscle cells to release fatty acids which are absorbed. The remnants of the VLDL, termed intermediate-density lipoprotein (IDL) and low-density lipoprotein (LDL), are recycled to the liver (Figure 1.19).

Metabolism in the Fed and Fasting States

In the fed state, most of our energy demands are met by the metabolism of glucose, or obtained from the bloodstream or from the digestion of glycogen (see Oligosaccharides and Polysaccharides). In the hours following a meal, the body gradually uses up these sources of glucose and must switch to alternative energy sources, predominantly fatty

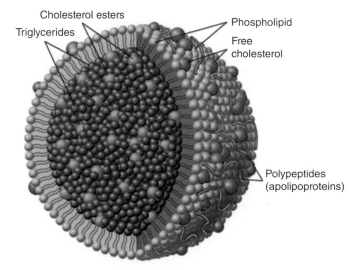

Figure 1.18 Absorption of lipids and packaging.

Cholesterol esters

Triglycerides

Phospholipid

Free cholesterol

Polypeptides (apolipoproteins)

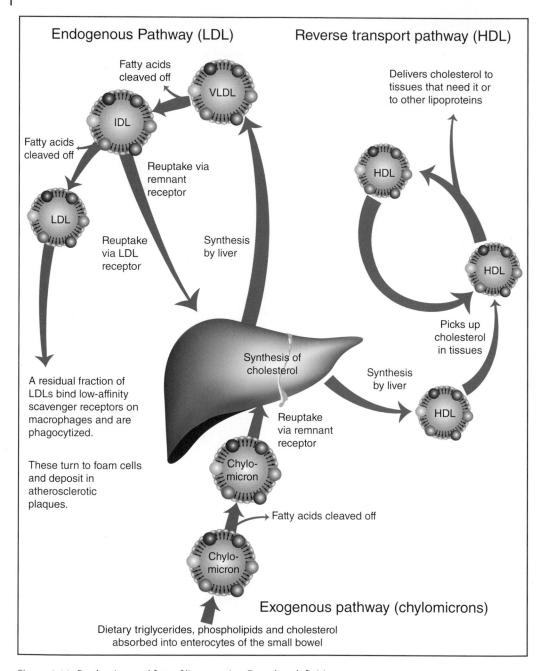

Figure 1.19 Production and fate of lipoproteins. For other definitions see text.

acids but ultimately other biomolecules such as amino acids. The levels of blood glucose are tightly controlled by two hormones secreted from the pancreas, **insulin** and **glucagon** (Feature box 1.6). When blood glucose levels drop, a high glucagon/insulin ratio stimulates the release of long-chain fatty acids from adipose tissue; these are absorbed by tissues such as muscle and converted, by a process called **beta-oxidation**, into acetyl-CoA which is then utilized in the TCA cycle to produce NADH and FADH$_2$

Feature box 1.6 Blood glucose homeostasis and diabetes

Maintenance of blood glucose levels is critical to prevent levels rising too high (hyperglycaemia) or too low (hypoglycaemia), both of which can be extremely dangerous. Glucose homeostasis is largely controlled by two hormones, insulin and glucagon, produced by the pancreas.

Diabetes results from the inability of the body to either produce insulin (type 1 diabetes mellitus) or respond (type 2 diabetes mellitus) to insulin, leading to poorly controlled blood glucose levels and resultant problems with vision, kidney failure and periodontal (gum) disease, among others.

(Figure 1.20). These reduced electron carriers subsequently enter the electron transport chain to generate ATP (see The TCA Cycle). In addition, low blood glucose in fasting conditions stimulates the release of glycerol from adipose tissue that can be utilized, in the liver, to generate glucose via **gluconeogenesis** (Figure 1.21). Gluconeogenesis is also able to synthesize glucose from other biomolecules such as amino acids, lactate (see Carbohydrates as a Fuel) and propionate, a short-chain fatty acid produced by the

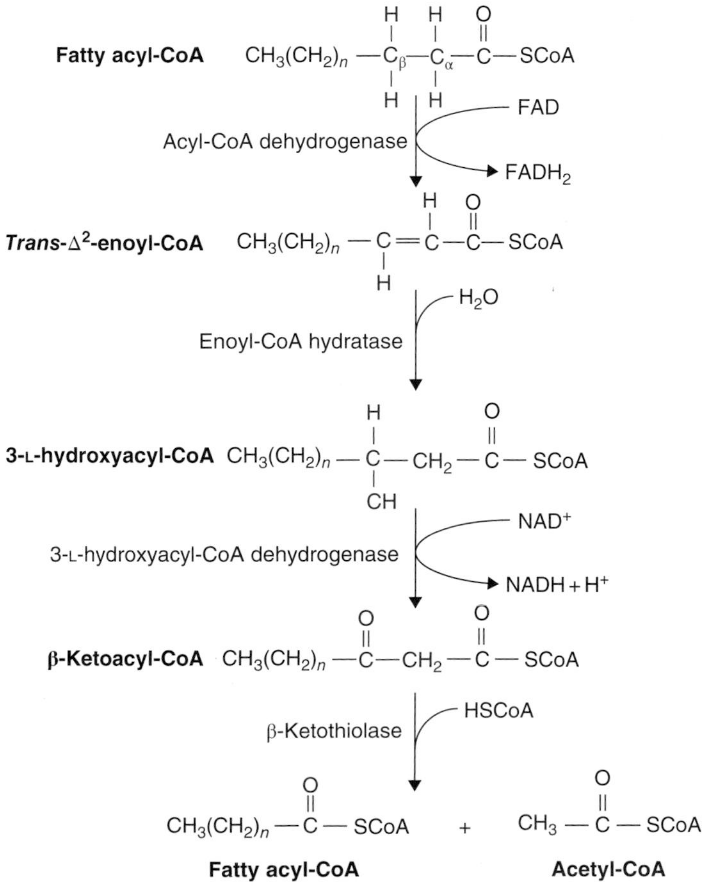

Figure 1.20 Fatty acid oxidation.

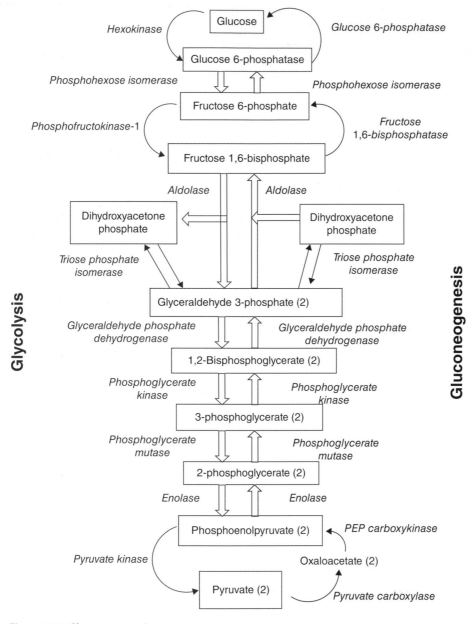

Figure 1.21 Gluconeogenesis.

bacterial fermentation of fibre in the gut, and is particularly important to supply tissues that rely on glucose as a metabolic fuel, such as the central nervous system. In conditions of starvation, after 2 or more days of fasting, the central nervous is also able to use a product of fatty acid oxidation, ketone bodies, produced by the liver.

2

Cell Biology

Daniel W. Lambert and Simon A. Whawell

School of Clinical Dentistry, University of Sheffield, Sheffield, UK

Learning Objectives

- To be able to describe the structure and function of cell membranes and membrane proteins.
- To be able to describe the role of subcellular organelles such as the nucleus, lysosomes and mitochondria.
- To be able to describe the basic events that occur in transcription and translation of genes.
- To understand the events that occur during the cell cycle and apoptosis and describe how they are regulated.

Clinical Relevance

Cell biology is another basic life science that underpins the structure and function of all living tissues including the many different cell types found in the head and neck. An understanding of cell biology is essential to appreciate normal physiology but also to understand how faults in these processes can result in diseases such as cancer. Given the rapid progress in research using cell-based therapies it is possible in the future clinicians will be administering such treatments.

Introduction

The body is composed of roughly 10 trillion cells, all doing the right things at mostly the right times, making up tissues as diverse as skin and brain. It is not just the whole organism that is complex, however; the cells that comprise the tissues are intricate in themselves. Although cells vary hugely in function and structure according to the tissue in which they reside (and in different organisms), eukaryotic cells have certain features in common.

It is not surprising, given their different modus operandi and environments, that eukaryotic and prokaryotic cells are a bit different. Prokaryotic cells, although bounded by a membrane, contain no distinct organelles.

Basic Sciences for Dental Students, First Edition. Edited by Simon A. Whawell and Daniel W. Lambert.
© 2018 John Wiley & Sons Ltd. Published 2018 by John Wiley & Sons Ltd.
Companion website: www.wiley.com/go/whawell/basic_sciences_for_dental_students

They do have ribosomes, but that is about it. They also have a peptidoglycan capsule, which acts as a defensive shield.

The Plasma Membrane

All eukaryotic cells are bounded by the **plasma membrane**. It is a **lipid bilayer** which acts as a barrier, selectively taking molecules up and ejecting molecules from the cell. It comprises two layers of **phospholipids**, arranged with their hydrophilic phosphate groups facing outwards and their hydrophobic tails inwards. In among these lipids are numerous proteins and **glycoproteins** (proteins conjugated to a carbohydrate moiety) and other lipids such as **cholesterol** (Figure 2.1).

The Structure of Membranes

Membranes are a critical component of all cells. They form the external barrier and encapsulate subcellular organelles. In this role they must regulate the movement of solvents and solutes into and out of membrane-bound compartments, be they cells or organelles. Membranes create a barrier to the movement of molecules, allowing the establishment of osmotic and electrostatic gradients. A number of different phospholipids exist in membranes, each with different structural or other cellular roles, such as acting as signalling molecules, relaying messages from outside of the cell to the inside. Some phospholipids are able to form lipid bilayers alone, whereas others require interaction with other lipids to do so. The lipids of the plasma membrane are not just phospholipids, however; there is also **cholesterol**, which plays a structural role and also helps to cluster membrane proteins together in cholesterol-rich regions of the membrane termed **lipid rafts** (Feature box 2.1).

Membrane Proteins

Take a look at a scanning electron micrograph of the surface of a cell and you will see that far from appearing an ordered structure, it appears as quite an uneven surface, with many protrusions (Figure 2.2). This is largely because of the presence of a wide variety of membrane proteins and the sugar groups attached to them. Proteins play a key role in the structure and function of the membrane and can be classed as either **extrinsic** (just on one or other surface) or **intrinsic** (generally spanning the membrane) (see Figure 2.1).

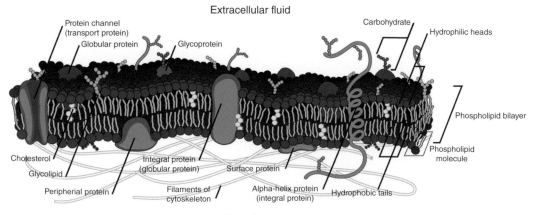

Figure 2.1 The basic structure of the plasma membrane.

Feature box 2.1 Lipid rafts in health and disease

Areas of the plasma membrane are thought to be enriched in certain lipids such as cholesterol and sphingolipids, forming discrete 'lipid rafts'. Although controversial, it is generally accepted that these areas of the membrane are more tightly packed and allow clustering of proteins which may otherwise be more evenly distributed in the membrane. This clustering of specific proteins is reported to alter their functions, such as transmitting signals from outside the cell. Changes in the nature or amount of lipid rafts has been linked to a number of diseases including Alzheimer's disease.

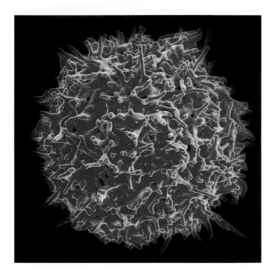

Figure 2.2 The cell surface.

One of the most important functions of membrane proteins is in regulating the entry and exit of materials from the cell; proteins involved in this can be classed as transport proteins. Membrane transporters regulate the movement of molecules by three major mechanisms: **facilitated diffusion** (distinct from diffusion, which does not require the presence of a protein), **gated channels** (opened or closed by ligand binding; see Chapter 5) and **active transport** (Figure 2.3). Active transport, which requires the presence of the cellular source of chemical energy, ATP, can be further broken down into primary active transport and secondary active transport. Primary active transport involves the pumping of a single solute against its concentration gradient whereas secondary active transport uses the electrochemical gradient generated by actively pumping one substrate to provide an electrochemical gradient to transport a different solute.

Another major class of membrane proteins is **receptors**. Membrane receptors bind specific molecules outside the cell, termed **ligands**, and translate this event, via interactions with other proteins, into **signals** within the cell, allowing the cell to adapt and respond to changes in the environment. These external signals may come from neighbouring cells (termed **juxtacrine** signalling), nearby cells (**paracrine**), distant cells elsewhere in the body (**endocrine**) or even the same cell (**autocrine**). There are many classes of receptor; some of the most commonly encountered are **ion channel receptors**, **heptahelical receptors** and **kinase-associated receptors** (Figure 2.4). Clinically, receptors are of great interest as many drugs mimic normal ligands to block the function of specific receptors; a good example of this is the anti-cancer drug, trastuzumab (sold as Herceptin).

The final class of membrane proteins we should consider is **membrane-bound enzymes**. There is not much that goes on in the body that doesn't involve membrane-bound enzymes, and they are the target of a myriad of drugs which inhibit their function. The major function of membrane-bound enzymes is to catalyse reactions involving passing substrates, or to modify the function of other proteins in the cell membrane or within the cell (Figure 2.5).

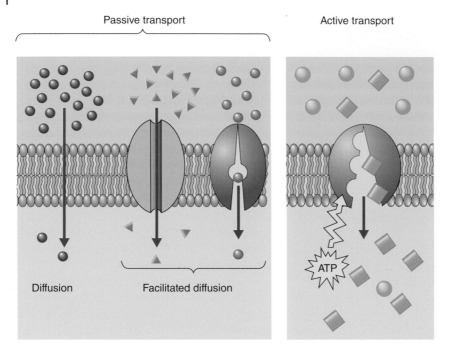

Figure 2.3 Types of membrane transport.

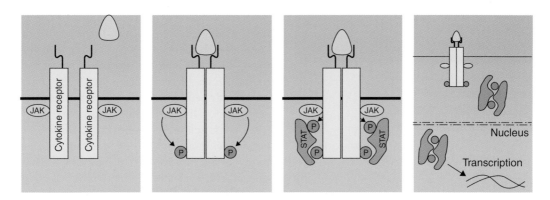

Figure 2.4 Membrane receptors. Diagram shows a kinase-associated receptor. Phosphorylation (P) of the intracellular domain causes recruitment of STAT proteins which are then able to move to the nucleus to cause transcription of specific genes

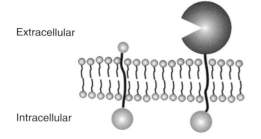

Figure 2.5 The diagram shows a membrane-bound enzyme (depicted as a Pacman shape) adjacent to its substrate, in this case also a membrane-bound protein, which can be cut ('cleaved') by the enzyme.

Subcellular Organelles

The membrane bounds the **cytoplasm**, a fluid environment containing a protein **cytoskeleton** and membrane-bound organelles. Each of these organelles has a particular function and their diverse structures reflect this.

The Nucleus

The **nucleus** contains the genetic material of the cell, in the form of **deoxyribonucleic acid** (**DNA**). The nucleus consists of a double phospholipid membrane with small gaps in it, termed pores (Figure 2.6). These **nuclear pores** allow things into the nucleus (mainly proteins needed for DNA replication and transcription), and things out (mainly RNA) in a controlled way. The membrane is continuous with another membrane that forms the endoplasmic reticulum. The nucleus also contains a region called the **nucleolus**: this is where the ribosomes, required for protein synthesis, are assembled.

DNA

DNA contains all the information required to produce and maintain all the components of a cell. It is comprises four bases – **adenine**, **guanine**, **cytosine** and **thymine** – each of which is bonded to a **deoxyribose**: each of these is termed a **nucleoside**. The nucleotides form a linear string along a **phosphate backbone** (each nucleoside bound to a phosphate is termed a **nucleotide**), and it is the sequence of these four nucleotides which determines the sequence of every protein in the cell, which determines the function of the cell. Two strands of nucleotides line up opposite each other, with each string going in the opposite direction; that is, one going 5′–3′ and one going 3′–5′ (Figure 2.7; see also Chapter 1). The structure of the bases only allows adenine to be opposite thymine, and guanine to be opposite cytosine; this allows the greatest number of bonds to form (actually, other combinations are possible, but this is generally undesirable). The two strands are coiled into a helix (called a **double helix**) as there are two strands. This structure is very stable, with the bases protected by the sugar phosphate backbone (this is one of the most important roles of DNA, just keeping things safe), but the cell has a problem. This molecule is big, really big: 6.8 billion base pairs, in fact (to give this scale, it would take you about 9.5 years to read it out). So it coils up more, wrapped around proteins called **histones** to

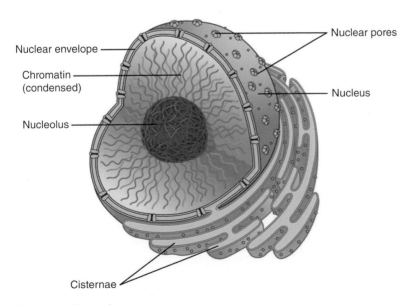

Nuclear envelope

Chromatin (condensed)

Nucleolus

Nuclear pores

Nucleus

Cisternae

Figure 2.6 The nucleus.

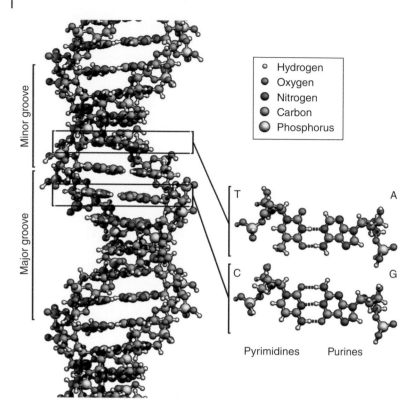

Minor groove

Major groove

○ Hydrogen
● Oxygen
● Nitrogen
● Carbon
○ Phosphorus

T   A

C   G

Pyrimidines   Purines

Figure 2.7 The structure of DNA.

form a **nucleosome**, and then lots of nucleosomes coil up to form a **solenoid**. All of this together is termed **chromatin**, which in a dividing cell condenses further around **scaffold proteins** to form **chromosomes** (each human diploid cell has 46 of these, termed 2*n*). When a cell is preparing to divide, it needs to copy all of its DNA. This is termed **DNA replication**, and is achieved by small sections of the DNA unwinding to form 'bubbles' that allow an enzyme, **DNA polymerase**, to copy each of the strands of DNA (Figure 2.8). The new strand of DNA is then paired with its template parental DNA strand and separates into the new 'daughter' cell.

Genes

So, we have covered DNA and the nucleus. But other than storage and replication, what does DNA do? Regions of the DNA provide the code to produce proteins (although considering this is arguably the main purpose of

DNA these regions make up a very small proportion of the whole human **genome**, about 1.5 %)). Each region encoding a protein, along with some sequence around it with a regulatory role, is called a **gene**. Diploid cells (all cells except egg and sperm cells which are termed **haploid**, *n*) contain two copies of each chromosome, and therefore each gene; the two copies of a gene are called **alleles**. Alleles are significant in both inheritance and disease. To produce **messenger RNA** (**mRNA**), which is then used as the template for synthesizing the protein, the section of DNA around the gene must unwind and the strands separate, allowing an enzyme, **RNA polymerase**, to get in and synthesize a strand of RNA with a sequence complementary to that of the template DNA strand. This is called **transcription** (Figure 2.9). The mRNA sequence is therefore an exact copy of the DNA sequence. The mRNA is then modified (sections of sequence called **introns** are

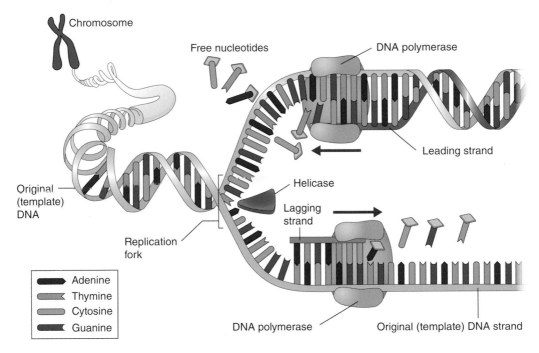

Figure 2.8 DNA replication.

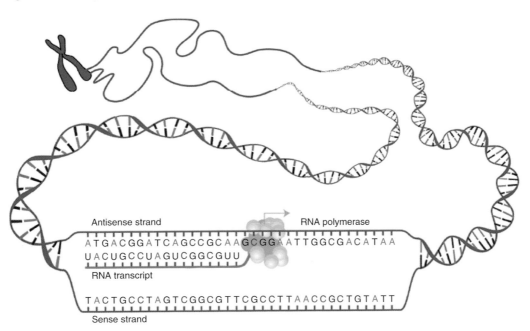

Figure 2.9 Transcription.

spliced out (removed) and a cap and a tail are put on it). The resulting mature transcripts are then exported from the nucleus through the nuclear pores and **translated** into proteins by **ribosomes**. Strings of amino acids (polypeptides) are formed by specific **transfer RNA** (**tRNA**) recognizing three-base **codons** on the mature mRNA; each

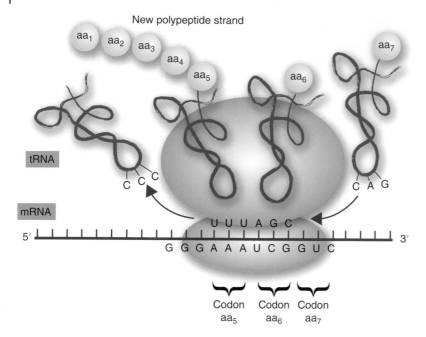

New polypeptide strand

tRNA

mRNA

5′   3′

U U U A G C

G G G A A U C G G U C

Codon aa₅   Codon aa₆   Codon aa₇

Figure 2.10 Protein translation.

codon specifies a tRNA molecule covalently bound to a specific amino acid. Because there are more possible three-base combinations than there are amino acids, there is some **redundancy** in this system, and some codons (**stop codons**) do not 'code' for an amino acid and therefore cause translation to cease (Figure 2.10). Peptide bonds form between the amino acids bound to the tRNA, forming a polypeptide, and when a stop codon is reached the entire ribosomal assembly dissociates and the polypeptide is released.

The Endoplasmic Reticulum and Golgi Apparatus

The nuclear membrane is connected to the membrane of the **endoplasmic reticulum** (**ER**) (Figure 2.11). The ER is a complex system of membranes which exists in two forms: rough and smooth. **Smooth ER** is involved in lipid synthesis and **rough ER**, which is studded with ribosomes, is involved in production and processing of proteins, in collaboration with another series of membranes known as the **Golgi complex**. Proteins synthesized in

the rough ER are transported to the Golgi complex in **vesicles** that are then modified and sent, again in vesicles, to either the plasma membrane for secretion or to **lysosomes**.

Lysosomes

Vesicles leaving the Golgi complex are coated with particular proteins which direct them to the appropriate destination. Lysosomes arise from their precursors, **endosomes** and contain hydrolytic enzymes, trafficked from the Golgi complex, which degrade proteins and other large molecules. The lysosomes also process materials brought into the cell by **phagocytosis**, **pinocytosis** and **receptor-mediated endocytosis** (Figure 2.12). A closely related structure, the **peroxisome**, degrades long-chain fatty acids and cholesterol.

Mitochondria

Finally, to **mitochondria**, the power stations of the cell. They oxidize fuel in their inner matrix and generate **ATP** across their inner membrane via the electron transport chain

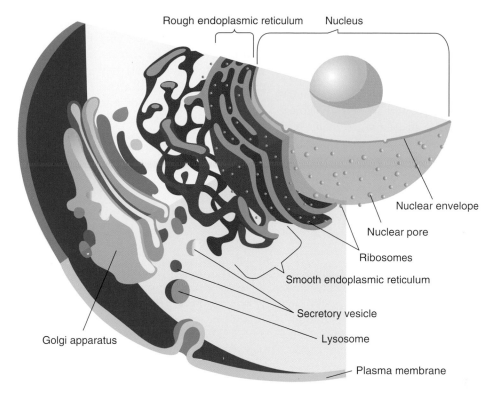

Figure 2.11 The endoplasmic reticulum and Golgi complex.

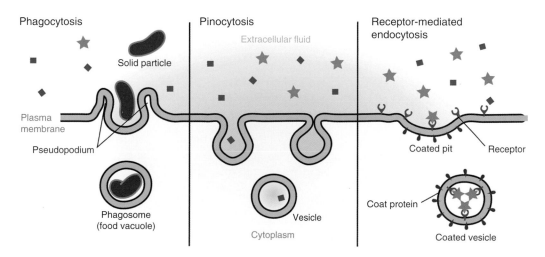

Figure 2.12 Endocytosis.

(see Chapter 1). The inner membrane is extensively folded to maximize the surface area for generating ATP; these folds are called **cristae**. Mitochondria are able to divide independently from the cell (see The Cell Cycle), thanks in part to them containing their own DNA, which encodes some of the proteins required to make new mitochondria. The lipids required to make new membranes are derived from the smooth ER.

The Cytoskeleton

The cytoskeleton of a cell is a network of **protein polymers** that provide mechanical support for the cell to maintain shape but are also intimately involved in cell and organelle movement and in cell division. These cytoskeletal proteins are made up from thousands of subunits and are characterized by their **dynamic** nature in that they are constantly assembling and disassembling. There are three types of cytoskeletal polymer: **actin filaments** (microfilaments), **intermediate filaments** and **microtubules** (Feature box 2.2). Actin filaments are concentrated beneath the cell membrane and are ubiquitous in eukaryotic cells. They are narrow, flexible and highly organized and form cytoplasmic extensions such as microvilli, lamellipodia and filopodia. Actin is intimately involved with phagocytosis and cytokinesis (splitting of a cell into two during division; see later in this chapter). **Myosin** proteins are molecular motor proteins that use ATP to generate force along actin filaments, providing the contractile forces in muscle. Intermediate filaments are nuclear and cytoplasmic meshworks made from high-tensile-strength 'rope-like' filaments and are crucial to tissue structure. **Keratin** is the most common intermediate filament in mammals and forms the most superficial layer of the skin along with hair and finger/toe nails. Finally, microtubules are hollow rigid polymers of tubulin and provide the cell with the strongest resistance to compression. The organization of microtubules differs from cell to cell; they have a critical role in mitosis and reorganize to form the mitotic spindle along with microtubule-dependent motor proteins (dynein). **Cilia** and **flagella** consist of long bundles of microtubules and interactions within these bundles provdes movement back and forth to allow the cell to move or fluid to pass over the cell surface.

Life and Death of a Cell

The Cell Cycle

Mitosis is the process by which two identical daughter cells are produced from one cell. It is one of the most important cellular processes and is required not only for growth and development but also the normal turnover of cells in a mature organism. The events leading up to cell division are ordered and tightly regulated and result in the formation of two identical daughter cells. DNA must be duplicated and equally divided between these cells that is distinct from meiosis, which occurs during gamete formation and which is not covered in this book.

The stages of the cell cycle are shown in Figure 2.13 and consist of two phases: the mitotic or **M phase** during which nuclear and cytoplasmic division occurs and the remaining phases which collectively are termed **interphase**. Interphase starts with Gap 1 or G_1 where the cell increases in size and synthesizes RNA and protein to prepare for chromosomal replication. During the

---

Feature box 2.2 Microtubule-interacting drugs

Paclitaxel (Taxol™), which can be found naturally in the Pacific yew tree, binds and stabilizes microtubules. This drug prevents mitosis and has been used in the treatment of breast and ovarian cancer. Colchicine, which can also be isolated from plant sources, disrupts microtubules and prevents the rearrangements necessary for cell migration including the recruitment of white cells to sources of inflammation. It has been used in the treatment of gout and oral ulcers.

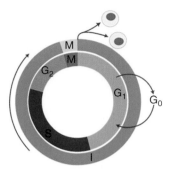

Figure 2.13 The cell cycle.

synthesis or **S phase** the DNA is duplicated and briefly the cell contains four pairs of chromosomes ($4n$). During the second gap or G_2 phase the cell continues to grow and synthesize protein in preparation for mitosis. There are times when a cell can permanently or temporarily leave the cell cycle and this is termed **quiescence** or G_0. The cell may not be completely dormant but retain other functions such as secretion. Most lymphocytes exist in G_0 but upon stimulation with an antigen can re-enter the cell cycle at G_1. **Terminally differentiated** cells such as keratinocytes in the upper layers of the skin never re-enter the cell cycle but continue their specialized functions until they die.

The mitotic phase of the cell cycle can be further divided into the phases shown in Figure 2.14 during which specific processes occur. The interphase cell enters a transition to the main starting point of mitosis, **prophase**, during which the cytoskeleton dis-

assembles, the nucleolus fades and chromatin condenses into chromosomes. During prometaphase the nuclear envelope breaks down and the spindle fibres elongate from the centrioles and attach to protein bundles on the chromosome called kinetochores. During **metaphase** tension is applied to these fibres and the chromosomes align in one plane in the centre of the cell. It is at this stage that mitosis can be obvious in a histological section of tissue as the dense concentration of DNA can be seen as a 'metaphase plate'. While not a pathological event the number and location of such cells displaying this feature may inform pathologists of the presence of disease. During **anaphase** the spindle fibres shorten and the chromosomes are pulled apart towards the cell poles. Finally, during **telophase** the chromosomes arrive at the poles, the spindles disappear and a contractile ring is formed that divides the cell in two (**cytokinesis**).

Control of the Cell Cycle

As with any cellular process, control and regulation are of paramount importance. The cell cycle is regulated by both extracellular signals such as growth factors and cell anchorage and intracellular **checkpoints** which can arrest the cell cycle if certain criteria are not favourable. This monitoring and surveillance occurs in particular at G_1 where appropriate growth, environment and lack of DNA damage determine entry into the S phase. During G_2 correct DNA replication is a prerequisite and

Prophase	Metaphase	Anaphase	Telophase

 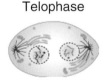

Microtubules appear chromosomes condense nuclear envelope disappears	Chromosomes align	Chromosomes separate	Chromosomes disperse nuclear membrane reforms two daughter cells formed with two nuclei

Figure 2.14 Phases of the cell cycle.

finally the transition between metaphase and anaphase is blocked if there is improper alignment of the spindle. Classic cell fusion experiments led to the discovery of the molecular events that control progression through the cell cycle. **Cyclin** proteins are highly conserved across animal species and the levels of these proteins oscillate according to the phase of the cell cycle. Cyclins work in conjunction with **cyclin-dependent kinase** (**CDK**) enzymes to trigger cell cycle transitions. CDKs are effectors that phosphorylate other proteins; their levels remain fairly stable during the cell cycle but they must bind the appropriate cyclin in order to be activated. CDKs are regulated by the availability of cyclins and by specific inhibitors of these enzymes.

Apoptosis

If we now move from cell division to cell death, a cell can either die as a result from an injurious agent causing necrosis or from **apoptosis** or **programmed cell death**. It is important to note that apoptosis is an important part of normal development, a classic example being resorption of a tadpole's tail as part of metamorphosis. The other essential task of apoptosis is the destruction of cells that pose a threat to the organism. Such cells can be those infected with a virus, immune effector cells to prevent such cells causing unnecessary tissue damage at the end of the response, and cells that have DNA damage and may thus become cancerous. Apoptosis can occur with the withdrawal of positive survival signals such as growth factors, cytokines or hormones, or on receipt of negative signals such as ultraviolet light.

In a similar way to the cell cycle, apoptosis consists of an ordered set of events including the morphological changes that occur in an apoptotic cell. This is characterized by **cell shrinkage**, cytoskeletal and **organelle disruption** and chromatin condensation. The nucleus is **fragmented** and

membrane **blebbing** occurs followed by cell fragmentation, leading to the formation of small membrane-bound '**apoptotic bodies**' which are phagocytosed by macrophages or neighbouring cells. It is important to remember that apoptosis is a process distinct from pathological cell death or necrosis. Unlike necrosis, apoptosis is a controlled process requiring ATP; it does not elicit an immune response, results in no scarring and is limited to single cells rather than large groups.

Control of Apoptosis

The molecular mechanisms of apoptosis are, in a similar way to the cell cycle, highly conserved with most recent understanding coming from the study of the nematode worm *Caenorhabditis elegans*. There are two major pathways, summarized in Figure 2.15. The **intrinsic pathway** (shown on the left in the figure) can act without external signals and is centred on the **mitochondrion**. Disruption of the integrity of the outer membrane causes the release of cytochrome *c*, which when in the cytoplasm interacts with the apoptotic factor Apaf-1 and caspase 9 in the presence of ATP. The formation of this complex, called the apoptosome, initiates a chain reaction that results in apoptosis. These caspases are cysteine proteases that follow a cascade of sequential activation culminating in the proteolysis of cellular substrates that lead to cell death. **Bcl-2**, which was first identified from B-cell lymphoma, is an oncogene (a cancer-causing gene) that promotes blood cell survival. It does this by binding to Apaf-1 on the mitochondrial outer membrane, preventing apoptosis in normal cells.

An alternative mechanism by which apoptosis is triggered is the **external pathway** (shown on the right in Figure 2.15), involving specific membrane receptors of the tumour necrosis factor family such as Fas and tumour necrosis factor (TNF)-receptor-1. These 'death receptors' bind Fas ligand or TNFα, for example, and lead to a conformational change in the receptor allowing interaction

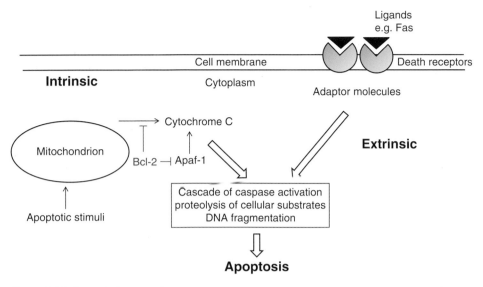

Figure 2.15 Control of apoptosis.

with adaptor molecules and initiation of the caspase cascade as described for the intrinsic pathway. The Fas–FasL interaction is one way in which cytotoxic T-cells induce their target cells to apoptose.

p53 and p27

As, broadly speaking, dysregulated cell growth results in cancer it is not perhaps surprising that many cell cycle-regulatory genes are tumour suppressors. p53 is a protein that functions to block the cell cycle if DNA is damaged. The absence of functional p53 through mutation thus leads to an increase in cells with DNA damage and is found in over half of all human cancers. p27 is a CDK inhibitor that blocks entry into S phase.

Reduced levels of p27 predict a poor outcome in breast and gastric cancer. These are just two examples; much research has been and will be done into control of the cell cycle and how it is related to disease.

Viruses, Apoptosis and Cancer

In the same way that promotion of cell division occurs in cancer, avoidance of apoptosis would lead to the same survival advantage. Human papilloma virus is a causative agent in cervical cancer that can bind and inactivate p53, thus preventing apoptosis. Epstein–Barr virus produces a molecule similar to Bcl-2 and enhances the production of this by the host cell, both of which leads to resistance to apoptosis.

3

Tissues of the Body

Daniel W. Lambert, Aileen Crawford and Simon A. Whawell

School of Clinical Dentistry, University of Sheffield, Sheffield, UK

Learning Objectives

- To be able to list the basic tissue types in the human body.
- To be able to describe the structure and histological appearance of epithelia, connective tissue and muscle.
- To be able to relate the structure of these tissues to their function.
- To define the term extracellular matrix, list some of its common components and understand the role it plays in tissue and cell biology.

Clinical Relevance

Following on from biochemistry and cell biology, tissue biology represents the next level of complexity in the human body. All the major tissue types are present in the orofacial region and thus there is considerable variation in their structure and function. Tissues are damaged or replaced during dental procedures and specific diseases arise within them. Thus a detailed knowledge of their structure and function is essential for patient care.

This chapter will detail the structure and function of the major tissues of the body normally classified as: epithelia, connective tissue and contractile tissue. The nervous system is dealt with in Chapter 5.

Epithelia

Epithelium covers the body surface as skin and it also lines all internal cavities and surfaces as a continuous layer. Embryonically it is derived from ectoderm (epidermis and enamel) or endoderm (gastrointestinal and respiratory tracts). Like all cells and tissues epithelia are adapted to their position and function in the body and therefore vary widely in their structure; however, there are some general characteristics which are common to all epithelia. Epithelia exist as continuous sheets of **densely packed** cells with minimal extracellular matrix. These tissues are also **avascular** (no blood vessels) and thus have to rely on the underlying connective tissue for supply of nutrients and physical support. Epithelia have a number of functions in the body including mechanical protection, secretion, absorption and filtration. They can be **polarized** whereby individual cells have a difference between their basal surface (adjacent to the connective tissue) and apical surface (in contact with the surface or lumen of a tubal system).

Classification of Epithelia

To aid in description of both histology and function epithelia can be classified according to various physical properties (Feature box 3.1). The number of epithelial cell layers present is one such property: **simple** epithelia have a single cell layer while those with multiple cell layers are called **stratified**. The shape of the cells can also vary, being cuboidal, columnar or squamous (flattened) (Figure 3.1). Some epithelia have specific cell modifications including cilia or microvilli or have other cells present such as mucus-secreting goblet cells. More than one classification system applies and thus a combination of these terms can be used to accurately describe all the specific modifications that an epithelium has. **Simple squamous** epithelium thus has a single flattened layer of cells and is found in the alveoli of the lungs where a short diffusion distance allows rapid and efficient transfer of respiratory gases. **Simple columnar** epithelium is found lining the gastrointestinal tract, the surface area for absorption of nutrients being considerably enhanced by the presence of microvilli and the transit of food being aided by the presence of mucus-secreting goblet cells. The respiratory tract is also lined by simple columnar epithelium but the orientation of cells is such that while all cells are in contact with the basal layer not all appear to reach the surface. Histologically it thus appears to have more than one layer and is referred to as **pseudostratified**. Goblet cells and cilia are present to maintain a moist environment and to trap and remove particulate matter and pathogenic organisms. **Stratified squamous** epithelium has multiple layers of cells the upper layers of which are flattened. Such a tissue is highly resistant to abrasion and thus forms the epidermis of the skin and the epithelium of the oral mucosa.

Oral Epithelium

The oral epithelium is similar in structure to the skin and consists of four main layers above the connective tissue (Figure 3.2); however, the additional structures found in skin (sebaceous glands, sweat glands and hair)

Feature box 3.1 Histology

Histology is the microscopic study of tissues where cells and ECM structure can be visualized within a tissue. To enable this to be carried out the tissue must go through a number of steps, starting with **fixation**. The tissue is fixed to preserve the architecture and morphology by increasing its mechanical strength and rigidity and also inactivates tissue-degrading enzymes and microorganisms. Chemicals such as formaldehyde are used, which crosslinks proteins and anchors soluble proteins to the cytoskeleton and ECM. **Dehydration** then takes place using alcohol where the water in the tissues is replaced with molten paraffin wax. This wax is allowed to cool so that a solid block containing the tissue is formed. This can then be finely **sectioned** on a microtome and placed on a glass slide. To enable the tissue features to be visualized more easily the section is often **stained** with agents such as **haematoxylin and eosin**. Haematoxylin is a purple basic dye which binds to DNA in the nucleus and also some carbohydrates in cartilage. Eosin is a pink acidic dye which binds to cytoplasmic and ECM proteins. Examples of the images obtained by observing such stained sections under light microscopy appear in this chapter.

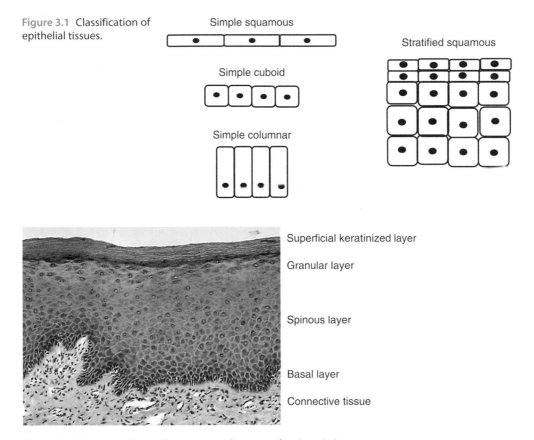

Figure 3.1 Classification of epithelial tissues.

Simple squamous

Simple cuboid

Simple columnar

Stratified squamous

Figure 3.2 Haematoxylin- and eosin-stained section of oral epithelium.

Superficial keratinized layer

Granular layer

Spinous layer

Basal layer

Connective tissue

are not present. The **basal layer** is where cell division occurs to supply replacement cells for those which are continually shed from the epithelial surface. Cells are attached to a specialized extracellular matrix called the **basement membrane** (basal lamina), which forms the junction of the epithelial layer and the connective tissue by a complex of adhesion proteins called **hemidesmosomes**. This junction is also undulating in skin and attached gingiva in particular to allow a larger surface for attachment of the epithelium, preventing it from shearing off as a result of physical forces. These epithelial projections are called **rete ridges**. As cells progress up the epithelial layer into the **spinous** (or **prickle**) **layer** they undergo **differentiation** whereby their proliferative capacity is lost as they take on more specific tasks related to the function of the tissue,

with eventual loss of cellular features such as nuclei. Cells are strongly linked together by **desmosomes** (Feature box 3.2). The **granular layer** contains cells with keratohyalin and membrane-coating granules important in waterproofing. Finally, the upper **superficial layer** of the epithelium contains dead cells and in some parts of the oral cavity, such as the hard palate, it also has a thick layer of **keratin** to act as a further protective barrier to abrasion. In other areas such as the buccal mucosa where the epithelium needs to be more flexible this keratin layer is absent.

Glands

When the capacity of an epithelium to secrete is not sufficient to achieve its functional requirements the epithelium in-folds to form a structure with a much larger surface

---

Feature box 3.2 Pemphigus vulgaris

Pemphigus vulgaris is an **autoimmune** disease characterized by the presence of ulcers, predominantly in the oral cavity, which are in fact multiple broken blisters. Components of desmosomes called desmogleins are targeted by autoantibodies which results in intra-epithelial blistering where the normally close attachment of epithelial cells breaks down.

Histological diagnosis can be achieved using immunofluorescence to visualize the presence of autoantibodies within the tissue and treatment is with corticosteroids. This serves to highlight not only the importance of epithelial integrity but also the role of oral healthcare professionals in the diagnosis of systemic diseases.

---

area called a gland. If communication with the overlying epithelium and external environment is via a duct through which the secretion is delivered this is referred to as an **exocrine gland**. Salivary glands are a good example of this kind of system and are covered in detail in Chapter 12 of this book. If a duct secretes its products into the bloodstream then the gland is called an **endocrine gland**. Examples include the thyroid, pituitary and adrenal glands.

Connective Tissues

One of the prime functions of connective tissues is to provide a structural framework for the body. Connective tissues hold together or keep separate the body cells, tissues and organs and provide protection for them. All connective tissues are composed of living cells embedded in an **extracellular matrix** (**ECM**). The ECM is a non-living, non-cellular component that is secreted by connective tissue cells and is vital for the function of the connective tissue. Compared to other tissues, such as epithelial tissues, connective tissues contain relatively few cells which are widely separated from each other by ECM. The ECM provides not only essential physical scaffolding for the cells and is responsible for the structural properties of connective tissue, it also provides crucial biochemical and biomechanical cues required for tissue formation (morphogenesis), differentiation and homeostasis. Fundamentally, the ECM of all connective tissues is composed of fibrous proteins (such as collagen) embedded

in 'ground substance' which is a viscoelastic gel-like substance composed of water and proteoglycans. However, the biochemical composition and biomechanical properties of the ECM vary greatly from one connective tissue to another. Therefore, it is important to remember that each connective tissue has an ECM with a **unique composition and structure** that is **essential to its function**. The ECM is a highly dynamic structure that is continually undergoing remodelling by the connective tissue cells.

Connective Tissue Cells

The major cell present in connective tissue is the **fibroblast**. The fibroblast is a long, thin cell often with protrusions (termed a 'spindle' shape) and their major job is to maintain the ECM and provide structural and nutrient support to nearby cells, such as the epithelium (as seen in Figure 3.2). Under certain conditions, such as when a tissue is wounded, fibroblasts may become **activated** to differentiate into **myofibroblasts**. Fibroblasts are attracted by chemokines into the wound bed of damaged tissue, and there become contractile, physically pulling the edges of the wound together, and secrete ECM, chemokines and cytokines to attract immune cells to clear debris and bacteria and epithelial cells to grow over the wound bed and repair the tissue. The myofibroblasts are then either removed from the wound or return to their normal state; in some circumstances, however, this doesn't occur, and myofibroblasts persist in a wounded area, continuing to secrete ECM and causing scarring.

Myofibroblasts are also sometimes found around cancers, and are thought to help tumours grow and spread. Fibroblasts differ in between tissue and sometimes have special features related to where they are found in the body, such as the fibroblasts of the periodontal ligament.

A number of other cell types may be found in connective tissue depending of the tissue: **endothelial** cells, **pericytes**, **smooth and skeletal muscle** cells, **neurones** and **immune cells**, among others, can be found performing specialist roles in connective tissues.

Composition of the ECM

The ECM of connective tissue comprises two main classes of macromolecule: fibrous proteins and proteoglycans. Water is also a major component.

Fibrous Proteins of the ECM

Collagen is the most abundant protein in the ECM and makes up about 30% of the total protein mass in humans. To date, 28 collagens have been identified in vertebrates and the fibril-forming collagens, particularly collagens of types I and II, are the main components of the ECM of connective tissues such as tendons, cartilage and bone. Type I and type II collagens are considered 'nature's rope'; the structure of these collagens endows them with excellent tensile properties so that they resist stretching and provide a structural framework and tissue strength to the tissues (see Feature box 3.3). In addition to its tensile properties, collagen also regulates cell adhesion, supports chemotaxis and is important in directing tissue development.

Elastin is an important fibrous protein found the ECM of some connective tissues.

Feature box 3.3 Collagens

Twenty eight collagens have been identified in vertebrates. Collagens are characterized by being composed of **three polypeptide chains** which intertwine around each other to form a **right-handed triple-helical region** in their tertiary structure. The length of the triple helical region varies between the different collagens. Fibrous collagens are the main structural collagens in the ECM of connective tissues. These collagens form long continuous regions of triple helix (over 1000 amino acids). These collagens form supramolecular aggregates that make fibrils which aggregate into larger fibres. Examples of **fibrous collagens** are collagen types I (found in bone, teeth, tendon, ligaments and cornea), collagen type II (found in cartilage, vitreous body of the eye, central portion of the vertebral discs), collagen type III (found in skin, vessel walls and the reticular fibres of most tissues). Some collagens contain a shorter sequence of triple helical structure and these form collagen-interlaced network structures. Examples of **network-forming collagens** are collagen type IV which forms an interlaced network in basement membranes such as the glomerular basement membrane, which is essential for the filtration function of the kidney. Other collagens (**f**ibril-**a**ssociated **c**ollagens with **i**nterrupted **t**riple helices, the **FACIT** collagens) have several domains of triple-helical regions which impart flexible hinge regions to the molecule. These collagens (e.g. collagen type IX) are found in association with the fibrous collagens and are important in controlling the fibre diameter of the fibrous collagens during fibril formation. Collagen molecules are synthesized inside the cell in a similar process to most proteins but may also undergo post-translational modifications such as hydroxylation of proline and lysine residues which are needed for crosslinking the collagen fibrils together to form larger fibres. Formation of collagen fibrils occurs **outside of the cell**. Molecules of collagen are secreted outside the cell and, after cleavage of terminal peptides on the ends of the molecules, the collagen molecules can self-assembly into collagen fibrils which are then enzymatically crosslinked at the hydroxylysine residues to stabilize the fibrils. The fibrils then self-assemble into larger collagen fibres.

Unlike collagen, elastin has a **low tensile strength** but has the critical property of **elasticity** and is an essential fibrous protein found in tissues that experience repeated stretch such as the lungs and arteries. It is the presence of elastin in these tissues that endows them with elasticity and resilience so that they can be repeatedly stretched and then undergo elastic recoil to return to their original size and shape.

Fibronectin and **laminins** are important fibrous proteins found in the ECM. Fibronectin has a crucial role in guiding the organization and structure of the ECM. Both fibronectin and laminins are important in **cell differentiation**, **cell migration** and **cell adhesion** to the ECM. Fibronectin and laminins can bind to both components of the ECM and integrin receptors on the plasma membrane of cells so anchoring the cells directly to the ECM.

The above proteins are the major structural protein components of the ECM but they are not the only proteins found in the ECM of connective tissues. Examples of other proteins found in the ECM include various growth factors, tenacins and fibrillins. The latter are found in elastic tissues and are important in the assembly of elastin into elastic fibres.

Proteoglycans of the ECM

Connective tissue cells synthesize a diverse group of proteoglycans. **Proteoglycans** are composed of a specific **protein core structure** to which long, unbranched **polysaccharide side chains** are **covalently attached**. The polysaccharide side chains attached to the core protein are made up of repeating disaccharide units and have come to be named **glycosaminoglycan (GAG)** side chains as the repeating disaccharide building blocks are made up of an amino sugar and a uronic acid or galactose moiety. Some proteoglycans may contain only one or two GAG chains and others, such as aggrecan, a proteoglycan found in articular cartilage, have over 100 GAG chains. Some GAGs (such as chondroitin and keratin sulphate found in

aggrecan) are sulphated. This means that the proteoglycans can carry a **dense negative charge** and so will bind water molecules to form a **hydrated gel** that can resist compressive forces when the proteoglycans interact with other ECM components such as collagen.

Proteoglycans have been classified according to their core proteins, localization and GAG composition. The interstitial class of proteoglycans found in the ECM of connective tissues is diverse, differing in size and GAG composition. However, they are critical components of the ECM and contribute to stabilizing and organizing collagen fibres. Examples of ECM proteoglycans include the family of small leucine-rich proteoglycans (SLRPs). These are abundant in tendons and essential in regulating the diameters of the collagen fibrils during fibrillogenesis. Their hydrophilic nature allows them to act as a lubricant, aiding collagen fibres to glide over each other. In articular cartilage the proteoglycan aggrecan is vital to enable the tissue to withstand compressive loading.

Categories of Connective Tissue

Connective tissues can be categorized according to the type of ECM they contain. These categories are as follows.

Embryonic connective tissues refer to the connective tissues found in the embryo. Embryonic connective tissues are classified as **mesenchymal** or **mucoid** and will not be considered further in this chapter.

Loose connective tissue is a soft, pliable tissue used for spacing and packing. It is found throughout the body and is composed of fine fibres of collagen (reticulin fibres) and elastin embedded in a substantial amorphous ground substance. Within the ECM are fibroblasts which secrete and maintain the ECM. This connective tissue helps to fill spaces between larger organs and forms loose sheets around blood vessels, nerves and tendons. Loose connective tissue also connects the muscle layer and skin. An example of a loose connective tissue is adipose tissue which

Figure 3.3 Histological section showing adipocytes embedded in loose connective tissue.

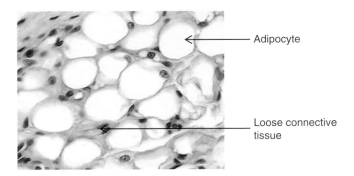

Adipocyte

Loose connective tissue

Figure 3.4 Histological section through the periodontium showing the collagen fibres of the periodontal ligament.

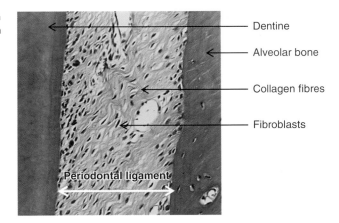

Dentine

Alveolar bone

Collagen fibres

Fibroblasts

Periodontal ligament

contains fat cells (adipocytes) distributed in a loose connective tissue of ECM and fibroblasts (Figure 3.3).

Dense connective tissue contains large, strong collagen fibres which impart considerable strength to the tissue. The collagen fibres are so numerous that there is little ground substance. The compact arrangement of collagen fibres resists stretching. A sparse population of fibroblasts is found attached along the axis of collagen fibres and is responsible for maintaining the ECM. The dense connective tissue comprises fascial membranes, the dermis of the skin, periosteum and capsules of organs. Dense connective tissue also comprises ligaments and joint capsules which connect bone to bone, and tendons, which connect muscles to bone. The periodontal ligament which holds the teeth in the tooth sockets are examples of classical ligaments. In this example the ligaments attach to the tooth dentine and

alveolar bone. In tendons and ligaments, the collagen fibres are arranged in a parallel fashion along the long axis of the tissue so that they can resist linear forces (Figure 3.4). Most ligaments and tendons need strength and inelasticity and so contain very few elastic fibres. However, in the neck and back some tendons and ligaments contain elastic fibres as flexibility and stretch are important functions of these tissues. The ligamentum flavum ligament connects the laminae of adjacent vertebrae in the spine and contains a high proportion of elastin fibres (60–70%).

Specialized connective tissues, as the name suggests, have very specialized functions in the body which are the direct result of the structure and composition of the ECM. Cartilage, bone, enamel, dentine and blood are examples of specialized connective tissues. In cartilage and bone the specialized nature of the ECM confers specific mechanical properties to the tissue.

Structure and Function of Cartilage

Cartilage is a specialized connective tissue and, unlike most tissues, it is avascular. Four types of cartilage are found in the body. These are discussed below.

Hyaline cartilage is characterized by a dense ECM rich in **collagen type II** fibres and ground substance. Embedded within the ECM are a sparse population of cartilage cells called **chondrocytes**. The chondrocytes are responsible for maintaining the ECM. Hyaline cartilage is the main component of the nasal septum and the C-shaped rings of cartilage found in the trachea (Figure 3.5). In these tissues the hyaline cartilage has a supporting function. Nasal septal cartilage gives shape to the nose and in the trachea the C-shaped cartilage rings prevent the walls of the trachea collapsing and so maintain an open airway.

Hyaline cartilage also covers the surfaces of the bones in synovial joints such as the knee and hip, where it is called articular cartilage. The functions of articular cartilage are to provide a smooth, near-frictionless surface to enable a gliding, pain-free joint motion and to be a biological 'shock absorber' to protect the bones from the forces generated during loading of the joint during joint motion such as walking. These functions of articular cartilage are completely dependent on the structure and composition of the ECM. The major components of the ECM of articular cartilage are a dense network of collagen type II fibres and ground substance. The ground substance of articular cartilage is composed largely of water and the highly sulphated proteoglycan, aggrecan, which forms large molecular complexes (molecular weight approximately 10^6 Da) with hyaluronic acid. As a consequence of their large size, the aggrecan–hyaluronic acid complexes are trapped within the stiff collagen network. Due to presence of the large number of negatively charged sulphate groups, aggrecan is very hydrophilic and binds water molecules which make the aggrecan molecules swell. Since the aggrecan complexes are trapped within the collagen network the degree of swelling is limited and the tissue develops a swelling pressure and becomes very turgid, forming a dense, viscoelastic gel that can resist compressive loading.

Fibrocartilage is characterized by a dense orderly arrangement of thick interlaced **collagen type I** fibres; there is relatively little ground substance compared to that found in hyaline cartilage. Fibrocartilage is found in the intervertebral discs, and at the insertion points of tendons and ligaments. Fibrocartilage also comprises the articular disc found in the temporomandibular joint and is essential for pain-free movement of the joint during speech and mastication (Figure 3.6).

Elastic cartilage, as it name suggests, has properties of elasticity. Histologically, elastic and hyaline cartilage look very similar in structure. However, in addition to ground

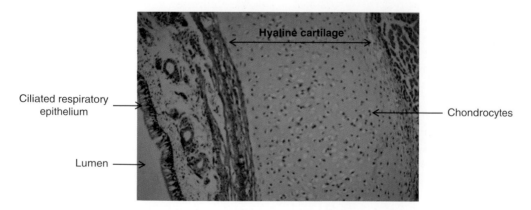

Figure 3.5 Histological section taken from the trachea showing part of the C-shaped hyaline cartilage ring.

Figure 3.6 Histological section
showing the structure of fibrocartilage.

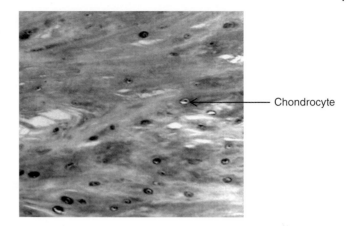

Chondrocyte

substance and collagen fibres the ECM of elastic cartilage also contains a network of fibres of elastin which enable elastic cartilage to have a rigid but elastic framework. Elastic cartilage functions to provide and maintain shape when the tissue is twisted or distorted. Elastic cartilage is found in the external structure of the ear, epiglottis and larynx.

Hypertrophic cartilage is an essential intermediate tissue in bone formation by the process of endochondral ossification that occurs during embryonic and foetal development. After birth, hypertrophic cartilage is found in growth plates and is formed during the repair of bone fractures. A 'template' of hyaline cartilage is first formed which is then remodelled by the chondrocytes into hypertrophic cartilage (Figure 3.7). The ECM of hypertrophic cartilage is characterized by fibres of collagen type X in addition to collagen type II. Also, the chondrocytes of hypertrophic cartilage are very large (around five times the size of chondrocytes in hyaline cartilage). After deposition hypertrophic cartilage is remodelled into bone by the process of endochondral ossification.

Figure 3.7 Histological section through the growth plate of a 5-week-old rat.

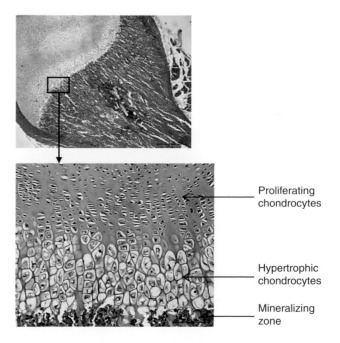

Proliferating chondrocytes

Hypertrophic chondrocytes

Mineralizing zone

Structure and Function of Bone

Bone is also classified as a specialized connective tissue; it is a **mineralized connective tissue** and is one of the hardest connective tissues when fully developed. The ECM of bone is comprised of 30% organic material composed mainly of fibres of **collagen type I** with small amounts of non-collagenous proteins. Some 45% of the ECM is made up of small, inorganic, plate-like crystals of **calcium hydroxyapatite** which is a hydrated form of calcium phosphate. It is the hydroxyapatite that gives bone its mechanical strength. Cementum, dentine and enamel are also mineralized connective tissues but the ECM of these tissues contains a greater percentage of hydroxyapatite compared to bone. The ECM of cementum contains 55% hydroxyapatite (by dry weight), much lower than the hydroxyapatite content of dentine and enamel, which are 70% and 90% respectively.

It is the ECM of bone which gives the tissue its mechanical strength and enables it to perform the **functions** of **support** for the body and **protection** of internal organs and tissues such as the brain, spinal cord, lungs, heart, pelvic viscera and bone marrow. The bones enable attachment of muscles so **enabling movement**; for example, movement of the legs and arms and chest cavity during ventilation of the lungs. The bones of the body contain 99% of the total body calcium in the ECM and therefore play an important role in **calcium homeostasis**. Serum Ca^{2+} levels are maintained by interplay between absorption in the intestines, renal excretion and skeletal mobilization or uptake of calcium ions in bone. The outer surfaces of all bones are covered by a layer of dense connective tissue called the periosteum. A thin cell-rich connective tissue called the endosteum lines the surfaces of bone facing the marrow cavity.

Types of Bone

There are three types of bone: **cortical bone**, **trabecular bone** and **woven bone** (Figure 3.8).

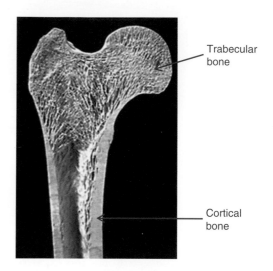

Trabecular bone

Cortical bone

Figure 3.8 Longitudinal section through a femur to show the cortical and trabecular bone.

Cortical bone: approximately 80% of the skeleton is composed of cortical bone which has a very characteristic dense structure, with no spaces or hollows visible to the naked eye. It forms the outer surfaces of all bones (Figure 3.9a). Cortical bone forms the thick-walled tube of bone forming the shaft (diaphysis) of long bones which surrounds the marrow cavity. A thin layer of compact bone also covers the epiphyses of long bones.

Trabecular bone has a porous 'lace-like' structure consistng of delicate bars and sheets of bone called trabeculae (Figure 3.9b) and which make up approximately 20% of bone in the body. Most trabecular bone is found in the axial skeleton (the bones of the skull, vertebrae and ribs). Although trabecular bone is weaker than cortical bone when tested by 'testing machines', overall bone strength is also dependent on the microstructure of trabecular bone. This aspect is highlighted in the disease condition osteoporosis where reduced oestrogen or androgen levels in the body result in an increase in bone resorption and in 'thinning' and loss of the trabecular bone. The consequence of this is an increased risk of bone fracture.

Woven bone (Figure 3.10) is the first form of bone to be laid down in bone formation during

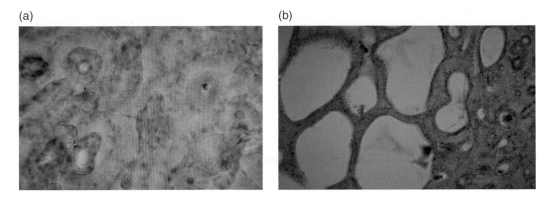

Figure 3.9 (a) Image of a ground section of mineralized cortical bone. The 'tree-ring'-like structures that arise are called Haversian systems. (b) Ground section image of mineralized trabecular bone.

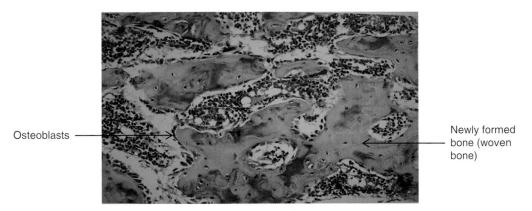

Osteoblasts — Newly formed bone (woven bone)

Figure 3.10 Histological section of demineralized woven bone formed by endochondral ossification. The blue-coloured regions are remaining areas of hypertrophic cartilage which are being remodelled into woven bone.

development of bone during embryogenesis, rapid growth and repair after fracture, and in response to certain anabolic factors. Woven bone has a higher density of cells, both osteoblasts and osteocytes, than cortical or trabecular bone and lacks the strength of mature bone (cortical or trabecular). The collagen is also in deposited in a random, interlacing fashion and is composed of thicker fibres. But it has the important advantage that it can be formed very quickly within weeks. Once formed, the woven bone is then remodelled in the body over a period of several months into cortical or trabecular bone as required.

Cell Types Found in Bone

In common with all connective tissues, bone tissue is dependent on bone cells in the ECM to maintain the structure and strength and metabolic functions of the tissue. Bone contains several cell types, all of which are necessary to maintain the integrity of the ECM and the principal cell types are listed below.

Osteoblasts are responsible for **synthesizing** and **mineralizing** bone ECM. The osteoblasts first form a cell layer at the sites of bone formation. A collagen-rich organic matrix is secreted first by the osteoblasts which is then mineralized by the cells.

When the cells are forming bone they become trapped in the bone matrix and either undergo apoptosis or differentiate into osteocytes (see below).

Osteocytes are found embedded in bone matrix; they are derived from osteoblasts that have become trapped in the matrix during ECM synthesis. Osteocytes have an important function of **sensing** the **mechanical loads** placed upon bone and are involved in the maintenance of the ECM and **calcium homeostasis**.

Osteoclasts are large, multinucleated cells which are responsible for **bone resorbtion**. These cells bind to the bone matrix and secrete hydrochloric acid and an enzyme, cathepsin K, which break down the ECM.

Osteoprogenitor cells are the precursor cells of osteoblasts. The osteoprogenitor cells are mesenchymal stem cells which are located in the periosteum and endosteum and can differentiate into osteoblasts when bone formation is required. Osteoclasts are derived from haemopoietic stem cells which are found within the bone marrow.

Muscle

Muscle is a contractile tissue essential for movement in animals. Three types of muscle that differ in their structure and function are found in the body; **smooth** muscle, **skeletal** muscle (also known as striated or voluntary muscle) and **cardiac** muscle (this is covered in Chapter 4). Smooth muscle is composed of small oval cell cells containing an irregular pattern of contractile protein fibres (this irregularity makes the muscle look smooth under the microscope, hence the name). Smooth muscle function is regulated by the autonomic nervous system and is capable of long, sustained contractions, such as those seen in visceral tissue like the gastrointestinal tract. Skeletal muscle is widespread throughout the body, often connected to bones; it is

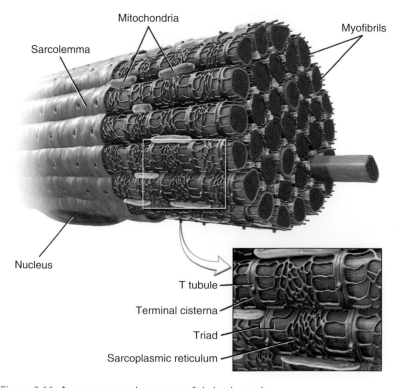

Figure 3.11 Appearance and structure of skeletal muscle.

composed of cells containing regular arrays of contractile proteins (mainly myosin and actin) which give skeletal muscle its characteristic striated (stripy) appearance (Figure 3.11). Skeletal muscle is controlled by the somatic nervous system and is capable of short, vigorous contractions.

Structure of Muscle

Muscle cells (sometimes called fibres) are largely composed of myofibrils, which are made up of actin- and myosin-rich myofibrils.

These form functional units (sarcomeres) in which myosin and actin fibres are interleaved; several of these join end to end to form the muscle fibre (Figure 3.11). There are two types of muscle fibre: type I (slow twitch) and type II (fast twitch). Slow twitch fibres contract slowly (hence the name) and contain a lot of mitochondria and are able to produce large amounts of energy slowly by aerobic metabolism and are resistant to fatigue. Fast twitch fibres, in contrast, produce large amounts of energy quickly, leading to rapid, strong contractions and early fatigue. They contain

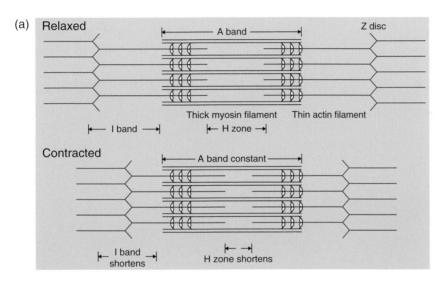

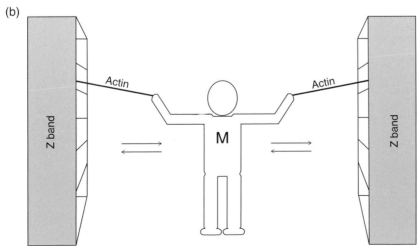

Figure 3.12 Structure of muscle and the sliding filament theory.

few mitochondria and produce energy for contraction largely through anaerobic respiration (see Chapter 1).

How do Muscles Contract?

Muscle contraction occurs when the actin and myosin fibres making up the sarcomeres slide over each other, causing the sarcomere to shorten (Figure 3.12). The coordinated shortening of many sarcomeres, stacked to form the striations visible under a microscope, causes the length of the muscle to change.

Control of Muscle Contraction

Skeletal muscle contraction is regulated by the somatic nervous system, with signals provided by motor neurones which may innervate one or many muscle fibres; this is collectively termed a motor unit. Large motor units, in which a single motor neurone may innervate thousands of muscle fibres, often control large, postural muscles; in muscles requiring very fine control, for example in the tongue, a motor unit may be composed of a much smaller number of muscle fibres innervated by a single motor neurone.

4

The Cardiovascular, Circulatory and Pulmonary Systems

Peter P. Jones

Otago School of Medical Sciences, University of Otago, Dunedin, New Zealand

---

Learning Objectives

- To be able to describe the structure of the heart and how blood flows through it.
- To understand the mechanism of heart contraction.
- To be able to describe the biological events that occur during a normal electrocardiogram.
- To be able to describe the circulatory system and structure of blood vessels.
- To be able to explain the regulation of blood flow and blood pressure.
- To be able to describe the pulmonary system and anatomy of the airways.
- To understand gas exchange and the mechanism and control of breathing.

Clinical Relevance

The cardiovascular system is an organ system where two organs work in cooperation and is a classic example of human physiology, homeostasis and control mechanisms. Healthcare professionals must be trained in medical emergencies including heart attack, fainting and choking, and therefore an understanding of the basic physiology is essential. As cardiovascular disease is one of the most prevalent in the developed world it is highly likely that a significant number of patients attending dental appointments will be taking medication to treat such conditions. A detailed medical history is thus essential prior to commencing treatment as such drugs can have a major impact on patient care; for example, the risk of undergoing dental extraction while on anticoagulant medication.

Introduction

The cardiovascular and pulmonary systems are not only essential for the efficient delivery of both metabolites and oxygen but also ensure the effective removal of carbon dioxide and waste products from all organs of the body. In order to achieve this function the flow of blood must be carefully controlled. Heart rate, blood flow and ventilation must be dynamically regulated to accommodate the demands of the body at rest, as it

Basic Sciences for Dental Students, First Edition. Edited by Simon A. Whawell and Daniel W. Lambert.
© 2018 John Wiley & Sons Ltd. Published 2018 by John Wiley & Sons Ltd.
Companion website: www.wiley.com/go/whawell/basic_sciences_for_dental_students

moves and as it responds to the external environment. Simplistically it may appear that all these systems work independently; the heart as a pump, the blood vessels as pipes and the lungs as spaces for gas exchange. However, all of these systems receive similar neuronal and hormonal input and must work together seamlessly. This chapter will describe the basic structure and function of cardiovascular and pulmonary systems and how they are controlled by both external and internal factors.

Cardiac System

The Heart as a Pump

The average human heart beats roughly 70 times per minute; therefore, during an average lifetime the heart will beat almost 3 billion times. Each and every one of these beats is critical and it only takes a few to be missed or ill-timed to lead to serious complications or death. Every beat of the heart ejects blood and forces it around the body. The volume of blood ejected per beat is known as the **stroke volume** (**SV**) and is typically around 70 mL at rest. However, a more important measure is the total volume of blood pumped out of the heart per minute; this is known as the **cardiac output** (**CO**). This measure takes into account both the SV and the **heart rate** (**HR**).

$$CO = SV \times HR$$

Therefore:

$$CO = 70\,mL \times 70\,beats/min = 4900\,mL/min$$

CO is dependent on body size as a larger person will have a larger heart and therefore a larger SV. In order for the heart to pump blood effectively it must contract in a coordinated manner.

Structure of the Heart

The heart is actually **two pumps** which work in **series**, with the right side of the heart pumping blood to the lungs and the left side of the heart pumping blood to the rest of the body. These two systems are known as the **pulmonary** and **systemic** circulations, respectively. Each side of the heart is further divided into two chambers, giving the heart **four chambers** in total. At the top of the heart are the right and left **atria** and below them are the right and left **ventricles**. The atria receive blood returning from the body (right atrium) or the lungs (left atrium) and are responsible for collecting and then pumping blood into the ventricles below. The ventricles pump blood out of the heart to the lungs (right ventricle) or the body (left ventricle). The left and right sides of the heart are divided by a piece of cardiac muscle known as the atrial or ventricular **septum** which ensures that blood flows in a single direction through the heart (Figure 4.1).

Blood Flow through the Heart

De-oxygenated, carbon-dioxide-rich blood returns from the systemic circulation via the **superior vena cava** (blood return from the head, arms and upper torso) or the **inferior vena cava** (blood return from the rest of the body) (see 1 on Figure 4.2). Both of these vessels flow into the right atrium. As the heart contracts blood is forced through the **tricuspid valve** into the right ventricle (see 2 on Figure 4.2). From here the blood is pumped up through the **pulmonary valve** (see 3 on Figure 4.2) into the **pulmonary artery** and into the lungs (see 4 on Figure 4.2). In the lungs the blood releases carbon dioxide and takes up oxygen. This oxygenated blood is delivered to the left atrium by the **pulmonary veins** (see 5 on Figure 4.2). As the heart contracts again the left atrium pumps blood into the left ventricle through the **bicuspid valve** (also known as the **mitral valve**) (see 6 on Figure 4.2). Finally contraction of the left ventricle ejects blood through the **aortic valve** into the **aorta** and to the whole body (see 7 on Figure 4.2).

Systemic versus Pulmonary Circulation

Although the left and right sides of the heart work simultaneously to pump blood to the body and lungs respectively the force of

Figure 4.1 The structure of the heart.

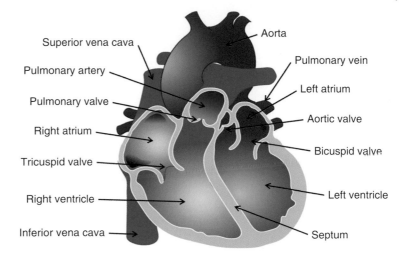

Superior vena cava

Pulmonary artery

Pulmonary valve

Right atrium

Tricuspid valve

Right ventricle

Inferior vena cava

Aorta

Pulmonary vein

Left atrium

Aortic valve

Bicuspid valve

Left ventricle

Septum

Figure 4.2 Blood flow and electrical conduction pathways in the heart.

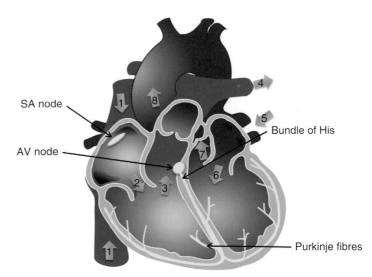

SA node

AV node

Bundle of His

Purkinje fibres

contraction and therefore the blood pressure that each side of the heart can generate differ considerably. The pulmonary circulation is a low-pressure system as it only perfuses the relatively delicate lungs. The peak pressure generated during contraction, known as **systolic pressure**, is roughly 2520 mmHg and the resting pressure between beats, known as **diastolic pressure**, is around 108 mmHg. In contrast the systemic circulation is a high-pressure system as it must pump blood to up to the head and around the rest of the body. Therefore the systolic pressure in the systemic system is typically 120 mmHg and the diastolic pressure is 80 mmHg. The thickness of muscle on each side of the heart reflects the systolic pressure generated with the left ventricular wall averaging 1.1 cm compared to just 0.35 cm in the right ventricle.

See Feature box 4.1.

Contraction of the Heart

Contraction of the heart is initiated by a group of cells known as **pacemakers**; these cells represent around 1% of cardiac cells. Pacemaker cells are small, round cells which contain little or no contractile protein and

---

Feature box 4.1 Structural defects

To maintain sufficient CO blood must flow through the heart in sequence. However, a number of structural defects in the heart can alter this pathway. Several defects observed are congenital and are identified *in utero* or shortly after birth. The most frequent congenital defect is commonly referred to as 'a hole in the heart' but is clinically defined as a ventricular or atrial septal defect. As the name suggests these defects lead to a hole in the septum separating the left and right sides of the heart. As the blood in the left side of the heart is at a much higher pressure this leads to oxygenated blood being forced into the right de-oxygenated side of the heart. This has two consequences; first the CO is decreased as blood is pumped back into the right side of the heart rather than out through the aorta and secondly the influx of blood into the right side of the heart increases pulmonary pressure, leading to a disease known as pulmonary hypertension. A common non-congenital defect is aortic obstruction. Here the tissue surrounding the aortic valve becomes enlarged and reduces blood flow into the aorta which reduces CO.

---

therefore do not contribute to the contraction of the heart. These cells are responsible for generating an **action potential**. Pacemaker cells are clustered in two regions known as the **sino-atrial (SA)** node and the **atrioventricular (AV)** node. As cells within the SA node have an **unstable** membrane potential they **spontaneously** generate an action potential roughly 100 times per minute. SA node cells are tightly electrically coupled to the neighbouring contractile cardiac cells (**myocytes**) via **gap junctions**; therefore the action potential generated by the SA node is rapidly propagated throughout the atria ($\approx 0.5\,\text{m/s}$). This action potential is the **electrical trigger** which signals the myocytes to contract. Once the action potential has propagated through the atria, causing atrial contraction, it progresses to the ventricles.

However, the structure of the heart only allows the action potential to reach the ventricles by passing through the AV node. Cells within the AV node **slow the transmission** of the action potential (to $\approx 0.05\,\text{m/s}$), leading to a brief **delay** between atrial and ventricular contraction. This delay ensures that blood is completely ejected from the atria before the ventricles contract. Once the action potential leaves the AV node it is very rapidly transmitted ($\approx 5\,\text{m/s}$) to the bottom of the ventricles through specialized conductive cells known as the **bundle of His** and **Purkinje fibres** (Figure 4.2). The action potential then propagates up through the ventricles ($\approx 0.5\,\text{m/s}$). This allows fairly **synchronous** transmission of the action potential and contraction throughout the ventricles.

See Feature box 4.2.

Feature box 4.2 Arrhythmias

The conduction of the action potential through the heart must be completely synchronized. If the action potential does not propagate uniformly it can lead to arrhythmias. Arrhythmias may cause different parts of the heart contract at different times, reducing the effectiveness of the pump and thus decreasing CO. Arrhythmias can occur in both the atria and ventricles with those occurring in the ventricles having the greatest impact. Many ventricular arrhythmias can be so severe that the CO is effectively zero, which rapidly leads to death. Arrhythmias are frequently caused by sections of non-conductive heart tissue formed due to ischaemia or by dying myocytes which have unstable membrane potentials and therefore form 'ectopic' pacemaker cells.

How do Action Potentials lead to Contraction?

Between beats the **resting membrane potential** (**RMP**) of myocytes is determined by the high membrane permeability of potassium. The loss of potassium from each myocyte gives the cell an electrical charge or **polarizes** the cell so that they have a RMP of –90 mV. For contraction to take place an action potential arrives from the pacemaker cells, which increases the membrane's permeability to sodium. The positively charged sodium rushes into the cell and rapidly increases the membrane potential of, or **depolarizing**, the cell. As the membrane potential becomes positive **voltage-gated** calcium channels open to allow an influx of calcium. This calcium induces more calcium release from the internal calcium store (**sarcoplasmic reticulum**) in a process termed **calcium-induced calcium release** (**CICR**). Calcium within the cell then binds to troponin which triggers contraction. This entire process is known as **excitation-contraction coupling**. Relaxation occurs when calcium dissociates from troponin and is cycled back into the sarcoplasmic reticulum or is extruded from the cell; at the same time potassium begins to enter the cell, causing repolarization to –90 mV.

The Electrocardiogram (ECG)

The **electrocardiogram** (**ECG**) is a body surface representation of the depolarization and repolarization of all of the cells in the heart. Typically 12 **leads** are attached to the arms, legs and chest, each electrode giving a measurement of electrical activity from a different part of the heart. The most commonly recognized ECG is generated by lead II. By monitoring the electrical signal from lead II the depolarization and repolarization of the atria and ventricles can be determined. A typical ECG contains five 'waves' (P, Q, R, S and T) (Figure 4.3). The **P wave** represents atrial depolarization, the Q, R and S waves, known together as the **QRS complex**, represent ventricular depolarization and the **T wave** represents ventricular repolarization

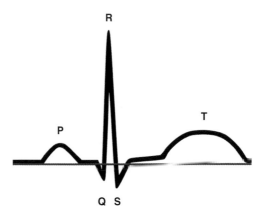

Figure 4.3 A typical electrocardiogram (ECG).

(note the repolarization of the atria is not observed as a wave as it is hidden in the QRS complex). An ECG gives a good indication of the electrical properties of the heart and can be used to determine a number of parameters and diseases. For example the **R–R interval** (time between sequential R waves) is used to calculate HR, and the **Q–T interval** indicates how long ventricular repolarization takes; this is important because an elongated Q–T interval increases the risk of arrhythmias. During arrhythmia the ECG becomes disrupted, and during ventricular arrhythmia the P wave is lost as the ventricles contract spontaneously. As arrhythmias increase in severity and progress towards **ventricular fibrillation** all of the waves can be difficult to discern and the ECG can often take on a saw-tooth pattern.

Extrinsic Control of the Heart

Although CO at rest is around 5 L/min, blood flow from the heart must vary considerably depending on the demands of the body. For example, during exercise the **metabolic activity** of muscle is increased and therefore so is its oxygen consumption. In order to meet this increased demand the heart must increase its CO. As CO is determined by both SV and HR a change of one or both of these variables can alter its magnitude. During exercise the heart receives an increased input from the **sympathetic** nervous system, which acts on **β-receptors** in the heart. This increased sympathetic drive reduces the time between action potential generation in the pacemaker cells, and in turn this leads to an increase in HR. This change in HR is termed a **chrono-tropic** response. Additionally, the sympathetic drive to the heart also increases the strength of contraction of each myocyte, and this leads to an increase in SV. This change in contractile force is termed an **ionotropic** response. The combined increase in both HR and SV significantly increases CO. In contrast, **parasympathetic** drive decreases both chronotropy and ionotropy reducing CO. Therefore, the CO of the heart at any given time is due to the balance of sympathetic and parasympathetic activity. At rest it is the parasympathetic drive that is responsible for reducing the frequency of action potentials generated by cells within SA node from 100 times per minute to approximately 70 times per minute to give us our normal resting HR.

See Feature box 4.3.

Intrinsic Control of the Heart

Extrinsic regulation of the heart also impacts on the intrinsic properties of the heart. An increase in chronotropy mediated by sympathetic input increases the ionotropy of the heart at the cellular level. This relationship is known as the **Bowditch**, **Treppe** or **Staircase** effect due to the stepwise increase in contractility of a cardiac cell as contraction frequency increases (Figure 4.4). The cellular mechanism by which this effect occurs is not completely understood but is thought to be due to an increase in calcium concentrations within the cell. Another intrinsic regulatory

mechanism of controlling the CO of the heart is the **Frank–Starling** response. The Frank–Starling law states that SV increases as the filling of the heart with blood increases. This means as blood pressure increases so does the volume of blood within the heart before a contraction. This increase in volume stretches the chambers of the heart which triggers a more forceful contraction, thus increasing SV (Figure 4.5). Combined, the

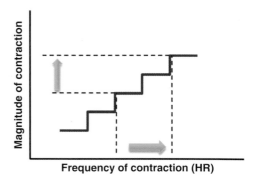

Figure 4.4 Bowditch, Treppe or Staircase effect.

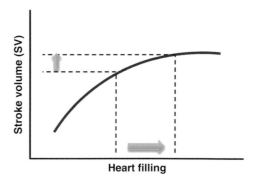

Figure 4.5 Frank–Starling response.

Feature box 4.3 β-Blockers

Heart disease commonly leads to an increase in sympathetic nerve activity; this in turn leads to a chronic increase in CO. Just like increasing the work of any other muscle over time this leads to an increase in muscle size. In the heart this is termed cardiac hypertrophy. As cardiac hypertrophy increases, the ejection of blood becomes less efficient, which can lead to insufficient blood supply to the body, particularly the heart itself. This decrease in blood perfusion of the heart is a common cause of heart attacks. Accordingly heart failure patients are often given β-blockers to decrease sympathetic input into the heart, preventing hypertrophy from occurring.

Bowditch effect and the Frank–Starling response work together as intrinsic mechanisms to amplify the effect of external sympathetic stimulation. Conversely, these mechanisms allow a greater reduction in CO due to parasympathetic stimulation as both HR and blood pressure are reduced.

Circulatory System

Anatomy

The movement of blood around the body is achieved by a vast network of blood vessels that deliver **oxygenated** blood to tissues and remove **carbon dioxide** for exhalation through the lungs. This dual function means the vasculature can be divided into two parts: (1) the **arterial system** which carries oxygenated blood from the heart and (2) the **venous system** which carries de-oxygenated blood back to the lungs. These two systems work in series to one another but within each system blood flows in **parallel**. In the pulmonary system blood flows from the heart to both lungs simultaneously. This ensures the blood is re-oxygenated efficiently rather than passing from lung to lung. Similarly in the systemic circulation blood flows to each organ in parallel, therefore all parts of the body receive oxygen-rich blood. The only major organ that is an exception to this is the **liver** as its function requires it to receive blood directly from the **stomach**, **intestines** and **pancreas** (Figure 4.6). It is important to note that although they oxygenate and pump blood, both the lungs and the heart themselves receive oxygenated blood from the systemic circulatory system.

See Feature box 4.4.

Different Types of Vessel in the Circulatory System

Blood leaves the heart through large-diameter **arteries** which primarily act as low-resistance **conduit vessels** delivering bulk blood flow at a high pressure. Arteries

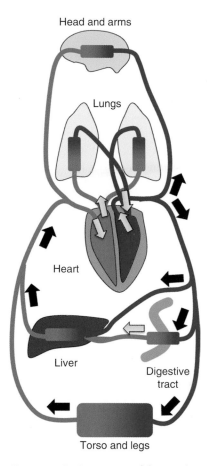

Figure 4.6 Basic anatomy of the circulatory system.

divide into smaller-diameter **arterioles** which offer more resistance, significantly reducing blood pressure before it reaches the delicate **capillaries**. Arterioles are also where the majority of blood pressure regulation occurs (see Blood Flow and Regulation). Capillaries are very narrow vessels ($<10\,\mu m$) which permeate almost all tissues to such an extent that barely any cells are more than a few cell widths ($\approx100\,\mu m$) away from their nearest vessel. This very short distance allows extremely efficient diffusion of gases, nutrients and waste products between cells and the blood. Capillaries turn into **venules** which continue to allow diffusion between the cells and blood. Venules then combine to form **veins** which like arteries are primarily a conduit system for returning blood to the heart (Figure 4.7).

Feature box 4.4 Coronary artery disease

The heart does not extract oxygen from the blood within its chambers; therefore it has a dedicated blood supply via the coronary arteries. Given the metabolic demand of the cardiac muscle it is imperative that this supply is maintained. Atherosclerosis is the thickening of the arterial wall due to the formation of plaques consisting of deposits of fat (particularly cholesterol), abnormal smooth muscle cells and connective tissue. When atherosclerosis occurs it begins to narrow the coronary vessels, increasing their resistance (see Blood Flow and Regulation) and decreasing blood flow. Although blood flow is reduced it typically does not stop completely: this occurs when the plaque ruptures. When a plaque ruptures a blood clot frequently forms on the surface which completely occludes the vessel. The area of the heart supplied by this coronary vessel becomes starved of blood (ischaemic) and begins to die. If the region affected is large enough this can alter the action potential propagation through the heart which can ultimately result in arrhythmias.

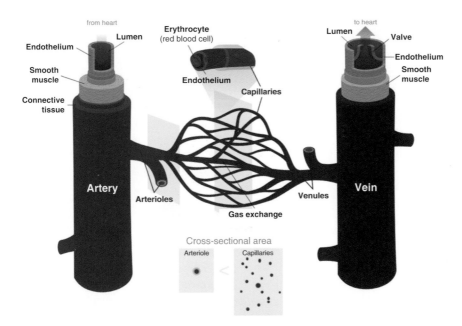

Figure 4.7 Structure and function of the different blood vessels.

Basic Structure of Blood Vessels

The structure of blood vessels largely reflects their function. The inside of vessels is called the **lumen**, which is always lined by **endothelial** cells. Endothelial cells are the internal layer of the **vessel wall** which, depending on the function and blood pressure experienced, can be formed by a single layer of cells or multiple thick layers of cells including muscle. The arteries leaving the heart experience the highest blood pressure so they have a relatively thick wall. Arterial walls are formed from a central layer of endothelial cells followed by many layers of **smooth muscle** cells and **connective tissue**, containing **elastin** and **collagen**, which run around the circumference of the vessels. These layers give the vessel strength, allowing it to resist the high blood pressure leaving the heart. As the blood pressure in artererioles is lower, less support is required and therefore these vessels are composed of endothelial cells surrounded by a much thinner layer of smooth muscle. Capillaries have the simplest structure and are formed by a single tube of endothelial cells. The very thin wall of capillaries allows the rapid diffusion of gases and nutrients into and out of the surrounding tissue. All of the venous system experiences a low pressure (less than 15 mmHg) and therefore all vessels in this system need much less structural support. This low pressure is enough to maintain unidirectional flow as in general these vessels are relatively large and offer little resistance. The presence of **unidirectional valves** also prevents any backflow and ensures unidirectional flow towards the heart. Venules are composed of endothelia surrounded by a thin layer of connective tissue, whereas the vessel wall of veins also contains a few layers of smooth muscle cells (Figure 4.7). This thin smooth muscle layer allows veins to contract and dilate, akin to arteries, to regulate blood flow back into the heart, which in turn alters the Frank–Starling response of the heart (see Intrinsic Control of the Heart).

Blood Flow and Regulation

Blood flow is dependent on the **pressure gradient** (ΔP) and the **resistance** (R) of the vessel through which the blood is flowing:

$$\text{Blood flow} = \frac{\Delta P}{R}$$

The pressure gradient through a vessel is **directly proportional** to the **force** and **frequency** of blood ejection from the heart (CO) and the resistance is **inversely proportional** to the **diameter** of the vessel. Therefore, blood flow is greatest as it leaves the heart where the pressure gradient is largest and the diameter of the arteries is largest. As blood moves away from the heart, large arteries branch into many, many smaller arteries and then arterioles. The smaller diameter of these vessels dramatically increases the resistance and reduces the pressure gradient and thus blood flow. Although blood flow within each vessel

decreases **total flow** (summation of flow in all parallel vessels) remains the same. Importantly, arteriole diameter can be altered due to the smooth muscle surrounding them; this allows the redistribution of blood towards or away from specific areas of the body at certain times. Vasoconstriction is achieved by activating the smooth muscle surrounding the vessels. This contraction of smooth muscle is normally mediated by sympathetic nerve activity and the release of the hormone adrenaline (epinephrine) from the sympathetic nerves which together activate smooth muscle **α-receptors**. Smooth muscle cells also contain β-receptors which trigger vasodilation but their density is much lower so the effect of α-receptors dominates. This explains why blood pressure is increased by stressful situations and exercise. Unlike cardiac muscle there is little to no parasympathetic innervation of arteriole smooth muscle so therefore vasodilation is mediated by a withdrawal of sympathetic stimulation. On the surface this vasoconstriction due to sympathetic nerve activity during exercise or stress would seem counterintuitive as although CO would increase so would vascular resistance, limiting blood flow to skeletal muscle. However, unlike most smooth muscle cells, those surrounding arterioles in skeletal muscle have a high density of β-receptors in addition to α-receptors. Therefore, the vasodilatory effect of these receptors dominates, leading to arteriole vasodilation in skeletal muscle. The result is that the resistance of arterioles in skeletal muscle decreases and elsewhere it increases. This diverts blood towards skeletal muscle increasing its blood supply to meet the metabolic demand (Figure 4.8).

See Feature box 4.5.

Auto-regulation of Blood Pressure

In addition to the diversion of blood flow to specific parts of the body during exercise and other stimuli the body must also regulate the overall blood pressure to keep it within a safe range. As blood pressure increases it stretches

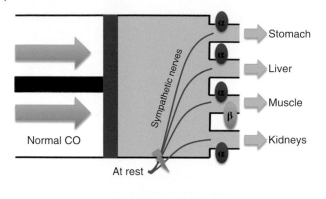

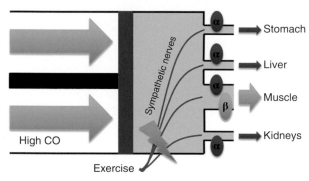

Figure 4.8 Mechanisms to redistribute blood flow.

Feature box 4.5 Clinical complications in the control of blood flow and pressure

Patients taking β-blockers may respond to anaesthetics containing adrenaline differently to other patients. Adrenaline is often included in local anaesthetics as it mimics the effect of sympathetic nerve activation and generally causes vasoconstriction. This helps reduce blood loss and prolong the effect of the anaesthetic. Adrenaline acts on both α-receptors and β-receptors of blood vessels so although the overall effect is vasoconstriction this is tempered by some vasodilatory action due to activation of the β-receptors. This small vasodilation response is abolished in patients using β-blockers which can lead to hyper-constriction and therefore severe hypertension (systolic pressure >200 mmHg), in turn leading to a range of symptoms from a headache to stroke.

---

the **carotid arteries** and the aorta. These vessels contain **baroreceptors** which like pacemakers can generate action potentials. As stretch increases the baroreceptors increase the rate at which they generate action potentials. The action potentials are transmitted to the **cardioregulatory** and **vasomotor centres** in the **medulla oblongata** in the brain stem via the **vagus** and **glossopharyngeal** nerves. This decreases sympathetic and increases parasympathetic input into the heart, reducing both chronotropy and ionotropy and thus CO.

At the same time sympathetic input into the blood vessels is also decreased, which causes **vasodilation**. The combination of a reduced CO and dilation of the blood vessels brings the elevated blood pressure back to normal (Figure 4.9). If blood pressure becomes too low all of these effects are reversed: sympathetic input into the heart and vessels is increased and parasympathetic input is decreased, together increasing CO and causing **vasoconstriction**.

See Feature box 4.6.

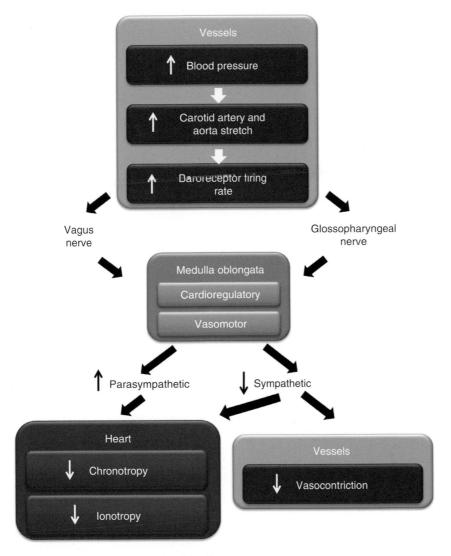

Figure 4.9 Maintenance of a stable blood pressure.

Feature box 4.6 Antihypertensive drugs

High blood pressure or hypertension is a major cause of morbidity and mortality. Antihypertensive drugs are designed to reduce blood pressure. A few drugs act to reduce blood volume by increasing water and salt loss through the kidneys. However, the majority of antihypertensive drug types work by reducing CO or inhibiting vasoconstriction. β-Blockers decrease sympathetic input to the heart, reducing CO; in addition, calcium channel blockers decrease CO and inhibit vasoconstriction and angiotensin-converting enzyme (ACE) inhibitors inhibit vasoconstriction. Combined, these effects either override the physiological pathway to increase blood pressure or act directly on the heart and vessels to decrease blood pressure.

Posture, Blood Volume and Blood Pressure

Although many blood vessels are supported by smooth muscle and connective tissue their walls are not rigid. Therefore, as **gravity** is a determinant of how much pressure is exerted on the vessel walls those vessels below the heart (both arterial and venous) are somewhat **distended** when standing. This is especially true for the **lower extremities** which can be 1 m or more below the heart. However, when lying down most of the vessels in the body are at roughly the same level as the heart. Consequently moving from a standing to sitting or supine position can have a profound effect on blood pressure in specific regions of the body. For example **standing** from a **supine** position shifts a large volume of blood into the leg veins potentially decreasing blood pressure, particularly to the head. To avoid this, baroreceptors must respond quickly to maintain adequate perfusion of the brain and prevent **fainting** or **syncope**. The body is tuned to the average position; that is, somewhere between lying and standing. This means that when standing the upper body experiences a low blood volume and responds with vasoconstriction. In addition to vasoconstriction movement is also important in moving blood up from the lower extremities. Muscle contraction during walking or other forms of leg activity squeezes the veins moving the blood. As veins contain unidirectional valves blood can only move towards the heart, driving blood up the body; this mechanism is known as the **skeletal muscle pump** (Figure 4.10). The requirement for skeletal muscle activity is one of the reasons lower leg blood pooling occurs during prolonged periods of sitting during international air travel. Conversely, when lying down the body responds with vasodilation as if it was experiencing hypertension. This is due to the increased blood volume in the torso and head. Although the body is normally tuned to the average position, extended periods of time in any position can cause the body to reset this set point; this is particularly problematic in patients who have long periods of 'bed rest' who are at a greater risk of insufficient brain perfusion when standing and other rapid positional changes.

The Pulmonary System

Anatomy of the Airways and Gas Exchange

Like the circulation system the respiratory system is formed by a large network, in this case of airways. When **inspiration** (inhalation) takes place, air rushes into the

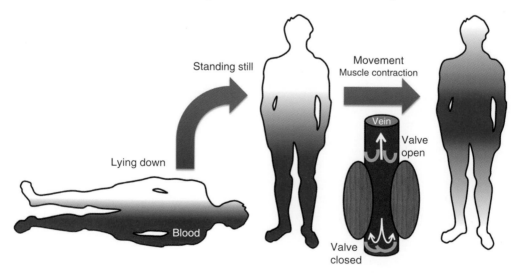

Figure 4.10 Effect of posture on blood distribution.

mouth or nose and into the **pharynx**, a cavity which links them together. From here air moves past the **hyoid bone** through the **larynx** (home of the vocal chords). Combined, the mouth, nose pharynx and larynx form the **upper airway**. After passing the larynx air moves down a **conduit** system composed of the **trachea** which subsequently branches into the left and right **bronchi** that direct air into the left and right lungs respectively. In the lungs the bronchi further divide into **bronchioles**. Air then moves from the conduit system into the **gas exchange** system of the lungs, which is composed of **respiratory bronchioles**, **alveolar ducts** and finally **alveolar sacs** and **alveoli** (Figure 4.11). Like a tree each division of the airway increases the number of branches. Starting with one airway, the trachea, the lungs ultimately contain approximately 10 million alveolar sacs. All of the gas exchange system of the lungs is covered by alveoli, which are small air-filled pouches lined with thin **squamous/ alveolar epithelial** cells. It is estimated that each lung has approximately 300 million alveoli giving a surface area of about 30 m^2! The exchange of carbon dioxide for oxygen takes place across the walls of the alveoli. In many places the epithelial cells of the alveoli fuse with the endothelial cells of

the capillaries; this means the gases only have to diffuse across the width of two cells, less than 0.5 μm.

Mechanics of Breathing (Inspiration and Expiration)

Inspiration is the movement of air into the lungs. In order for air to move into the lungs they must be at a negative pressure compared to the atmospheric pressure. This negative pressure is primarily due to the **active** contraction and downward movement of the **diaphragm** (Figure 4.12). At the same time the intercostal muscles contract which causes the ribs to move upwards. Combined, these two motions increase the volume of the **thorax**. As the thorax enlarges, the pressure of **intrapleural fluid** which surrounds the lungs decreases. As the fluid surrounding the lungs is now **sub-atmospheric** the difference in pressures (ΔP) between the atmosphere and the intrapleural fluid overcomes the **elasticity** of the lungs and leads to the movement of air into the lungs, causing them to inflate. As the lungs inflate the pressure difference between the atmosphere and the intrapleural fluid decreases until it is in equilibrium with the elasticity of the lungs and therefore inspiration ends. A large factor in determining the

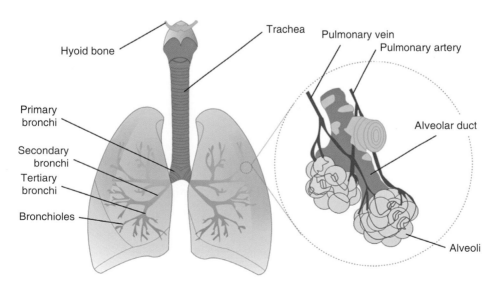

Figure 4.11 Basic anatomy of the lungs.

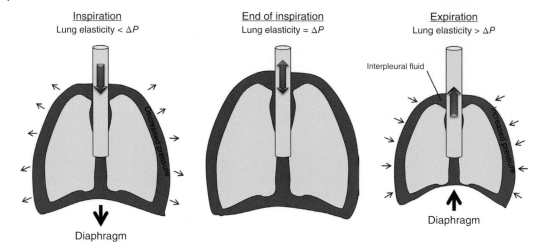

Figure 4.12 Mechanics of expiration and inspiration.

elasticity of the lungs is the **surface tension** of the alveoli. To aid in the expansion of the lungs the alveoli contain **type II cells** which secrete a **surfactant**. This fluid coats the alveoli and significantly reduces the surface tension.

Expiration is the movement of air out of the lungs. As inspiration finishes both the diaphragm and the intercostal muscle begin to relax. This causes both muscles to recoil to their resting positions. The decreasing volume of the thorax increases the intrapleural pressure which reduces the pressure difference between atmospheric and the intrapleural fluid. The elasticity of the lungs can now overcome this pressure difference and the lung volume decreases. As the alveoli begin to compress the air moves out of the lungs (Figure 4.12). As expiration only requires muscles to relax the whole process is

a **passive** one governed by the rate of relaxation and the atmospheric pressure.

The purpose of breathing is **ventilation**. Ventilation is the exchange of gas between the atmosphere and the alveoli. Like blood, air moves from a region of high pressure to a region of low pressure and the flow is inversely proportional to the resistance.

$$\text{Air flow} = \frac{\Delta P}{R}$$

During ventilation the pressure gradient is between the pressure in alveoli and the atmospheric pressure ($P_{\text{Alv}} - P_{\text{Atm}}$). Therefore, when atmospheric pressure is greater than alveolar pressure air flow is negative which leads to an inward movement of air (inspiration). When the converse is true air flow is positive and air is expelled (expiration).

See Feature boxes 4.7 and 4.8.

Feature box 4.7 Pneumothorax

As inspiration is completely dependent on the generation of a negative pressure within the thorax anything that hinders this has a major impact on lung inflation. A chest injury which penetrates the thorax will allow air to enter the intrapleural cavity. When this happens the intrapleural fluid is no longer kept at a negative pressure relative to the atmosphere. The elasticity of the lungs therefore causes the lungs to collapse. This phenomenon is known as a pneumothorax. To inflate the lungs a tube connected to a vacuum pump is used to decrease the intrapleural pressure before the puncture is repaired.

Feature box 4.8 Asthma

In patients with asthma, the airways are prone to periodic narrowing due to inflammation and spasm of the smooth muscle surrounding the airways. As with blood flow, air flow resistance is inversely proportional to the diameter of the airway. Therefore, as the diameter decreases the resistance increases, making breathing more difficult. Asthma is often treated with drugs that either reduce the inflammation or relax the smooth muscle cells directly, thus increasing airway diameter.

Exchange of Gas between the Atmosphere, Alveoli, Blood and Tissues

Once air enters the lungs during inspiration oxygen must move across the alveolar membrane into the capillaries then into the blood. At the same time carbon dioxide must move in the opposite direction. Gases, like fluids, move down their pressure gradients. The pressure of a specific gas (e.g. oxygen) in a mixture of gases (e.g. air) is called the **partial pressure** (P_x) and is calculated from the total pressure multiplied by the percentage that specific gas represents. Therefore, at sea level the partial pressure of O_2 (P_{O_2}) is:

$$P_{O_2} = 760 \text{ mmHg} \times 21\% = 160 \text{ mmHg}$$

In the alveoli the P_{O_2} is around 100 mmHg, in the blood the P_{O_2} is lower (90 mmHg) so oxygen moves down its P_{O_2} gradient into the capillaries. Finally oxygen diffuses out of the blood into tissue as the P_{O_2} of most tissues is less than 40 mmHg. The same process occurs in reverse for the diffusion of carbon dioxide out of tissue into the blood, alveoli (Figure 4.13).

Control of Breathing

During stress and exercise the amount of gas exchange occurring in the lungs must increase to match the increase in muscle metabolism. Breathing is controlled by signalling from the brain. This is because inspiration is governed by the contraction and downward movement of the diaphragm along with the upward movement of the ribs which rely on a neuronal input from the **motor neurones**. These neurones are controlled by the medulla oblongata in the brain. Within this region of the brain lies a group of pacemaker cells known as the **pre-Botzinger complex** which act in a similar way to cells in the SA node of the heart. At rest the rate of breathing is controlled by periodic signals from this complex to the diaphragm via the motor neurones. During exercise the

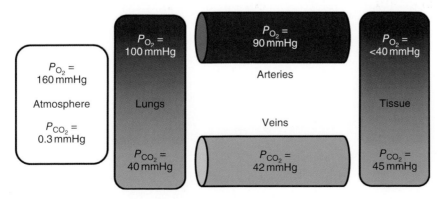

Figure 4.13 Diffusion and partial pressures of gases.

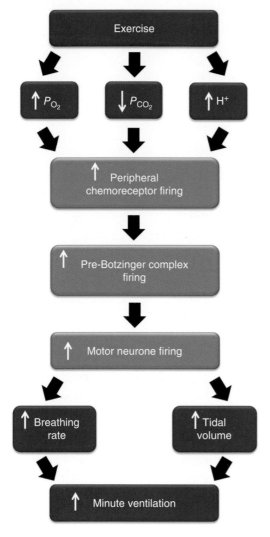

Figure 4.14 Control of breathing rate.

expiration allows the breathing rate to increase further as the lungs no longer have to rely on passive relaxation of the muscles. In addition to increasing the rate of breathing, exercise also increases the volume of air entering the lungs during a single breath (**tidal volume**). At rest the tidal volume of an adult is about 500 mL, but during exercise or deep breathing this can increase to over 3000 mL. Combined, the breathing rate and tidal volume give the **minute ventilation** which is the amount of air moved in and out of the pulmonary system each minute. In a typical adult at rest the minute ventilation is around 6000 mL:

Minute ventilation
= breathing rate (12 breaths/min)
  × tidal volume (500 mL)
= 6000 mL/min

During exercise, when both the breathing rate and tidal volume increase, the minute ventilation also increases. During strenuous prolonged exercise the minute ventilation can increase by more than 20 times. Although it is well established that the firing of the pre-Botzinger complex increases during exercise it is not fully understood why this occurs. It is proposed to be a combination of a decrease in P_{O_2}, an increase in P_{CO_2} and an increased acidification of the blood. All of these changes are a direct result of increased muscle metabolism. These changes stimulate the **peripheral chemoreceptors** located in arteries in the neck and aorta. When stimulated these receptors send action potentials to the pacemaker cells in the medulla oblongata, increasing minute ventilation as described above (Figure 4.14).

frequency of action potentials increases **breathing rate**. In addition to increasing the rate of inhalation another group of neurones can also trigger 'forced' expiration. Forced

5

The Nervous System

Fiona M. Boissonade

School of Clinical Dentistry, University of Sheffield, Sheffield, UK

Learning Objectives

- To be able to list the subdivisions and structural components of the nervous system.
- To be able to describe the role of neurones and glia.
- To understand the principles of membrane and action potentials and of synapses and neurotransmitters.
- To be able to describe the anatomy of neuronal axons, the spinal cord and the brain.
- To be able to describe the features of the autonomic nervous system and sensory and motor pathways.

Clinical Relevance

It is essential for dental care professionals to have detailed knowledge and understanding of neuroanatomy and physiology. Dental pain will be the most likely presenting symptom of urgent appointments, and sensation, taste, salivary flow and reflexes are all mediated by the nervous system. Many drugs including the various constituents of local anaesthetics work via their influence on different components of the nervous system.

Introduction

The nervous system transmits information around the body extremely rapidly. It receives and integrates input from the external and internal environment and formulates appropriate responses. The system also controls execution of these responses by coordinating voluntary and involuntary actions.

Subdivisions of the Nervous System

On a functional and anatomical basis the nervous system can be subdivided into the central nervous system (CNS) and the peripheral nervous system (PNS). The CNS consists of the brain and spinal cord; the PNS is made up of peripheral nerves, which transmit information to and from the CNS.

Basic Sciences for Dental Students, First Edition. Edited by Simon A. Whawell and Daniel W. Lambert.
© 2018 John Wiley & Sons Ltd. Published 2018 by John Wiley & Sons Ltd.
Companion website: www.wiley.com/go/whawell/basic_sciences_for_dental_students

The PNS is further subdivided into the somatic nervous system and the autonomic nervous system (Figure 5.1).

The somatic PNS contains afferent (sensory) components, carrying sensory information into the CNS; and efferent (motor) components, carrying outputs from the CNS (Figure 5.1). The afferent components convey information mainly from the external environment, and the efferent components control skeletal muscle involved in voluntary (and some reflex)

actions. It comprises 31 pairs of spinal nerves and 12 pairs of cranial nerves (Figure 5.2).

The autonomic nervous system is discussed in more detail in a later section. It controls the internal environment and maintains homeostasis by regulating involuntary action of smooth muscle, secretion from glands and regulation of organ function. It can be further divided into two components: the sympathetic system and the parasympathetic system.

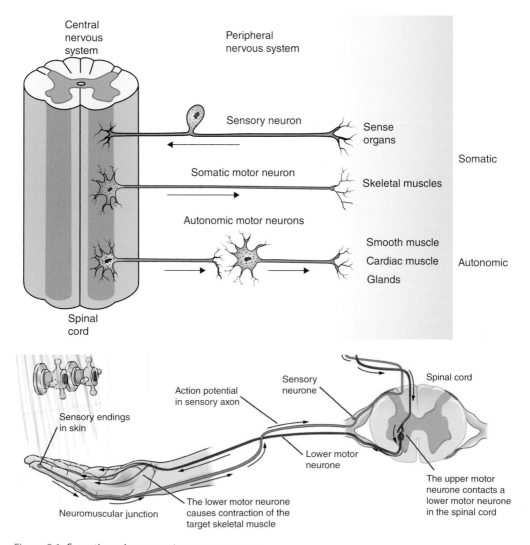

Figure 5.1 Somatic and autonomic nervous systems.

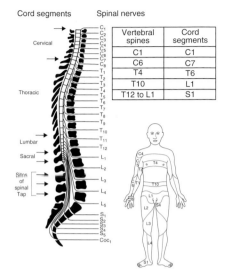

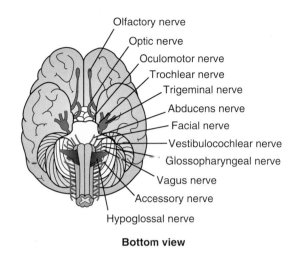

Bottom view

Figure 5.2 Spinal and cranial nerves.

Structural Components of the Nervous System

The nervous system contains a number of distinct components, namely neurones, synapses and glial cells. The functional units of the nervous system are the neurones (nerve cells), which carry information as electrical signals, often over considerable distances. These cells are not in electrical continuity but are separated by specialized cell junctions called synapses. Information is carried from one neurone to the next (across the synapse), by chemical messengers known as neurotransmitters. Neuronal function is supported and modulated by a variety of glial cells.

Neurones

Structure
Neurones are highly specialized to enable conduction of electrical impulses over long distances without attenuation of the signal. They are complex cells with widely varying morphology but can be divided into three major parts: cell body (or soma), axon and dendrites.

The cell body contains the nucleus and a number of cellular organelles (Figure 5.3). The majority of neuronal RNA is found in the nucleus, and most proteins are produced from mRNAs that are located in the cell body in close proximity to the nucleus. The axon is a single process that is often extremely long. For example, a motor neurone supplying the foot would have its cell body in the spinal cord and its axon would be approximately 1 m in length. Where the axon reaches its target it divides into a number of terminals where synaptic transmission takes place. Neurones also have other processes known as dendrites, which can be highly branched and may form extensive 'dendritic trees'. They receive incoming signals via synaptic transmission from other neurones and play a major role in integrating these inputs.

Membrane Potential
The ability of neurones to carry electrical impulses is vital to their function and arises as a consequence of specific properties of their cell membranes. Neuronal cell membranes contain specific ion channels and receptors that precisely control ionic movement across the membrane (Figure 5.4a).

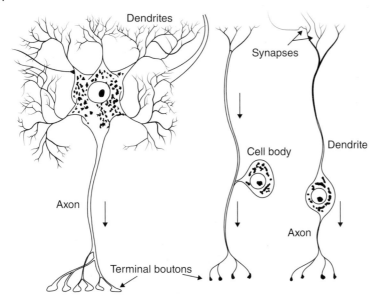

Figure 5.3 Neuronal morphology.

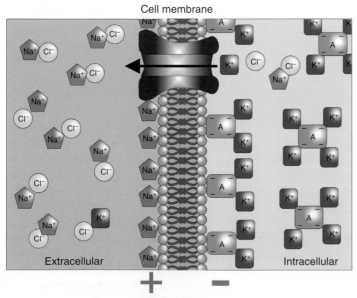

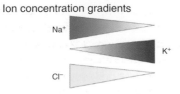

Figure 5.4 (a) Neuronal cell membranes.

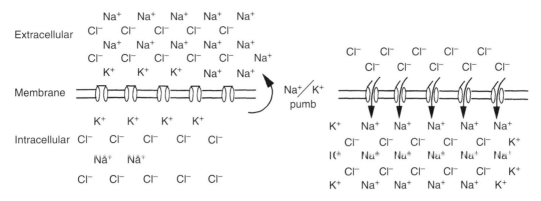

Figure 5.4 (b) Membrane and action potential.

They also contain specialized ion pumps that regulate ionic movement and concentration. This results in a significant potential difference (voltage difference) across the membrane, with the inside of the neurone being negatively charged with respect to the extracellular environment by −70 mV. The membrane potential (Figure 5.4b) is produced by the difference in concentration of ions on opposite sides of the membrane. This arises as a consequence of selective permeability of the membrane to a number of ions including sodium, potassium and chloride ions along with a number of large intracellular anions from a variety of sources, including proteins. At rest the cell membrane is permeable to potassium (K^+) and chloride (Cl^-) ions but relatively impermeable to sodium (Na^+) ions and other intracellular anions (A^-). The inside of the cell contains high levels of K^+ ions and A^- ions, and the outside of the cell contains high levels of Na^+ ions and Cl^- ions. This causes the K^+ ions to diffuse down their concentration gradient, leaving negatively charged ions that cannot cross the membrane inside the cell. The difference in ion concentration is maintained by the **sodium/ potassium pump**. This pump exchanges three Na^+ ions from inside the cell for two K^+ ions from outside the cell, giving a net movement of one positive charge from inside to outside, so contributing to the membrane potential.

Action Potential

The action potential consists of a rapid and transient reversal of the membrane potential which results from sudden opening of specific sodium channels in the cell membrane, allowing sodium ions to rush into the neurone creating a positive charge inside the cell. These sodium channels are voltage-gated, which means that whether they are open or closed depends on the membrane potential in the vicinity of the channel. The stimulus for action potential initiation can come from activation of a specific receptor (responding to light, sound, touch or other sensory stimuli) or synaptic activation. If the membrane is depolarized to a certain level, referred to as the **threshold**, the voltage-gated sodium channels open; sodium ions will rush into the neurone reversing the membrane potential and depolarizing the cell. The sodium channels only remain open for a fraction of a millisecond before closing again. Potassium channels then open and potassium ions rapidly leave the cell, which returns the membrane potential to its resting state. However, immediately after the action potential there is a brief negative shift in the membrane potential known as an after-hyperpolarization. As the membrane depolarizes, further sodium channels in adjacent sections of membrane open and by this means the action potential is propagated along the axon.

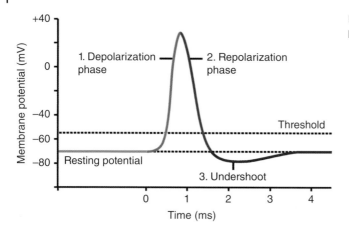

Figure 5.5 Generation of an action potential.

The action potential is an 'all or none' response (Figure 5.5). If the stimulus exceeds the threshold an action potential will be generated; if it is below the threshold no action potential will be generated. The action potential produced by any particular neurone is always of the same amplitude. See Feature box 5.1.

Synapses

Structure
Where the axon reaches the dendrites of another neurone it bulges to form a **terminal**, also known as a **synaptic bouton**, which forms part of the synapse (Figure 5.6). The synapse consists of three components: the presynaptic component (the synaptic bouton), the synaptic cleft and the postsynaptic cell. Thus axons are separated from their targets by a synaptic cleft that prevents electrical conduction of the action potential between cells. To enable the impulse to cross the cleft, neurotransmitters (which are stored in vesicles in the presynaptic terminal) are released from the presynaptic membrane; these cross the cleft and bind with receptors on the postsynaptic cell. These receptors are ligand-gated (i.e. opened by a specific molecule binding to the receptor).

Transmitter Release and Activation of the Postsynaptic Neurone
At the presynaptic terminal the membrane has a high density of voltage-gated calcium

---

Feature box 5.1 Blocking action potentials

Action potential generation and propagation can be prevented by a range of molecules that block sodium channels. Sodium channel blockers include naturally occurring toxins such as tetrodotoxin (TTX) found in fish from the Tetraodontiformes order, which includes pufferfish. TTX is extremely poisonous: ingestion of very low levels causes loss of sensation and paralysis of voluntary muscles, including the diaphragm and intercostal muscles, which stops breathing with fatal consequence. However, sodium channel blockade can also be used therapeutically; local anaesthetics such as lignocaine are sodium channel blockers that are widely used in medicine to enable surgical procedures to be carried out in conscious patients. These are used routinely in dental practice and have contributed significantly to modern-day dental and other surgical practice. More recently, blockers of very specific subtypes of sodium channels have been developed. These are being tested for the treatment of a range of chronic pain conditions that are associated with increased expression of specific sodium channel subtypes.

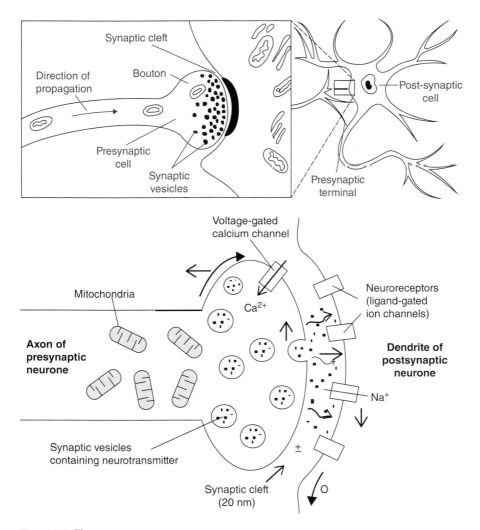

Figure 5.6 The synapse.

channels. When the action potential reaches the terminal these channels are opened and calcium ions enter the cell. This triggers a cascade of events that results in release of transmitter from the synaptic vesicles in the presynaptic membrane by exocytosis. The transmitters diffuse across the cleft and bind to their receptors on the postsynaptic membrane. The receptors are ligand-gated ion channels (i.e. opened by the binding of the ligand). Some neurotransmitters have an excitatory effect on the postsynaptic cell and others have an inhibitory effect. For example,

if the ligand–receptor interaction results in sodium channel activation this will cause an influx of Na^+ ions, which will make the inside of the postsynaptic neurone more positive and increase the chance of depolarization. This subthreshold depolarization is known as an excitatory postsynaptic potential (EPSP) (Figure 5.7a). However, if the ligand–receptor interaction results in chloride channel activation an influx of Cl^- ions will occur, causing a hyperpolarization of the cell and shifting the membrane potential further away from the threshold. This is known as an

(a)

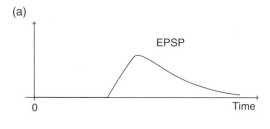

EPSP

0   Time

(b)

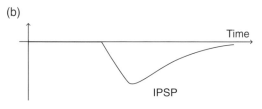

Time

IPSP

Figure 5.7 Effects of neurotransmitter binding on postsynaptic membrane potential.

inhibitory postsynaptic potential (IPSP, Figure 5.7b). Whether or not the postsynaptic neurone is activated sufficiently to produce an action potential depends on the balance of excitatory and inhibitory signals.

Glia

Neurones only make up about 10% of cells in the nervous system; the other cells are glial cells, which play a supporting role and are involved in insulation, nutrition and defence of neuronal cells. There are several different types of glial cell: some are present only in the PNS whereas others are found only in the CNS.

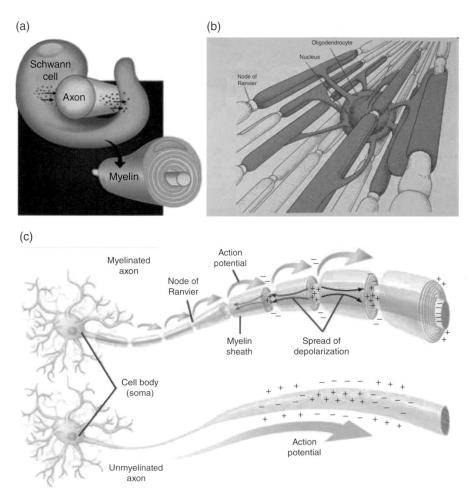

Figure 5.8 Myelination. (a) Schwann cell myelinating axon of peripheral neurone. (b) Oligodendrocytes myelinating axons of central neurones. (c) Action potential conduction in myelinated and unmyelinated axons.

Insulating Glia (Schwann Cells and Oligodendrocytes)

There are two types of glial cell that have an role in insulating neurones: **Schwann cells**, found in the PNS, and **oligodendrocytes**, found in the CNS. These cells wrap their membranes around the neuronal axons in numerous layers, producing the myelin sheath that insulates the axons. Each myelinating Schwann cell is only associated with one neuronal axon and only produces the myelin sheath for that part of the axon. However, each oligodendrocyte is associated with several neuronal axons and produces parts of the myelin sheath for a group of axons (Figure 5.8a&b).

Not all neurones have this sheath; those that do are known as myelinated neurones, while those that do not are known as unmyelinated neurones. Schwann cells and oligodendrocytes myelinate short sections of axon, and there are gaps between these segments known as nodes of Ranvier. The ion channels of myelinated nerves are located at these nodes and the action potential 'jumps' between the nodes (Figure 5.8c): this is known as saltatory conduction. This allows myelinated neurones to conduct impulses much faster than unmyelinated neurones. The speed of impulse conduction (known as conduction velocity) is also affected by the size of the axon, with small-diameter axons conducting more slowly than large-diameter axons. The fastest-conducting neurones are large-diameter myelinated neurones; the slowest are small-diameter unmyelinated neurones.

Astrocytes and Microglia

Astrocytes are star-shaped glial cells found only in the CNS (Figure 5.9). They are the most abundant cells in the brain. They are involved in many processes including nutrition of CNS neurones, repair and scarring following injury and disease, control of ion balance in the extracellular space and support of endothelial cells in the blood–brain barrier. Astrocytes are connected to each other by gap junctions, and some types of

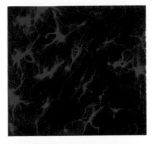

Figure 5.9 Immunofluorescent detection of astrocytes (shown coloured red).

astrocyte are able to communicate using calcium ions.

Microglia are defensive cells and are similar to macrophages that are found in peripheral tissues. They act as the first and main form of immune defence in the CNS, scavenging the CNS for damaged cells and infectious agents. Microglia destroy foreign and damaged material using cytotoxic and phagocytic mechanisms.

In addition to their protective effects, astrocytes and microglia have also been implicated in the development of a range of pathologies that affect the CNS.

Anatomical Organization of Peripheral Somatic Nerves and Spinal Cord

Within the nervous system individual neurones are grouped together to form a range of different structures. In the PNS these groupings form peripheral nerves and ganglia, whereas in the CNS they form nuclei and tracts.

Peripheral Nerves

Mammalian nerves contain several hundred or thousand individual axons (Figure 5.10). The nerves that leave the CNS at the level of the spinal cord are called spinal nerves, and those which leave at the level of the brain are termed cranial nerves (see later in this

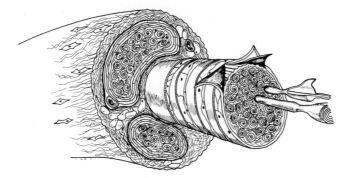

Figure 5.10 The structure of peripheral nerves.

section). Each of these nerves supplies a specific region of the body.

Epineurium, Perineurium and Endoneurium

The neuronal axons within the nerve are bound together by connective tissue sheaths, termed the epineurium, perineurium and endoneurium. The epineurium is the outermost layer and encircles the entire nerve trunk. Within a nerve there are several groups of axons bound together in fascicles; each fascicle is surrounded by a layer of perineurium. Each individual axon and its associated myelin sheath is enclosed in a layer of endoneurium, also known as the endoneurial sheath or endoneurial tube.

When peripheral nerves are injured the severity of the injury and the likelihood of recovery can be linked to the degree of damage to these sheaths. Lesions that just damage the endoneurium are less severe and more likely to recover than those involving damage to the perineurium and epineurium. Injuries to the trigeminal nerve (supplying the mouth and face) can occur as a consequence of dental and maxillofacial surgery, the most common cause being the removal of lower third molars. If these injuries are serious the nerve may have to be surgically repaired; this can be achieved by suturing the epineurium layer together.

Spinal and Cranial Nerves

As described earlier the PNS consists of spinal and cranial nerves. There are 31 pairs of spinal nerves and 12 pairs of cranial nerves. These nerves vary in their composition in terms of the axon type within them. The spinal nerves carry sensory axons that carry impulses arising from receptors located in peripheral structures (e.g. skin) to the CNS, and motor axons carrying impulses from the spinal cord to the muscles. Some nerves also carry autonomic fibres (the autonomic system is described in more detail later in this chapter). The cranial nerves are more variable in composition; some are mixed, some are purely motor and others carry information related to the special senses of sight, hearing and taste.

Connections to the Spinal Cord: Dorsal and Ventral Roots, Dorsal Root/ Trigeminal Ganglion

Spinal nerves are mixed nerves containing both motor and sensory axons. However, the motor and sensory components are segregated before they join the spinal cord. As they approach the spinal cord, spinal nerves divide into motor and sensory components (Figure 5.11). The sensory axons join together to form the **dorsal root** and the motor axons form the **ventral root**. The terms dorsal and ventral refer to their position relative to each other. Dorsal is derived from the Latin *dorsum*, meaning back, and ventral from *venter*, meaning belly. Thus the dorsal root is the root that enters the cord on the side closest to the back (think of the dorsal fin on a fish).

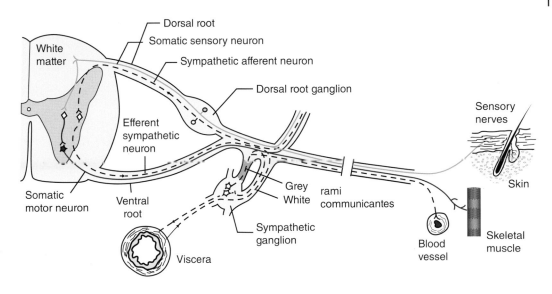

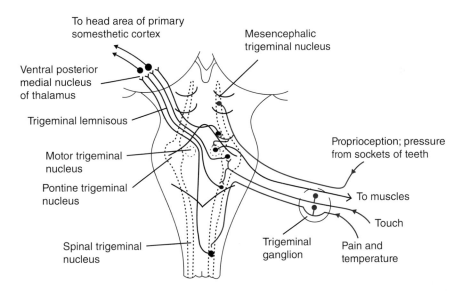

Figure 5.11 Dorsal and ventral roots, dorsal root ganglion and the trigeminal ganglion.

Sensory neurones are **pseudounipolar**; this means that they have an axon that has two terminals, one of which is located in the periphery and the other in the spinal cord. The cell body or soma lies between the two terminals, within the dorsal root in a specialized region called the dorsal root ganglion. The dorsal root ganglion contains all the cell bodies of the sensory axons entering the spinal cord at that particular level. The sensory neurones *do not* synapse here, but continue through the dorsal root and enter the spinal cord, where their central terminals synapse with central neurones in the dorsal horn of the spinal cord (described later). Axons supplying the orofacial region are carried in the **trigeminal nerve** (a cranial nerve). The trigeminal nerve enters the CNS at the level of the pons (see later). As for the spinal nerves the sensory and motor axons are

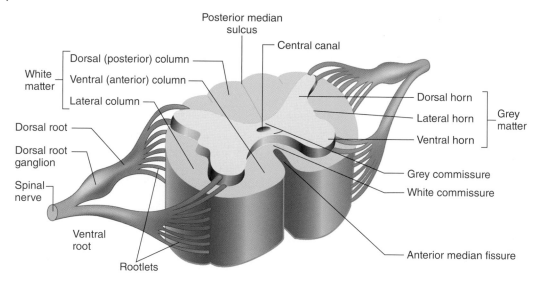

Figure 5.12 The spinal cord.

separated into motor and sensory roots as they enter the CNS. The cell bodies of the sensory neurones are located in the trigeminal ganglion.

The cell bodies of the motor neurones are also grouped together, and in the case of spinal nerve motor neurones are located in the CNS in the ventral horn of the spinal cord. The cell bodies of the trigeminal motor neurones are located in the trigeminal motor nucleus in the brainstem.

The Spinal Cord

White Matter, Grey Matter, Dorsal and Ventral Horns

The spinal cord is divided into white and grey matter (Figure 5.12). These descriptions relate to the colour that different regions appear in anatomical specimens. The white matter appears white because it consists of myelinated axons forming ascending or sensory (to the brain) pathways, and descending or motor (from the brain) pathways. The grey matter contains cell bodies, dendrites and synapses.

In a cross-section of the spinal cord the white matter is found peripherally and surrounds an 'H' or 'butterfly' shape of grey matter centrally (see Figure 5.12). The grey matter is subdivided into dorsal and ventral horns. As described earlier, the sensory neurones of the peripheral nerves enter the CNS through the dorsal root and synapse with CNS neurones in the dorsal horn of the spinal cord. The cell bodies of the motor neurones are located in the ventral horn, and their axons run in the ventral roots to join the peripheral nerves. In between the dorsal and ventral horns there is a third region of the grey matter known as the lateral horn. The lateral horn contains the cell bodies of the presynaptic neurones of the sympathetic division of the autonomic nervous system (described in more detail in the next section).

The Autonomic Nervous System

The autonomic nervous system controls **internal bodily functions** and operates largely below the level of consciousness. It has wide-reaching effects within most systems and organs of the body including the **respiratory** and **cardiovascular** systems, the **gastrointestinal** tract, the **skin** and the **eye**.

It has two divisions: the **sympathetic** and **parasympathetic**. These divisions are functionally, anatomically and pharmacologically distinct.

Functions

The autonomic nervous system acts locally on specific organs and systems to meet functional demands and maintain homeostasis. However, it can also act on the whole body to produce a coordinated response to particular stresses. A good example of this is the 'fight-or-flight' response, a physiological reaction occurring in response to a perceived harmful event, attack or threat to survival that is brought about by widespread activation of the sympathetic nervous system. It produces effects that include increased heart rate, dilation of bronchioles and pupillary dilatation; these effects prepare the body to fight or flee. In contrast, the parasympathetic system can be described as having actions that are consistent with 'resting and digesting' (e.g. increased secretion and motility in the gastrointestinal tract, slowing of heart rate).

Anatomy and Pharmacology

Both sympathetic and parasympathetic systems employ two neurones to carry a signal from the CNS to the peripheral target (see Figure 5.13). One neurone has its cell body within the CNS and its axon passes from the CNS to a specialized ganglion outside of the CNS, termed an **autonomic ganglion**. Within these ganglia the neurones synapse with the cell bodies of the second neurone. The axon of the second neurone then carries the signal to its target. The neurones with their cell bodies in the CNS that carry the signal to the ganglia are known as preganglionic neurones. The neurones with their cell bodies in the ganglia that carry the signal to the target are known as postganglionic neurones.

There are distinct anatomical differences between the parasympathetic and sympathetic systems (see Figure 5.14). The cell bodies of the preganglionic parasympathetic neurones are located in the brainstem and the sacral spinal cord. The presynaptic neurones located in the brainstem leave the CNS and their axons travel within cranial nerves III, VII, IX and X. Those in the sacral cord leave via the sacral nerves. These neurones synapse within parasympathetic ganglia that lie very close to or within the target organ.

The cell bodies of the preganglionic sympathetic neurones are found within the lateral horn of the thoracic and lumbar spinal cord, between segments T1 and L3. The ganglia where these neurones synapse with the postganglionic neurones form chains lying either side of the spinal cord, known as the sympathetic chains (Figure 5.14).

Irrespective of the division of the autonomic nervous system the neurotransmitter that is released by autonomic preganglionic neurones is acetylcholine.

Note that (as described earlier) postganglionic parasympathetic neurones (with cell bodies in the parasympathetic ganglia) are very close to or within their target organ, whereas the cell bodies of postganglionic sympathetic neurones are some distance from their target. The axons of these neurones reach their targets by a variety of routes; they may rejoin spinal nerves, they may run along arteries or, rarely, they may form specific sympathetic nerves.

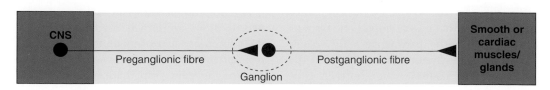

Figure 5.13 Signal transmission from CNS to periphery.

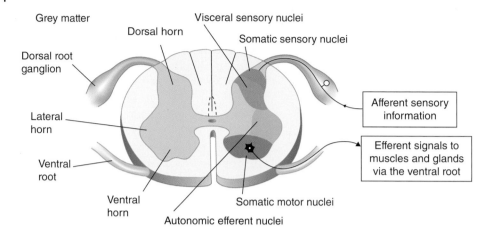

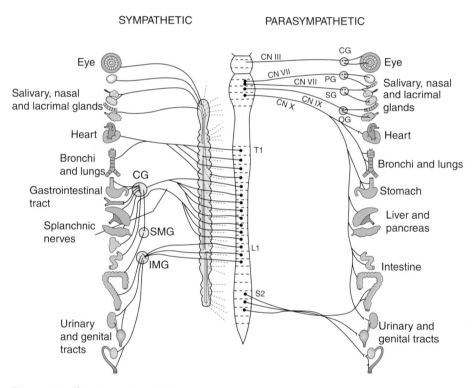

Figure 5.14 The autonomic nervous system.

The difference between the ganglion sites of the parasympathetic and sympathetic systems means that in the parasympathetic system the preganglionic neurones are long and the postganglionic neurones are short; in contrast, in the sympathetic system the preganglionic neurones are short and the postganglionic neurones are long (Figure 5.15).

The functional differences between the two divisions are largely mediated through the different neurotransmitters that are released by the postsynaptic neurones. In the case of the parasympathetic system this is acetylcholine and in the sympathetic system it is noradrenaline (norepinephrine). These neurotransmitters activate cholinergic or

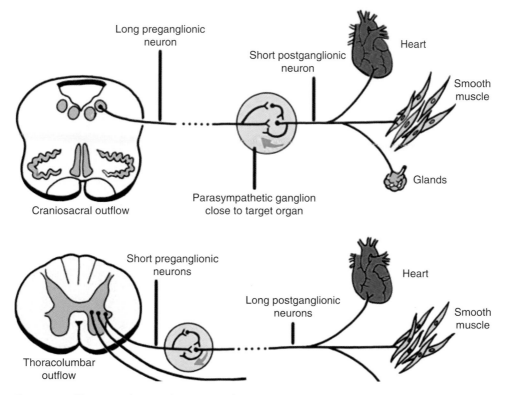

Figure 5.15 The sympathetic and parasympathetic nervous systems.

Feature box 5.2 Clinical considerations related to autonomic function

- Nervous patients experience sympathetic stimulation; this leads to increased heart rate, sweating, pallor of facial skin, and dilated pupils. It may also precipitate fainting.
- Most local anaesthetics contain noradrenaline, which produces localized vasoconstriction and has a number of beneficial effects. These include increasing the duration of anaesthesia and reducing bleeding during surgical procedures. However, inadvertent injection into blood vessels can cause skin blanching, fainting or occasionally a serious increase in heart rate, which may be dangerous, particularly in patients with a history of heart disease.
- Many drugs work via actions on the autonomic nervous system. One effect of some of these drug types is inhibition of salivation, producing dry mouth (xerostomia). This may lead to more rapid onset of dental caries, periodontal disease and mouth infections, and can cause difficulty with swallowing and speech.

---

adrenergic receptors and it is activation of these different receptors in the target organs that mediates the different effects of parasympathetic and sympathetic activation. See Feature box 5.2.

Anatomy of the Brain

The brain can be divided into three regions; the forebrain, the midbrain and the hindbrain (Figure 5.16).

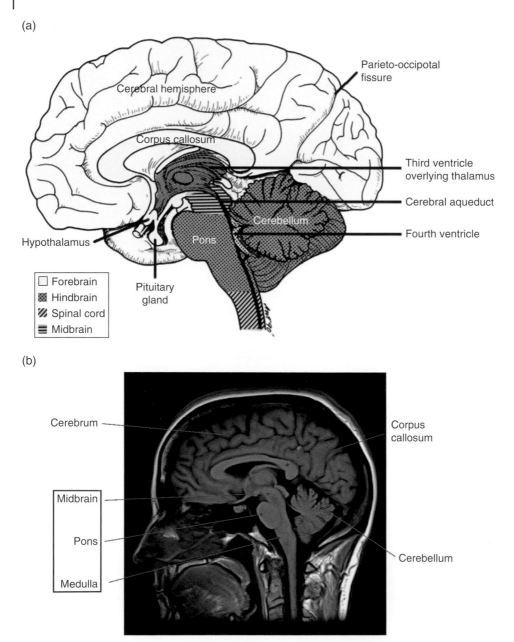

Figure 5.16 (a) Anatomy of the brain. (b) MRI normal T1 sagittal section scan of the human brain.

The Hindbrain (Rhombencephalon)

The hindbrain (Figure 5.17) consists of the pons, the medulla and the cerebellum; together these components support a number of vital functions.

The Medulla

The medulla is the most caudal part (i.e. towards the lowest part of the body) of the hindbrain and its caudal end is continuous with the spinal cord. It contains the nuclei of the 7th to 12th cranial nerves,

Figure 5.17 Anatomy of the hindbrain.

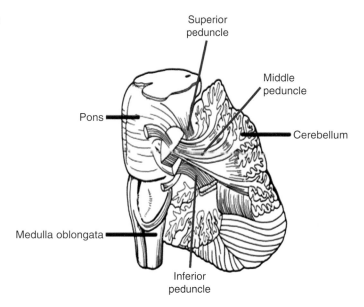

Superior peduncle

Middle peduncle

Pons

Cerebellum

Medulla oblongata

Inferior peduncle

the cardiovascular and respiratory centres and a number of ascending and descending tracts. It plays a major role in the control of a range of vital autonomic functions including breathing, heart rate, swallowing, digestion, vomiting and sneezing. It houses the spinal nucleus of the trigeminal nerve which plays a major role in the processing of sensory information from the mouth and face and is extremely important in the processing of inputs related to pain and temperature from the orofacial region. The medulla also acts as a conduction pathway for all nerve tracts passing from the spinal cord into the higher levels of the brain.

Damage to the medulla is potentially serious as it can compromise cardiovascular and respiratory function. The medulla is very vulnerable to damage by compression caused by any head injury or disease that causes raised intracranial pressure. As the cranial cavity is closed, any increase in intracranial pressure causes the brain to be displaced downwards: if severe this can cause compression of the medulla as it is forced into the spinal canal; this is known as 'coning'. This leads to loss of function of the cardiovascular and respiratory centres and is life threatening.

The Pons

The pons is the most rostral part (i.e. towards the uppermost part) of the hindbrain and is continuous with the medulla caudally and the midbrain rostrally. It contains the main sensory nucleus and motor nucleus of the trigeminal nerve (5th cranial nerve) and the nucleus of the 6th (abducent) cranial nerve. It also contains other nuclei that connect motor pathways to the cerebellum and ascending and descending tracts connecting higher brain structures to the medulla and spinal cord. It contributes to the control of a number of autonomic functions, relays sensory information between the cerebrum and cerebellum, and is important in arousal and sleep.

The Cerebellum

The cerebellum is positioned at the back of the brain below the cerebral hemispheres and behind the pons and medulla. *Cerebellum* is Latin for 'little brain', and this structure plays a major role in movement coordination, precision and accurate timing. It does not initiate movement but integrates inputs from the spinal cord and other parts of the brain and allows fine-tuning of motor activity. Thus cerebellar damage does not produce paralysis but causes disorders of fine control of movement, posture and motor learning.

The cerebellum is connected to the medulla, pons and midbrain by three stalks or peduncles. Inputs to and outputs from the cerebellum are carried within fibre bundles that run through the peduncles. The cerebellum has three functional subdivisions.

- **Vestibulocerebellum:** this is the oldest part of the cerebellum in evolutionary terms and participates in balance and spatial orientation. Its primary connections are with the vestibular nuclei and damage to this region causes disorders of balance and gait.
- **Spinocerebellum:** this part functions to fine-tune body and limb movements. It receives proprioceptive inputs from muscles and joints from the dorsal columns of the spinal cord and the trigeminal nerve, and input from the visual and auditory systems. It sends outputs to both the cerebral cortex and brainstem and provides fine control of descending motor systems.
- **Cerebrocerebellum:** this is the largest functional division of the human cerebellum. It receives input from the cerebral cortex and sends output to the thalamus. It is involved in the planning and timing of movements and also plays a role in cognitive functions.

If the cerebellum is diseased or damaged motor movement becomes inaccurate; this is known as cerebellar ataxia.

The Midbrain (Mesencephalon)

The midbrain sits at the rostral end of the pons and plays important roles in vision, hearing, motor control, alertness and temperature regulation. Its major structures include the superior and inferior colliculi, the cerebral peduncles, the red nuclei and the substantia nigra. The 3rd (oculomotor) and 4th (trochlear) cranial nerves arise from the midbrain.

Superior and Inferior Colliculi

These appear as distinct bumps on the posterior surface of the midbrain, with the superior colliculi positioned rostrally (Figure 5.18). The superior colliculi receive input from the retina and vision-related areas of the cortex; they are involved in visual processing, in particular in the control of eye movements. The inferior colliculi receive input from brainstem auditory nuclei and the auditory cortex. They integrate inputs to localize the source of various sounds and identify them as coming from a specific direction; they can also initiate head and body turning to orientate towards sound sources.

Cerebral Peduncles

Positioned in the anterior part of the midbrain, the cerebral peduncles connect the hindbrain and spinal cord to the cerebrum. They contain the large ascending and descending tracts that run to and from the cerebrum and thalamus; including descending fibres of the corticospinal and corticobulbar tracts, and ascending fibres of spino- and trigemino-thalamic tracts.

Red Nuclei and Substantia Nigra

There are two important pairs of nuclei in the anterior part of the midbrain: the **red nuclei** where information from the cerebellum joins motor pathways and the **substantia nigra** (Latin for 'black substance'), which play an important role in movement, reward and addiction. Both regions are subcortical centres of the motor system. In lower vertebrates the red nucleus controls gait; however, in species where the corticospinal tract is dominant (e.g. primates) the red nucleus does not play such a significant role in gait, but does play a role in movement of the shoulders and arms related to gait (e.g. arm swinging in normal walking). It also acts as an important relay for information from the cerebellum.

The substantia nigra's dark colour comes from high levels of neuromelanin in dopaminergic neurones (neurones containing the

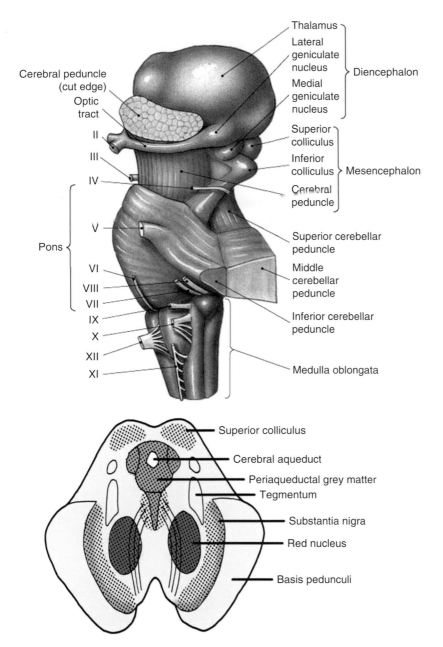

Figure 5.18 Anatomy of the midbrain.

neurotransmitter dopamine). It is part of a larger system known as the basal ganglia. The substantia nigra provides an input to the basal ganglia circuit, supplying the striatum with dopamine. It also provides an output from the basal ganglia, conveying signals to a variety of other brain regions.

Through its dopaminergic input the substantia nigra has effects that inhibit unwanted movement and amplify desired movement. In the neurodegenerative disorder Parkinson's disease, dopamine is deficient as a consequence of the death of nigral dopaminergic neurones. The symptoms that occur in this disease include tremor at rest and poverty of movement, such as slowness in the initiation of movement.

The Forebrain (Prosencephalon)

The forebrain can be further divided into the telencephalon and the diencephalon. The telencephalon or cerebrum (pair of large cerebral hemispheres) consists of the cerebral cortex and other subcortical structures including the basal ganglia (see later); the diencephalon consists of a group of structures deep within the cerebrum including the thalamus and the hypothalamus.

The cerebral cortex can be divided into four lobes: frontal, parietal, temporal and occipital. These lobes were originally identified on the basis of macroscopic anatomical features but also relate to functional differences. A more detailed subdivision of cortical areas was described in 1909 by Brodmann, based on the structure and organization of the cells in each region (Figure 5.19a). Brodmann's areas have been refined and renamed but are still the most widely used cytoarchitectural organization of the human cortex. All cortical regions have a six-layer structure, but the precise architecture and thickness of each layer varies between the different regions; this is related to functional differences. Functionally the different regions of cortex can be broadly classified as motor (controlling voluntary movement), sensory (receiving and processing information from specific senses) or association (integrating information from several sources and allowing interpretation of signals). Some examples of the differing structure of these regions are shown in Figure 5.19.

Since their original designation based on neuronal organization, Brodmann's areas have been found to correlate closely with highly specific functional areas. For example, areas 1, 2 and 3 make up the primary somatosensory cortex, area 4 is the primary motor cortex, area 17 is the primary visual cortex and the primary auditory cortex relates closely to areas 41 and 42.

Somatotopic Representation

In the sensory and motor cortices the body is represented in its anatomical layout. In this somatotopic map the size of different body parts reflects the relative density of their innervation rather than their actual size, so that areas with lots of sensory innervation or complexity of movement such as the hands and lips have huge areas representing them (see Figure 5.19c). The arrangement of anatomical regions on the cortex is also upside down (the feet are uppermost) and, due to the decussation (or crossing) of the motor and sensory pathways (see later), body regions are represented on the contralateral side of the cortex.

Sensory and Motor Pathways, Motor Nerve Injuries, Basal Ganglia

Sensory Pathways

There are a number of routes by which information carried by primary afferent fibres can reach the cortex. Examples of two well-described pathways are shown in Figure 5.20. The spinothalamic pathway (shown in blue) carries and processes sharp, pricking pain and dropping temperature (cool/cold) information from the body. The medial lemniscal pathway (shown in red) carries and processes discriminative touch and proprioceptive information from the body. Both of these pathways consist of three neurones: a primary sensory neurone carrying impulses from a receptor to the spinal cord or medulla; a second-order neurone from the spinal cord or medulla to the thalamus; and a third-order neurone from thalamus to cortex.

The **spinothalamic pathway** carries input from pain and temperature afferent fibres, which synapse at the level of the spinal cord. The second-order neurone crosses (decussates) at the level of the spinal cord and then ascends to the thalamus in the spinothalamic tract (hence the name of the pathway). The third-order neurone ascends from the thalamus to the somatosensory cortex.

The **medial lemniscal pathway** carries information from the afferent nerves

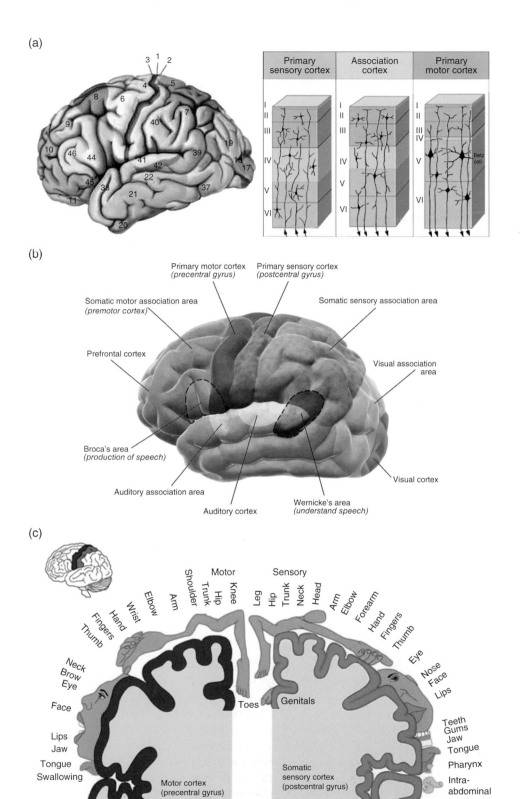

Figure 5.19 The forebrain. (a) Brodmann's areas. (b) Motor and sensory regions of the cerebral cortex. (c) Somatotopic map showing the areas of the body laid out on the sensory and motor cortices.

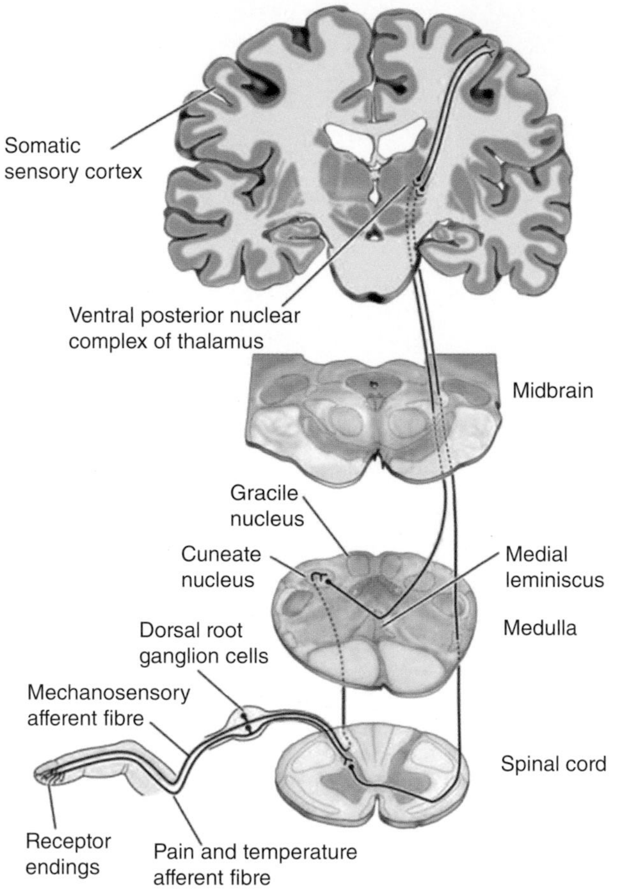

Figure 5.20 Sensory pathways.

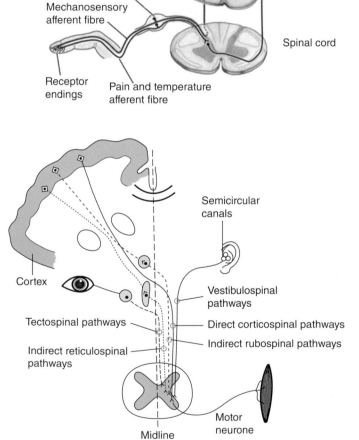

Somatic sensory cortex

Ventral posterior nuclear complex of thalamus

Midbrain

Gracile nucleus

Cuneate nucleus

Medial leminiscus

Dorsal root ganglion cells

Medulla

Mechanosensory afferent fibre

Spinal cord

Receptor endings

Pain and temperature afferent fibre

Figure 5.21 Motor pathways.

Semicircular canals

Cortex

Vestibulospinal pathways

Tectospinal pathways

Direct corticospinal pathways

Indirect rubospinal pathways

Indirect reticulospinal pathways

Motor neurone

Midline

responding to touch, which do not synapse in the spinal cord but ascend in the spinal cord to the cuneate and gracile nuclei in the medulla, where they synapse. Here second-order fibres decussate and travel in a tract known as the medial lemniscus (hence the name of the pathway) to the thalamus. As with the spinothalamic pathway the third-order neurone ascends from thalamus to the somatosensory cortex.

Motor Pathways and Motor Nerve Injuries

Motor pathways are very complex. The crucial distinction to draw is between (a) upper motor neurones, any neurones carrying information *within the CNS* making up (descending) motor pathways, and (b) lower motor neurones, neurones conveying motor information from brainstem (cranial nerves) or spinal cord (spinal nerves) to voluntary muscle, essentially the motor component of peripheral nerves.

Each lower motor neurone lying in the ventral horn of the spinal cord may receive information from several descending motor pathways (see Figure 5.21):

- direct corticospinal pathways (fine movement),
- indirect corticospinal pathways (postural movement; receiving input from the cerebellum),
- tectospinal pathways: from eyes via midbrain (position in relation to the environment),
- vestibulospinal pathways: from the semicircular canals in the inner ear (for balance).

Note that *all* upper motor neurones follows a similar course: direct corticospinal, indirect corticospinal and tectospinal pathways. *All* cross to the **contralateral** side in the medulla at the pyramidal decussation. Any injury to upper motor neurones therefore causes problems with movement of the contralateral side of the trunk and limbs. The effects of motor nerve injuries are different depending on whether upper or lower motor neurones are damaged.

If a lower motor neurone is injured, no signal from any source can get to the muscle. The muscle goes 'limp' (flaccid paralysis). If the motor neurones do not regenerate, muscle wasting occurs (atrophy) after about 6 months; and after about 12 months the muscle is replaced by fibrous tissue causing a contracture.

If upper motor neurones are damaged there is still one intact source of information acting on the muscle. However, this input cannot be modified by the brain, leading to spastic paralysis (in which the muscle is contracted), and hyperreflexia of the trunk and limbs occurs.

Basal Ganglia

The basal ganglia consist of large nuclei of grey matter in the depth of the cerebral hemispheres plus the substantia nigra in the midbrain. They connect the sensory areas of the brain to motor areas by highly complex loop systems. They suppress unwanted movement and amplify the intended movement. Damage to or disease of the basal ganglia produces dyskinesia (abnormal movement). This may manifest as chorea (dance-like movement), athetosis (slow, writhing movement) or tremor as seen in Parkinson's disease.

Summary of Brain Anatomy and Function

- There are three major divisions of the brain, the forebrain, the midbrain and the hindbrain.
- The hindbrain controls autonomic functions and movement.
- The midbrain controls body movement and is a relay station for auditory and visual information.
- The forebrain controls perception, memory, language and all other higher cognitive functions.
- Sensory pathways are the routes by which information is passed from the periphery to the cortex.
- Sensory pathways have sequences that are made up of three neurones, first- (or primary sensory neurone), second-, and third-order neurones.

- Motor pathways are very complex.
- The crucial distinction to draw is between:
Upper motor neurons – any neurones carrying information within the CNS making up (descending) motor pathways.

Lower motor neurons – neurones conveying motor information from brainstem (cranial nerves) or spinal cord (spinal nerves) to voluntary muscle – essentially the motor component of peripheral nerves.

6

Introduction to Immunology

John J. Taylor

School of Dental Sciences, Newcastle University, Newcastle upon Tyne, UK

Learning Objectives

- To be able to list the physical and chemical barriers that the body has to infection.
- To be able to describe the molecular and cellular components of the innate immune system.
- To understand the role of the cells and antibodies of the adaptive immune system.
- To be able to explain the role of the major histocompatibility complex and antigen processing.
- To be able to describe the key events that occur during inflammation and the immune response to infection.

Clinical Relevance

The immune system is essential to carrying out surveillance and initiating removal of infectious and damaging agents and abnormal cells from the body through the innate and adaptive systems. Inflammation is also a prerequisite to successful wound healing. The oral cavity is a common site for bacterial, viral and fungal infections and an understanding of the immunological processes that are stimulated by such challenges is essential to understanding both disease progression and treatment strategies.

Introduction

The study of the immune system (immunology) is fundamental to healthcare practice in a worldwide arena. Vaccination programmes have all but eliminated serious human diseases such as smallpox and polio. Also, the annual effort to develop effective influenza vaccines saves millions of lives and has a profound economic impact by preventing many lost hours of work. Exciting recent developments include vaccination against human papilloma virus (HPV) which has proven efficacy in the prevention of cervical cancer and may eventually be an efficacious prophylactic measure against HPV-associated oral cancer. Anti-inflammatory and immunosuppressive pharmaceuticals are widely used and their development requires knowledge of immunology.

Basic Sciences for Dental Students, First Edition. Edited by Simon A. Whawell and Daniel W. Lambert.
© 2018 John Wiley & Sons Ltd. Published 2018 by John Wiley & Sons Ltd.
Companion website: www.wiley.com/go/whawell/basic_sciences_for_dental_students

Immunology is especially relevant to good practice in dentistry. The oral cavity is a unique anatomical structure involving the juxtaposition of soft and hard tissues which is continuously challenged by the external environment and foreign material. The pathogenesis of many common disorders of the dental clinic, for example dental abscesses, involves immunological processes. Disease due to primary oral infections such as caries and periodontal disease are common and oral disease secondary to systemic disease, for example oral candidiasis, due to acquired immunodeficiency may also be seen in the dental clinic. The dental practitioner is required not only to identify and treat these disorders but also to have an understanding of the principles of the underlying disease processes as these are increasingly used as the basis for diagnostic and therapeutic strategies. The increasing emphasis on cross-infection control in all public healthcare environments gives the dental practitioner added professional responsibility to understand prophylactic measures such as vaccination.

This chapter aims to help the student understand and appreciate the main features of the molecules, cells and tissues of the human innate and adaptive immune system and how they are integrated to provide effective immunity. The immune mechanisms involved in host defences to bacterial, viral and fungal pathogens will be explored and the immune processes which underpin inflammation – the most obvious pathological feature immune-mediated disease – described. Defects in immune function which result in immunodeficiency, autoimmunity and hypersensitivity will be outlined as many of these are clinically important and common conditions. Finally, the principles of vaccination as a healthcare measure in both individuals and populations will be discussed. This material is fundamental to the understanding of host responses in caries, periodontal disease and candidiasis discussed later in this chapter and also in gaining a perspective on how systemic immunopathologies can impinge on oral health.

Physical and Chemical Barriers to Infection

There are a number of intrinsic **anatomical and physiological elements** which, in addition to their other functions, have a critical role in the host defence against infection (Table 6.1). These elements form the first **barriers** against microbial pathogens and provide day-to-day protection against infectious disease. Only when these defences are breached do the specialized elements of innate and adaptive immunity come into play. Compromised barrier function after cuts or abrasions to the skin can lead to localized infections with bacteria such as *Staphylococcus aureus* but extensive loss of skin due to severe burns can lead to bacteraemia with life-threatening consequences such as sepsis. The **mucosal tissues** of the respiratory system, the gastrointestinal (or GI) tract and the urogenital tract also have elements to protect against microbial infection (Table 6.1). When these defences are breached they lead to serious diseases of the lung (e.g. tuberculosis) and the gastrointestinal tract (e.g. cholera). The abnormally thick (and, hence, ineffective) mucous that patients with cystic fibrosis secrete is one precipitating factor that leads to serious lung infections (e.g. with *Pseudomonas aeruginosa*). Also, the chronically damaged respiratory epithelia characteristic of a long-term smoking habit can lead to conditions such as chronic obstructive pulmonary disease, a major risk factor for respiratory infections such as pneumonia and lung abscesses. The mouth is also lined with mucosal tissue where **saliva** is a key component of the host defence against infection (Table 6.2, Feature box 6.1). Indeed, patients with 'dry mouth' (xerostomia) are highly susceptible to dental caries. **Gingival crevicular fluid** is a serum exudate in the crevice between the tooth and the gingiva that is increased in conditions of gingivitis and periodontitis and carries mediators of host protection against subgingival plaque bacteria.

Table 6.1 Physical barriers and chemical agents against infection and their properties.

Barrier	Properties	Function
Skin	Keratinized epithelium	Dry surface inhibits bacterial reproduction; keratin layers and tight cell–cell junctions prevent microbial penetration; sloughing of cells and high turnover rate prevent colonization
	Lactic acid and fatty acids from sweat and sebaceous glands respectively	Low pH inhibits bacterial growth
Mucosal tissue	Secreted mucins	Form mucus with water; coagulates particulate matter, preventing attachment and facilitating ejection
	Ciliated epithelium (e.g. in trachea)	Works with mucus layer to physically eject particulate matter
	Flow of air (airways) and fluid (e.g. in the urogenital tract)	Prevents attachment and washes out microbes
Gastrointestinal tract	Acid environment in stomach (also in kidney and bile)	Low pH inhibits bacterial growth
	Digestive enzymes	Inhibit bacterial growth
Paneth cells in small intestine	Antimicrobial peptides, lysozyme and phospholipase	Destroy bacterial cells

Table 6.2 Host defences in the saliva.

Innate factor	Examples	Function
Antimicrobial peptides	Defensins, cathelicidin, histatins, statherin	Disrupt bacterial membranes and enveloped viruses
Adhesive proteins	Mucin, agglutinin, $\beta_2$microglobulin, proline-rich proteins (PRPs)	Bacterial agglutination in the fluid phase and prevention of attachment but PRPs can promote adhesion to teeth
Metal ion chelators	Calprotectin, lactoferrin (also in gingival crevicular fluid (GCF))	Scavenge Zn^{2+} (and Mn^{2+}) and Fe^{3+}
Protease inhibitors	Cystatin	Prevent nutrient acquisition by bacteria
Bacterial cell wall disruptors	Lysozyme (also in GCF), phospholipase	Osmotic lysis of the cell membrane
Fluid flow and swallowing action		Prevents attachment, clears particulate material

Microbiological Barriers to Infection

Non-pathogenic **commensal microflora** (on the teeth, the mucosal surfaces and in the gastrointestinal tract) successfully compete with pathogens for nutrients, attachment sites and living space; if this interaction is disrupted then pathogens can profit and cause disease. For example *Clostridium difficile* infection (which causes a severe diarrheal disorder) develops in some patients undergoing treatment with broad-spectrum antibiotics; these drugs will kill much of the

| Feature box 6.1 | Saliva as a diagnostic fluid |

The diagnosis and monitoring of many diseases rely on traditional clinical examinations which, although they define the current status of the disorder (which is a reflection of historical progress of the disease), often fail to objectively determine patient susceptibility, current disease activity and potential response to treatment. The management of the chronic inflammatory disorder periodontitis certainly falls into this category. However, our increased understanding of the pathogenesis of human disease has allowed us to identify candidate 'biomarkers', molecules that when assayed in biological fluids may reflect present activity and predict disease progress. Studies of saliva are particularly advantageous for oral diseases as this fluid comprises the secretions of salivary glands mixed with inflammatory mediators present in gingival crevicular fluid and at the oral mucosal surface. Also, saliva is easy, painless and cheap to collect. Although we have identified several candidate biomarkers for periodontitis including proinflammatory cytokines (e.g. IL-1β) and destructive enzymes (e.g. matrix metaloproteinases), more substantial clinical trials are needed to confirm their efficacy.

commensal microflora in the gut but allow pathogenic *C. difficile* to proliferate.

Gut microflora constantly stimulate the colonic epithelial cells to provide a balanced state of **physiological inflammation** that is protective in nature. The inflammatory bowel disorder Crohn's disease, a chronic condition of excessive and damaging inflammation in the gastrointestinal tract, is caused by mutation in nucleotide-binding oligomerization domain (NOD) proteins which regulate host–bacterial interaction in epithelial cells. In the gingival tissues low numbers of mainly commensal, non-pathogenic plaque bacteria maintain a physiological inflammation associated with low but measurable levels of proinflammatory cytokines and tissue neutrophils. This stable and protective situation is disrupted as the result of ecological shifts in dental plaque resulting in a pathogenic microflora, gingivitis and eventually periodontitis. There are some obvious and important anatomical differences between the periodontium and the gut epithelium which are reflected in different mechanisms of immune homeostasis in these tissues but there is a common principle of a balanced interaction between commensal microbiota and host immune responses maintaining tissue health.

Molecular Elements of Innate Immunity: Antimicrobial Peptides and Complement

If the aforementioned barriers are breached microbial pathogens will encounter specific elements of immediately available (or quickly produced) host defences which are part of the **innate immune system**. It is very important to appreciate that the categorization of the immune system into 'innate' (thus intrinsic and not elaborated as the result of infection experience) and 'adaptive' (thus able to modified and improved as the result of infection or antigen exposure) helps us understand some fundamental differences in the mechanism of action of individual elements of the immune response in mammals (and their evolutionary significance) but, in terms of the holistic function of the immune defences, these two systems are highly integrated and mutually supportive. Importantly, we know through studies of human immunodeficiency disorders and gene knockout models in mice that incorrect development or function of one or another of these systems has adverse consequences for the duration, intensity and spread of infections.

Feature box 6.2 Cytokines: what's in a name?

There are over 100 molecules in human cells that be classified as cytokines the basis of their biological action in the immune system and in immune-mediated diseases. There are over 50 individual cytokines called interleukins grouped into families according to structural homologies (see Table 6.5 for examples). Cytokines such as TNF α, oncostatin-M, the colony-stimulating factors (e.g. GM-CSF) and the interferon family are also cytokines even though they are not called 'interleukins'. This simply reflects a historical nomenclature based on the experiments by which these molecules were first discovered. TNF-α, for example, has many similar biological activities to IL-1β even though they are structurally

distinct molecules. Recently, it has become clear that many other molecules have cytokine-like activity in addition their more-established roles outside the immune response: these include growth factors (e.g. TGF-β) which also regulate development, tissue growth and repair and mediate disease pathogenesis (e.g. cancer), adipokines (e.g. leptin) which are hormone-like molecules synthesized by adipose tissue that physiologically regulate food intake and metabolism and neuropeptides (e.g. vasoactive intestinal peptide) which are involved in nerve function. These findings reflect the functional integration of the immune response with other physiological systems.

A wide range of **antimicrobial peptides** and **antimicrobial enzymes** are produced by skin, at mucosal surfaces and by **neutrophils**; these are all important elements of innate immune defences and in particular the saliva (Tables 6.1 and 6.2). In addition to a direct action on microbial pathogens, antimicrobial peptides also have wider functions in the immune response: they stimulate chemotaxis, cytokine secretion and antigen presentation (Feature box 6.2). Also, inflammatory disorders such as Crohn's disease, psoriasis and ulcerative colitis are all associated with aberrant antimicrobial peptide secretion.

The **complement system** is a group of some 30 blood and tissue fluid proteins that, when activated, have numerous effector functions central to innate immunity but which also greatly enhance ('complement') adaptive immunity (Figure 6.1). Patients with congenital complement deficiencies suffer from recurrent infections from extracellular pathogens such as *Streptococcus pneumoniae*. It is intriguing to note the similarities of the complement system with antimicrobial peptides: both appeared

early in the evolution of host defences, they are activated by proteolytic cleavage, have numerous antimicrobial effector functions and have evolved several other functions beyond these fundamental innate defence processes. With regard to the latter, it is now known for example that complement activation is associated with heightened T-cell responses.

Cellular Elements of Innate Immunity

Phagocytosis (and concomitant intracellular destruction) is a fundamentally important process in eliminating pathogen infections. Phagocytes (Table 6.3) are ever present in the tissues and blood stream, are stimulated to migrate to sites of infection during innate responses but, critically, their development and function is greatly enhanced by the adaptive immune response. **Neutrophils** are the professional phagocyte of immune responses which migrate into tissues in response to chemokine gradients, increased localized vascular flow

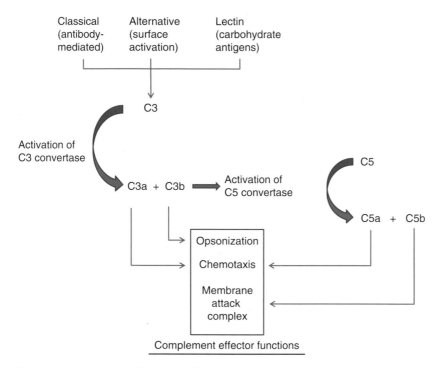

Complement activation pathways

Figure 6.1 Activation and function of the human complement system. The complement system is activated by the recognition of protein and carbohydrate antigens on pathogen surfaces (often interacting with antibody molecules) and comprises a series of interacting pro-enzymes (zymogens) that form a proteolytic cascade of activation leading to the localized production of a limited number of effector molecules which attempt to eliminate the pathogen. Cleavage of the complement component C3 by activation of the enzyme C3 convertase is the common endpoint for all three activation pathways. The products of this reaction (C3a and C3b) are key complement effector molecules. C3b also activates C5 convertase which cleaves C5, producing further effector molecules (C5a and C5b). Complement effector pathways comprise binding to antigen to enhance neutrophil phagocytosis (opsonization), stimulating movement (chemotaxis) of neutrophils into sites of tissue inflammation and formation of a membrane attack complex which punctures the bacterial cell membrane, causing lysis.

Table 6.3 Phagocytic cells of the immune system and their function.

Phagocytic cell type	Anatomical location	Immune function
Macrophages	Connective tissues (e.g. lamina propria of the gingivae); major organs (e.g. lung); immune tissue (e.g. lymph nodes).	Phagocytose pathogens to initiate signalling of neutrophils and T-cells via cytokines; antigen presentation to T-cells; scavenge dead cells (e.g. neutrophils)
Neutrophils	Bone marrow and blood	Short-lived, highly effective phagocytes for pathogen clearance; multiple killing pathways including enzymes, antimicrobial peptides and reactive oxygen species
Dendritic cells	Connective tissues and lymph nodes	Phagocytosis and antigen uptake; antigen presentation in secondary lymphoid tissues (lymph nodes, Peyer's patches)

and enhanced adhesion molecule expression in vascular endothelium of infected tissues. Neutrophils recognize pathogens coated with complement and/or antibodies ('**opsonization**') by virtue of membrane-bound complement and immunoglobulin F_c receptors respectively, facilitating phagocytosis of pathogens; once internalized the neutrophils have a wide armory of intracellular mechanisms for pathogen destruction (Table 6.3). **Macrophages**, unlike neutrophils, are long-lived resident cells of tissues with a wide distribution, in particular in lymphoid tissues such as the spleen and lymph nodes as well as in the mucosal tissues. These cells have a sentinel function responding early to infections, phagocytosing pathogens and signalling other elements of innate and adaptive immunity through secretion of cytokines and chemokines as well as presenting antigen to T-cells. In this regard, macrophages are the supreme multitasking cell of the immune system. During infection, macrophage tissue numbers can be enhanced by emigration of blood monocytes (the precursor cell of the macrophage).

Natural killer (NK) cells are central in the host defence against **viral infections** and exert their effector function by killing infected host cells. NK cells are large granular lymphocytes present in the circulation and in the tissues. NK receptors are complex and diverse and regulate NK function through both activating and inhibitory signals received through recognition of altered levels of major histocompatibility complex (MHC) class I molecules on host cells. NK cells also have F_c **receptors**; this pathway results in cell destruction by **antibody-dependent cell-mediated cytotoxicity (ADCC)** and serves as another example for the integrative function of innate and adaptive immunity. Another important function of NK cells is to secrete interferon-γ (**IFNγ**; type II interferon), which serves to activate CD8+ T-cells, which have an antigen-specific cytotoxic function.

Innate Immune Signalling: Pattern Recognition, Chemotaxis and the Interferon Response

It is fundamentally important that the immune system can recognize the presence of pathogen ('non-self') molecules and respond by eliminating (or, at least, attempting to eliminate) the infection. Signalling adaptive immunity is also of critical importance as this will greatly enhance the effectiveness of the host defences and provide memory of disease experience so second encounters with the same pathogens can be more immediate and efficient. The initial interaction of pathogens with host cells is mediated by an array of so-called **pattern-recognition receptors (PRRs)** (Table 6.4).

PRRs recognize a wide range of molecular structures associated with microbes (but not found on host cells) often described as **pathogen-associated molecular patterns (PAMPs)** or microbe-associated molecular patterns (MAMPs) in acknowledgement of the fact that these structures are found in commensal and pathogenic microorganisms alike. The best characterized PRRs are the **Toll-like receptors (TLRs)**, which consist of some 10 different cytoplasmic and cell-surface molecules expressed in macrophages, dendritic cells, B-cells and some non-immune cells such as epithelial cells and fibroblasts. In general terms, cell-surface TLRs detect extracellular pathogens (and their products) and endosomal TLRs detect phagocytosed pathogens or those in the intracellular milieu (Table 6.4). Signalling through TLRs is often mediated by activation of the classical proinflammatory transcription factor **nuclear factor kappa-light-chain-enhancer of activated B-cells (NF-κB)** and leads to enhanced secretion of **cytokines**, **chemokines** and antimicrobial peptides. Thus, cytokines such as **interleukin-1β (IL-1β)**, **IL-6 and tumour**

Table 6.4 Pattern-recognition receptors and the ligands (and microorganisms) they recognize.

Pattern-recognition receptor (PRR)				
Family	Examples	Cell expression	Ligand (PAMP)	Associated microorganisms
Toll-like receptors	TLR-2/TLR-1 and TLR-2/ TLR-6 heterodimers	Cell surface of monocytes, dendrtitic cells, mast cells	Lipomanans	Mycobacteria
			Lipoproteins	Gram-negative bacteria
			Lipotechoic acids	Gram-positive bacteria
			β-Glucans	Bacteria and fungal cell walls
	TLR-3	Endosomes of NK cells	Double-stranded RNA	Viruses
	TLR-4	Cell surface of macrophages, dendritic cells	Lipopolysaccaride	Gram-negative bacteria
			Lipotechoic acids	Gram-positive bacteria
	TLR-7	Endosomes of plasmacytoid dendritic cells, NK cells, B-cells	Single- stranded RNA	Viruses
	TLR-9	Endosomes of plasmacytoid dendritic cells, B-cells	Unmethylated DNA	Bacteria and herpes viruses
NOD-like receptors	NOD1 and NOD2	Surface or intracellular vesicles of epithelial cells, macrophages, dendritic cells	Peptidoglycans and their breakdown products	Gram-negative bacteria
RIG-like helicases	RIG-1	Widely expressed in the cytoplasm of cells	Singe-stranded intracellular viral RNA	Viruses

necrosis factor-α (**TNF-α**) (so-called **pro-inflammatory cytokines**; Feature box 6.3) stimulate vascular endothelium causing increased blood flow and neutrophil emigration into the tissues. The chemokine **CXCL-8** (also known as IL-8) has a chemotactic effect on neutrophils attracting them into the site of tissue infection. Mutations in the elements of the signalling pathways lead to immunodeficiency and recurrent bacterial infections and these proteins are important targets for anti-inflammatory drugs. Activation of TLR pathways by viral molecules leads to an antiviral response mediated by transcription factors of the interferon regulatory factor (IRF) family. The consequence of IRF activation is secretion of **type I interferons** (**IFNα** and **IFNβ**) which cause resistance to viral replication and activation of NK cells.

There are at least 100 molecules with cytokine activity and they are grouped in families generally according to peptide sequence (Table 6.5). Individual cytokines

Feature box 6.3 Cytokine networks

Most studies of cytokines have been on individual molecules, the pathways they activate and the consequence for immune responses. In the real world though there is a 'cytokine milieu' comprising a soup of many different cytokines which is variable depending on the tissue context and the environmental exposure (especially the presence of microbes). Also, we know that different combinations of cytokines elicit different responses in cells and many individual cytokines have opposing effects. How can we get to grips with this complexity? Measuring many cytokines simultaneously is expensive but now feasible. We can now identify 'signatures' of response and function which comprise multiple mediators divided into discrete functional groups that are coordinately regulated along with the receptors and signalling molecules necessary for their function. How do we use these experimental data to gain a holistic understanding of the immune response? This is where the science of bioinformatics steps in: immunologists are using these data and applying network theory to model immune responses. Such models recognize that changes in the levels of individual elements may not have predictable effects on function and that there may be novel, emergent properties of the network not obvious from the investigation of individual elements. These developments will also help us to understand what happens to the immune response when we perturb the system with a novel element such as a microbial virulence factor or a pharmacological agent.

Table 6.5 The major families of cytokines and their functions.

Cytokine family (members)	Key members	Main functions
Interleukin-1	IL-1α (IL-1F1)	Promotes inflammation, intracellular stress responses, fever
	IL-1β (IL-1F2)	Promotes inflammation, T-cell activation, fever
	IL-1Ra (IL-1F3)	Antagonizes IL-1α, IL-1β
	IL-18	Stimulates IFNγ secretion by T-cells and NK cells, activates CD4+ T_H1 cells
Interleukin-2	IL-2	T-cell proliferation and activation
	IL-4	B-cell activation, CD4+ T_H1 cell differentiation, Ig class switching to IgE
Interleukin-6	IL-6	B-cell differentiation, acute-phase protein induction, fever
	Granulocyte colony-stimulating factor (G-CSF)	Neutrophil development
Interleukin-10	IL-10	Suppresses both macrophage function and CD4+ T_H1 cell differentiation
Interleukin-12	IL-12	CD4+ T_H1 cell differentiation, NK cell activation
	IL-23	CD4+ T_H17 cell differentiation
Interleukin-17	IL-17A	Promotes inflammation and in particular cytokine production by a wide range of cells
Type I interferon	IFNα/IFNβ	Antiviral responses, promotes MHC class I expression
Type II interferon	IFNγ	Macrophage activation, promotes MHC class I expression, suppression of CD4+ T_H2 cell differentiation
Granulocyte-macrophage colony-stimulating factor	GM-CSF	Granulocyte, monocyte and dendritic cell differentiation
Tumour necrosis factor	TNF-α	Promotes inflammation
Transforming growth factor	TGF-β	Modulates cell growth and inhibits immune responses

are pleiotropic and have overlapping functional attributes; thus, there is a degree of functional 'redundancy'. Cytokines drive specific immune cell development, activate immune cell subsets during specific infections and mediate immune cell effector functions. Specific combinations of cytokines have important synergistic activities and the 'cytokine milieu' is an important determinant of immune cell function. The cytokines IL-1β, IL-6, IL-12 and IL-18 have various roles in **lymphocyte activation**. NK cells, activated by type I interferons, themselves secrete type II interferon (IFNγ), which in turn activates antiviral responses mediated by T-cells. The aforementioned innate responses are very much limited to the immediate site of infections, but another important function of the macrophage-derived cytokines IL-1β, TNF-α and IL-6 is to stimulate hepatocytes to secrete **acute-phase proteins** into the circulation. These proteins, which include C-reactive protein (CRP) and mannose-binding lectin, serve to activate complement and enhance neutrophil phagocytosis.

Adaptive Immunity I: B-cells and Antibodies

In very general terms the effector functions of adaptive immunity are mediated by **B- and T-cells** (i.e. lymphocytes) but these cells are part of a complex network involving many other cellular (and molecular) elements. B-cells are fundamentally important in host defence against infection: in human primary immunodeficiency disorders such as Bruton's X-linked agammaglobulinemia gene mutations result in arrested B-cell development, reduced antibody levels, B-cell deficiency and consequent recurrent bacterial and viral infections. Central to the function of B-cells is their unique ability to synthesize **immunoglobulins (Igs)**, which are adapted to recognize and bind to specific molecular structures (antigens) expressed by pathogenic organisms (Figure 6.2). Immunoglobulin

molecules function initially as cell-surface receptors on B-cells, recognizing soluble antigens and activating differentiation and division (i.e. expansion) of B-cells into antibody-secreting **plasma cells**. Antibodies are the soluble form of the Ig molecule expressed by individual clones of B-cells; these molecules recognize the same antigens associated with the infection and mediate effector functions, the nature of which will vary depending on the form and anatomical location of the infections. Antibodies serve to neutralize toxins, for example, or prevent pathogens binding to (and invading) cells as in the case of viral infections. Antibodies also target antigens to other elements of the immune system such as neutrophils (for phagocytosis of opsonized antigen), the complement system (activation of complement effector functions through the classical pathway), NK cells (killing of infected cells through antibody-dependent cell-mediated cytotoxicity) and **mast cells** (activation of acute inflammation and physiological responses through release of histamine, prostaglandins, serotonin and other mediators). Structural differences in the Ig variable regions determine specificity for specific antigens (Figure 6.2). The enormous variation in potential antigens that may be encountered by host tissues is matched by the range of Ig peptide structures made by B-cells; this is made possible by complex molecular genetic **rearrangements of Ig genes** that take place during B-cell development (Figure 6.3) and are elaborated during the course of the initial infection. The function of antibody molecules made by individual clones is determined not by the **variable regions** of Ig molecules, but by the **constant regions** that, as their name implies, have limited heterogeneity (Table 6.6). In addition to improving the antigen-binding capability of antibodies during the course of an infection by a process of **somatic hypermutation** of variable region genes, the class of antibodies synthesized by B-cells can be altered to meet functional requirements by another molecular genetic process called **class switching**. Thus, the antibody molecules produced in

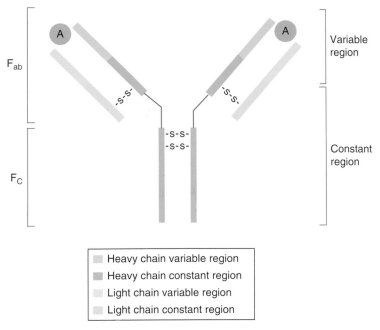

Figure 6.2 Structure of a typical antibody molecule. Antibodies are the soluble form of immunoglobulin (Ig) molecules and are large proteins with a complex 3D (globular) structure. The F_{ab} (antigen-binding fragment) of different Ig molecules has a highly variable (clonal specific) amino acid sequence. The F_c (crystallizable fragment) has a limited variability and functions to bind to F_c receptors on phagocytes and NK cells. These fragments are joined by a flexible hinge region. The precise region of F_{ab} which binds antigen (A) is formed by the combination of variable region peptides on the heavy and light chains of the Ig molecule. The heavy and light chains have contiguous non-variable regions (constant regions) which are joined together by disulphide bonds. The constant heavy chain peptide forms the F_c region of the Ig molecule and defines the antibody class (Table 6.6). T-cell receptors (the antigen-specific receptors on T-cells; TCRs) have a similar globular structure and subunit composition (comprising TCRα and TCRβ chains or TCRγ or TCRδ chains).

the initial stages of infection may be rather heterogeneous with respect to their precise molecular structure but will evolve during the infection to become less diverse but more effective. In addition to antigen specificity and improvement during immune responses, a third, critical, property of adaptive immunity is **immunological memory**, which allows lymphocytes to mount more rapid, more vigorous response on subsequent encounters with the same antigens. Immunological memory is mediated by long-lived, senescent cells called **memory B-cells**. B-cell memory is exploited by vaccination; vaccines are only effective if they generate effective initial B-cell responses and immunological memory (although the most effective vaccines also generate T-cell memory).

Adaptive Immunity II: Antigen Presentation and T-cell Activation

Effector T-cells directly contribute to pathogen clearance (e.g. CD8+ T-cells kill virally infected host cells) and they serve to activate and enhance other immune cells such as macrophages and B-cells. The intensity of cell- and antibody-mediated effector functions therefore also depend on activation of T-cells. The process by which T-cells are activated (and subsequently recognize target infected cells) is the interaction of antigen receptors on the surface of T-cells (so-called **T-cell receptors, TCRs**) and fragments of antigen 'presented' to the TCR in the context of **major**

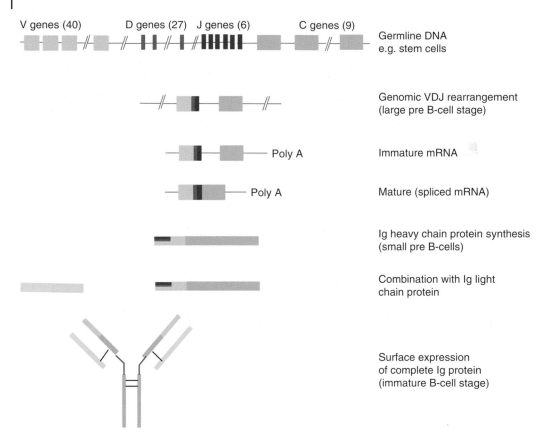

V genes (40)   D genes (27)   J genes (6)   C genes (9)

Germline DNA
e.g. stem cells

Genomic VDJ rearrangement
(large pre B-cell stage)

Poly A   Immature mRNA

Poly A   Mature (spliced mRNA)

Ig heavy chain protein synthesis
(small pre B-cells)

Combination with Ig light
chain protein

Surface expression
of complete Ig protein
(immature B-cell stage)

Figure 6.3 Structure and recombination of Ig genes. The constant region of the Ig heavy chain is encoded by one of nine possible constant (C) genes in the genome depending on the class or subclass of antibody to be synthesizes. The variable region of the Ig heavy chain peptide (Figure 6.2) is encoded by a combination of three genes: one variable (V) gene, one diversity (D) gene and one joining (J) gene. The human genome has multiple variants of each of these genes, but only one of which contributes to Ig synthesis in each individual B-cell clone; the possible combinatorial variations of Ig heavy chain variable region genes contribute to potential diversity of antigen-binding sites on Ig molecules. DNA containing the specific combination of VDJC genes necessary for Ig synthesis is produced as the result of a somatic recombination process that takes place in maturing B-cells. The Ig heavy chain peptide is combined with Ig light chain peptide (produced via a similar process) in immature B-cells to produce the Ig molecule ready for export. T-cell receptors are synthesized in developing T-cells by analogous processes.

histocompatibility complex (**MHC**) molecules (Figure 6.4). Class I MHC molecules are found on most cells and present viral antigens to CD8+ cytotoxic T-cells. Class II MHC molecules are only found on 'professional' antigen-presenting cells (APCs) such as macrophages, dendritic cells and B-cells; this interaction activates the various subsets of effector CD4+ T-cells. These stringent requirements for initial naïve T-cell activation are in place to prevent aberrant activation of T-cells and therefore inappropriate immune responses. One danger the immune system faces is the possibility of T-cell reactions against the body's own ('self') antigens and the onset of autoimmune diseases (such as type I diabetes mellitus), common disorders which are characterized by tissue destruction and loss of function. Fortunately, we have evolved a number of elaborate mechanisms to prevent autoimmunity and maintain a state of self 'tolerance' (Table 6.7).

Phenotypic diversity of T-cells is driven by the nature of the APCs as well as the cytokine

Table 6.6 Function of immunoglobulin classes and subclasses.

Ig class/ subclass		Structure	Function	Sphere of activity
IgA	IgA$_1$ IgA$_2$	Monomeric/ dimeric	Prevents attachment, neutralizes antigens (e.g. toxins), passive immunity to the newborn	Mucosal surfaces, breast milk (dimer), extracellular spaces (monomer)
IgD		Monomeric	Not fully understood	Coexpressed with IgM on B-cell surface during B-cell activation
IgE		Monomeric	Sensitizes mast cells	Extravascular sites in skin and mucosa
IgG	IgG$_1$ IgG$_2$ IgG$_3$ IgG$_4$	Monomeric	Neutralizes and opsonizes antigens, targets NK cells, activates complement and provides passive immunity to the foetus. Functional profile varies between subclasses	Blood, extravascular sites, across placenta
IgM		Pentameric	Early in immune response, low affinity for antigen but multivalent and activates complement effectively	Blood and lymph

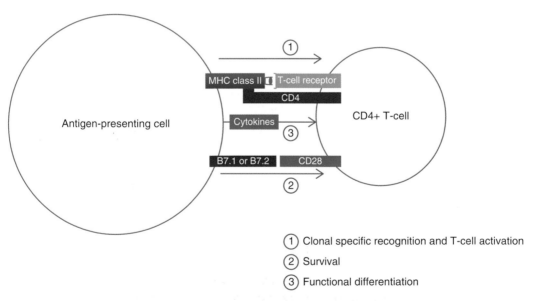

Figure 6.4 Activation of antigen-specific T-cells by antigen-presenting cells. T-cell receptors on naïve T-cells recognize fragments of macromolecules produced as the result of 'processing' and 'presentation' in the context of MHC molecules in APCs such as dendritic cells. Other important connections take place at the surface of T-cells and APCs. Thus, the CD4 molecule on one T-cell subset (CD4+ T-cells) serves to cooperate with TCRs in their interaction with MHC class II molecules on APCs (signal 1). Conversely, CD8+ T-cells (which do not express CD4) interact exclusively with MHC class I molecules (not shown). The intercellular binding of so-called co-receptors such as B7.1 or B7.2 on APCs with CD28 on T-cells (signal 2) is required in the initial stages of infection where naïve T-cells, which have never encountered their cognate antigen before, are activated (for example, in a lymph node). Subsequent encounter with antigen/MHC molecules on target cells at the site of infection does not require this secondary signal. Activation of T-cells also requires cytokines such as IL-6, IL-12 and TGF-β derived from the APC (signal 3); the precise combination of cytokines influences T-cell differentiation and therefore the effector phenotype of the T-cell (see Table 6.8).

Table 6.7 Processes which lead to self tolerance.

Process		Features
Central tolerance		Occurs in the thymus where during development, self-reactive T-cells are eliminated by apoptosis
Peripheral tolerance	Anergy	Inactivation through inadequate signalling in secondary lymphoid tissues
	Action of regulatory T-cells (T_{reg})	Suppression of T-cell function by IL-10 and TGF-β
	Immune deviation	Changing CD4+ phenotype
	Antigen sequestration	Barrier to access to self-antigens in some tissues (e.g. thyroid gland)

Table 6.8 CD4+ T-cell subsets and their immunological function.

CD4+ T-cell subset	Differentiation signal 3 from APC	Effector functions: expand to type of pathogens	Infections eliminated	Effector cytokines
T_H1	IL-12, IFNγ	Activate macrophages	Intracellular bacteria (e.g. *Mycobacterium tuberculosis*)	IFNγ
T_H2	IL-4, IL-6	B-cell help especially switch to IgE, mast cell activation	Parasitic infections at mucosal surfaces (e.g. helminth worms)	IL-4, IL-5, Il-13
T_H17	TGF-β, IL-6	Promote neutrophil activity	Fungi (e.g. *Candida albicans*), extracellular bacteria (e.g. *Streptococcus penumoniae*)	IL-17
T_{reg}	TGF-β	Inhibit T-cell responses	N/A	TGF-β, IL-10
T_{FH}	IL-6	B-cell help and class switching in lymphoid follicles	All	IL-21, ICOS (a cell-surface molecule)

milieu (Table 6.8) and is regulated within the cell by specific transcription factor expression. Thus, during immune responses T-cell functions become increasingly polarized in response to positive and negative regulation by cytokines. CD4+ T-cells in particular have considerable functional diversity and their functions are defined by the cytokines they produce (Table 6.8). T-cell subsets comprise a complex network of interacting cells providing a flexible and dynamic effector function which may shift during the course of an infection to meet host defence requirements and which may mirror fluctuating signs and symptoms of human diseases with an immune pathogenesis. Thus, cytokines from one T-cell subset can suppress the development of other subsets. Also, activation of CD8+ T-cells by dendritic cells can be 'licensed' by help from CD4+ T-cells. Functional T-cell subsets may not be terminally differentiated cells but may be functionally 'plastic', switching between different effector and memory functions.

It is important to map individual cell–cell interactions and phenotypes to the dynamic of infections to gain a holistic understanding of human disease and to design appropriate therapies. This is a challenging task given the great heterogeneity of human microbial pathogens and their mode of infection and even more so for polymicrobial diseases such as periodontitis in which the aetiological factor is a complex and dynamic biofilm.

Some generalizations are, however, possible. Thus antigens are often taken up in the periphery by **dendritic cells** and transported to secondary lymphoid tissues such as Peyer's patches (for antigens taken up in the gut) or lymph nodes (for antigens taken up in the tissues). Alternatively, antigens are transported directly from the tissues via the lymphatic system. Processed antigens are then presented to naïve CD4+ or CD8+ T-cells that express their cognate TCRs

Inflammation

Inflammation is often one obvious symptom of infection but underpinning this are ongoing immune responses (Table 6.9). **Acute inflammation** is the primary response to a range of injuries including, but not limited to, infections. Thus, other causes of inflammation include physical agents such as trauma, ionizing radiation, extremes of temperature, chemicals (e.g. strong acids and alkalis), tissue necrosis (e.g. as in an ischaemic infarction) and inappropriate immune responses as evident in **hypersensitivity reactions** and **autoimmune diseases**. Inflammation is a tissue response that is indicative of increased tissue blood flow to combat the injurious agent (e.g. a microbial pathogen). This process facilitates entry of

Table 6.9 Physical characteristics of acute inflammation.

Symptom (Latin term)	Cause
Redness (*rubor*)	Dilation of blood vessels
Heat (*calor*)	Increased blood flow and systemic fever
Swelling (*tumour*)	Oedema and increased mass of inflammatory cells
Pain (*dolor*)	Pressure and stretching of tissue/chemical mediators (e.g. prostaglandins)
Loss of function	Movement inhibition by pain, immobilization by swelling

elements of the immune response (e.g. neutrophils) to the site of infection, delivers important nutrients and oxygen (for metabolically active neutrophils), dilutes damaging bacterial products such as toxins and promotes fibrin formation and thus coagulation as part of tissue repair. **Gingivitis** is one example of acute inflammation and is induced by accumulation of dental plaque at the margin of the tooth and the gingivae. Another, potentially more serious acute inflammatory response is a **dental abscess** which is a lesion caused by complex mixtures of bacteria that may penetrate the periodontium through deep carious lesions extending through the tooth root. The abscess itself comprises an accumulation of pus (dead bacteria and neutrophils caused by a persistent infection) walled off from the tissue by fibrous (repair) tissue. The swelling abscess causes pain but may progress to cellulitis (inflammation of tissue fascia) and eventually sepsis. Acute inflammation is often resolved, especially if the causal agent is removed. However, persistence of the pathogenic organism can lead to a state of **chronic inflammation**. One example of this is the progression of gingivitis to **periodontitis**. Gingivitis is reversible but periodontitis is an effectively irreversible chronic inflammation of the periodontium manifested by tissue destruction and compromised tooth function. Chronic inflammation is a common feature of infections with 'successful' pathogens: thus infection with *Mycobacterium tuberculosis* can lead to lesions in called **granulomas** that may become necrotic, resulting in loss of lung tissue function.

Immune Responses During Infection

In the face of all the diverse elements and functions of the immune response it is often difficult to appreciate how they are coordinated to effectively remove pathogens and prevent future damaging infections. Although the fundamental and common properties of responses to particular pathogens can be defined, in reality the course of infection and immunity is variable between individual hosts. Some of this variety is the direct consequence of the evolution of a highly polymorphic immune response exemplified by the staggering genetic polymorphism within MHC genes; this confers our population with diversity in antigen-presenting function that is clearly advantageous for the human species. Other individual-specific factors influence the course of human infections: these include general health (including coexisting infections), age and nutritional state. We know these factors are important because the disease experience of different groups of the same societies are variable; for example

there are well-defined susceptibility groups for influenza infection which include the elderly, pregnant women, young children and immunocompromised individuals. Also, whereas many viruses, bacteria and fungi share common properties and life cycles, individual infections and infection events vary in terms of the exposure to, and 'dose' of, the infective agent, the route and mode of transmission and the intrinsic properties of the pathogen itself.

The fundamental stages of infection in terms of the host response are well characterized (Figure 6.5) even if new details of the molecular and cellular mechanisms continue to be revealed and existing knowledge revised and updated by immunologists. A critical stage in the progress of an infectious disease

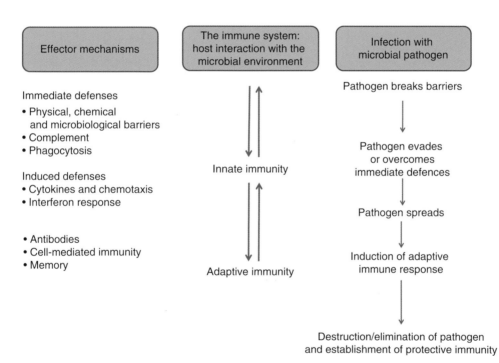

Figure 6.5 Holistic scheme illustrating the immune response to infection. Illustration of the dynamic of the host response to infection with a microbial pathogen. The immune system has several layers of effector mechanism which integrate to achieve destruction and/or elimination of pathogenic microorganisms. These are often categorized into innate and adaptive immunity although this is not always useful as these elements are highly integrated and mutually dependent. The exact nature of the host response and the stage at which the infection is halted is dependent on the site of infection, the exposure and the nature of the pathogen itself. Understanding the diverse elements of the immune response and their interaction is critical to the development of prophylactic measures (e.g. vaccines, allergen avoidance), therapies (anti-inflammatory and immunosuppressive drugs) and novel approaches to clinical management (biomarkers).

is the spread of pathogens from the initial site of infection; factors such as adherence, penetration and colonization of tissues are important and the innate and adaptive immune system combines to inhibit these processes. The nature of the immune response is determined by the properties of the individual pathogen and the anatomical location of the infection. Activation of innate immunity is essential in the early stages of the immune response and this is achieved by recognition of PAMPs by macrophages and dendritic cells. This promotes innate immune effectors and drives the development of the more effective, long-lasting adaptive immune response by stimulating antigen presentation and providing the necessary cytokine milieu for the development of an appropriate T-cell effector response.

Thus, **extracellular bacteria** (e.g. *S. pneumoniae*) are phagocytosed by neutrophils and macrophages, a process enhanced by the combined action of complement and antibody (humoral immunity). Traditionally, CD4+ T-cells of the T_H2 subset were viewed as central to the regulation of antibody responses but increasingly T follicular helper cells (T_{FH}) in lymph nodes are viewed as the most important cells in providing generic B-cell help (Table 6.8). Thus, T-cells recognize cognate antigen presented by B-cells and provide 'help' to B-cells in the form of specific cytokines (e.g. IL-4, IL-5 and IL-6) which promote B-cell differentiation and the development of antibody-secreting plasma cells (Table 6.8). Effective immunity to **extracellular parasites** such as helminth worms depends on the action of T_H2 cells which help B-cells to switch IgE secretion that activates mast cells at mucosal barriers (Table 6.8).

Immune responses against **intracellular bacteria** (e.g. *M. tuberculosis*) are effected by cell-mediated immunity in which CD4+ T-cells of the T_H1 subset activate phagocytic cells such as macrophages, promoting intracellular killing of bacteria taken up by these cells (Table 6.8); this 'help' is mediated by specific cytokines and soluble ligands and in

particular IFNγ and CD40L. Another effect of increased IFNγ is the increased differentiation of tissue macrophages from the pool of circulating of monocytes. T_H17 cells activate neutrophil function which also promotes clearing of extracellular infections. Similar mechanisms are central to effective immunity to **intracellular parasites** such as the protozoan *Leishmania*.

Bacteria in the mouth take the form of a complex and dynamic biofilm, which effectively has its own ecosystem. The unique anatomy of the mouth represents some unusual ecological niches; for example, the gingival crevice (or sulcus) between the tooth and the gingiva is not protected by salivary components such as mucin or IgA antibodies. Also, the junctional epithelium which attaches the tooth to the gingiva is unusually porous, representing an opportunity for tissue invasion by periodontal pathogens. Prevention of potentially damaging inflammation in the mouth is a challenging task for the immune system.

Immune responses to **viral infections** involves both antibody- and cell-mediated immunity commensurate with the life cycle of viruses which involves phases of intracellular replication (and possibly senescence) and extracellular spreading. Antibodies bind to viral particles, preventing their attachment and uptake by target cells. If viruses do invade host cells then the so-called interferon response ensues, mediated by IFNα and IFNβ secreted by infected cells. These cytokines signal neighbouring cells to activate a number of pathways that inhibit viral replication. Among the other effects of IFNα and IFNβ is to increase MHC expression on infected cells and activate the aforementioned NK cells which are capable of killing virus-infected cells. NK cell activity is not sustained and the task of cell killing is taken over by antigen-specific CD8+ cytotoxic T-cells which are activated by recognition of cognate antigen on APCs. IFNα and IFNβ promote CD8+ T-cell responses by activating macrophages and dendritic cells and by promoting lymphocyte recruitment through localized chemokine secretion. The mechanisms by which CD8+ T-cells kill virally infected cells are similar to NK cells but they are highly effective as they are targeted to infected cells by recognition of cognate antigen presented by class I MHC molecules.

A number of viral infections cause oral lesions which may be observed on the dental clinic. These include human herpes viruses (HHV) such as herpes simplex (HHV1) that is associated with cold sores and varicella zoster virus (HHV3) that causes both chicken pox (the symptoms of which may include lesions on the oral mucosa) and recurrent shingles (in which lesions on the head and neck region are rather common). The often red lesions, which may become fluid-filled and then scab over when broken, are the result of destruction of infected host tissues by the action of CD8+ cytotoxic T-cells. Other viral lesions that may be observed intra-orally are papillomas associated with HPV. It is known that some types of HPV (e.g. HPV-16 and -18) are associated with both papillomas and oral cancers (as well as genital cancers).

Fungal infections are of particular interest to the dentist as, in humans, they often affect the oropharyngeal region. We know the immune system is very important to prevent fungal disease as although as many as 50% of the population are actually infected with yeast (usually *Candida albicans*) few of us suffer any harmful effects. However, in conditions of immunosuppression, for example, as the result of chemotherapy for cancer or human immunodeficiency virus (HIV) infection, *Candida* infection can lead to candidiasis, a serious inflammatory condition of the mucosal tissues. *Candida* infection is suppressed by antimicrobial peptides and lactoferrin. The action of IgA in inhibiting adherence is critical (indeed patients with xerostomia, and therefore lacking salivary IgA, are much more likely to have candidiasis). If fungal cells do penetrate the tissues then phagocytosis by neutrophils (which often have to 'gang up' to combat large fungal cells, especially if they are budding) is an

important defence mechanism. Fungi may be recognized by PRRs (such as TLR2, TLR4 or TLR9) on myeloid cells (e.g. macrophages and dendritic cells) which can serve to activate cell-mediated immunity through the secretion of IL-12 which favours the activation of CD4+ T-cells of the T_H1 subset, further enhancing cell-mediated immunity. T_H17 cells also play a role in anti-fungal immunity through their neutrophil-activating function (Table 6.8).

The immune system is compromised by the ability of individual species of viruses and bacteria to mutate, exchange genetic material and thereby evolve surprisingly sophisticated mechanisms to subvert immune responses for their own gain. Thus, the development of a highly regulated mammalian immune response, which exhibits great diversity, functional redundancy and complexity, is the result of our coevolution with microbial pathogens. Investigation of these phenomena not only helps identify therapeutic targets and informs vaccine development but also helps us to comprehend the importance of individual immune pathways in host defences.

Genetic variation in some bacteria (e.g. *Salmonella*) is manifested by the existence of numerous 'serotypes' characterized by variation in cell-surface molecules that generate unique antibodies meaning that primary infections with one serotype do not confer protective immunity against secondary infections with other serotypes. Many viruses mutate gradually, exhibiting so-called 'antigenic drift', meaning that different 'strains' predominate at different times and in different populations. Influenza virus is one example of a pathogen that exhibits antigenic drift on an almost annual basis requiring new vaccine programmes and often resulting in limited epidemics. A major concern is 'antigenic shift' when a more radically different strain appears often as the result of recombination of different influenza genomes; depending on infectivity and virulence, these new strains have the potential to cause pandemics; hence, the health authorities are constantly monitoring disease outbreaks.

In contrast, smallpox virus exhibits no genetic variation and therefore vaccination programmes were highly effective in eradicating this virus from the population. A combination of a high replication rate and frequency of mutation in HIV severely compromises the effectiveness of host immune responses not to mention vaccine development (and also results in the development of antiviral-drug-resistant strains). Viruses have the greatest variety of mechanisms that subvert host immune responses as their life cycle is critically dependent on interactions with host biosynthetic and metabolic processes. Herpes and pox viruses subvert immune responses by inhibiting specific aspects of immune function; for example, both cytomegalovirus and herpes simplex virus inhibit MHC class I expression, a critical stage in host recognition of virally infected cells. Latency is an important strategy to avoid immune surveillance for many viruses including HIV and herpes simplex. Herpes simplex evades the immune system by infecting neuronal tissue, for example the trigeminal nerve in the face; this tissue expresses only low levels of MHC class I molecules and so is hidden from immune surveillance by cytotoxic T-cells and remains in a latent state. Herpes simplex re-emerges at times of 'stress' such as during hormonal changes, exposure to sunlight and coexisting infections and infects epithelial tissue, causing cold-sore lesions. Bacteria can also subvert host responses by a variety of pathways. Some 'hide' from immune effectors; thus *M. tuberculosis* inhibits phagosome/lysosome fusion in macrophages, preventing intracellular destruction.

Malfunctions of the Immune System

The immune system occasionally has intrinsic failings that result in inadequate and inappropriate function, leading to disorder and disease. **Immunodeficiency disorders** (Table 6.10) may either be 'primary' – that is, the result of inherited or spontaneous mutations in genes critical for immune cell development – or otherwise they are disorders secondary to acquired factors. There are over 100 different **primary immunodeficiencies** but individual disorders are very rare. The major symptoms are persistent and recurrent infections and the only treatment is often bone marrow transplantation. Mapping defective genes, signalling pathways and cells in diverse primary immunodeficiencies to the types of infection suffered by these patients continues to reveal much about the processes that underpin human immune responses. Primary immunodeficiencies often have other complex and variable symptoms, a number of which are relevant to dental practice; for example, in hyper-IgE syndrome (commonly caused by mutations in the STAT3 gene which encodes a transcription factor central for immune cell development) patients have abnormalities in tooth eruption and succession leading to the appearance of abnormal dentition.

More commonly, immunodeficiencies are caused by secondary (acquired) factors (Table 6.9). **Acquired immunodeficiency syndrome** (**AIDS**) caused by HIV is a major global health issue and these patients have well-defined oral symptoms including oral candidiasis and (less commonly) necrotizing ulcerative gingivitis (NUG). Cross-infection awareness and control are major issues as many people with HIV are unaware of their infection.

Autoimmune diseases are rather common (some 5% of people in Western populations suffer from autoimmune disease) and are characterized by aberrant immune responses to self-antigen (breakdown of self-tolerance; see Table 6.7) leading to tissue and organ damage and compromised physiological function (Table 6.11). The autoimmune processes are mediated by auto-reactive T-cells and so-called 'autoantibodies' and are similar to those seen in persistent infections in which chronic inflammation is a feature. The self-antigen cannot be eliminated and therefore the

Table 6.10 Conditions of immunodeficiency, their cause and symptoms.

Immunodeficiency	Cause	Symptoms
Primary immunodeficiencies		
Severe combined immunodeficiences (SCIDs)	Inherited gene mutations resulting in deficiency of proteins (e.g. IL-2 receptor) critical for (usually) T-cell development	Severe and generalized susceptibility to infection due to lack of T-cell, NK cell and antibody function
Bruton's X-linked agammglobulinemia (XLA)	Mutation in B-cell signalling proteins resulting in arrested B-cell development	Recurrent infections with extracellular pyogenic bacteria and chronic viral infections due to lack of antibodies
Common variable immunodeficiencies (CVIDs)	Diverse and many; mutation in cell signalling molecules	Often no symptoms or only mild symptoms (e.g. hyper-IgE syndrome and IgA deficiency)
Complement deficiencies	Gene mutation leading to deficiency in individual complement components	Recurrent infections with extracellular pyogenic bacteria
Secondary immunodeficiencies		
Age-related immune senescence	Nutritional deficiencies, in particular micronutrients, e.g trace elements and vitamins	Compromised immunity and increased susceptibility to infections
Trauma (burns, surgery, injury, etc.)	Compromised anatomical integrity, leading to increased spread of infection	Bacteraemia and sepsis due to disseminated infection
Drugs (e.g. cyclosporine)	Interference with immune cell signalling, regulation and function	Side effects of therapeutic immunosuppression (e.g. increased susceptibility to infections and some cancers); deleterious effects on non-target cells (e.g. cyclosporine-induced gingival overgrowth)
Cancers (e.g. chronic lymphocytic leukaemia)	Dysregulation of haematopoiesis, leading to compromised leukocyte development	Increased susceptibility to opportunistic infections
Infections (e.g. HIV)	Progressive destruction of specific leukocyte populations by virulent pathogen	Increased susceptibility to opportunistic infections and rare tumours

autoimmune disease, once manifested, persists for life and treatment is targeted at the symptoms (which often involve intermittent inflammation and endocrine hormone deficiency). Although much of the pathogenesis of autoimmune disease is well understood, the aetiological factors remain cryptic. We do know that most autoimmune diseases have a degree of genetic susceptibility and polymorphic genes encoding immune response molecules such as MHC, NOD and cytotoxic T-lymphocyte antigen 4 (CTLA-4) are known to be particularly important. It is possible that autoimmune diseases are triggered in the genetically susceptible host by acute infections, for example by viruses. A number of autoimmune diseases are important for oral health: **Sjogren's syndrome** is manifested by loss of salivary gland function and oral lesions are

Table 6.11 Some autoimmune diseases and their characteristics.

Disease	Pathogenesis	Abnormality
Organ-specific		
Type I diabetes mellitus	Autoimmune T-cells reacting against antigen in β-cells of the pancreatic islets	β-Cell destruction, diminished insulin production and loss of glycaemic control
Crohn's disease	Intestinal inflammation is response to commensal bacteria	Fluctuating symptoms including diarrhoea, pain, fatigue
Multiple sclerosis	Autoimmune T-cells against brain antigens (e.g. myelin basic protein)	Weak muscles, ataxia, paralysis
Graves' disease	Autoantibodies against the thyroid-stimulating receptor in the thyroid gland	Excessive, dysregulated production of thyroid hormones (hyperthyroidism: weight loss, hyperactivity, goitre)
Non-organ-specific (systemic)		
Rheumatoid arthritis	Autoimmune T-cells against antigens in the synovium of the joints	Cartilage damage, bone erosion leading to chronic pain and compromised function
Systemic lupus erythematosus	Autoantibodies and autoimmune T-cells against numerous nuclear antigens (e.g. DNA)	Vasculitis, glomerulonephritis, erythema (red rash) often seen on the face
Primary Sjogren's syndrome	Autoantibodies and autoimmune T-cells against ribonucleoprotein antigens	Loss of exocrine gland function (salivary and lacrimal glands) leading to dry mouth and eyes; possible systemic effects including muscle and joint pain
Pemphigus vulgaris	Autoantibodies against cadherin in the epidermis	Blistering of skin including lips and mouth

seen in patients with **phemphigus vulgaris** and **systemic lupus erythematosus**.

Hypersenstivity reactions are also common and are characterized by excessive, damaging immune responses to environmental component that are often harmless to the remainder of the population. The signs and symptoms of certain hypersensitivity reactions are similar to acute inflammatory responses including those seen in microbial infections. Hypersensitivity disorders are classified into four types depending on the nature of the triggering molecule and the chronological progression of the immune response (Table 6.12). **Type I hypersensitivity** reactions are acute inflammatory responses (often called 'allergies') that have a wide range of symptoms. Thus, temporary, local-ized irritation and oedema of the nasal mucosal tissues (allergic rhinitis or hayfever) is caused by certain, but not all, pollens. Serious acute, systemic responses ('anaphylaxis') including occlusion of the trachea and circulatory collapse can be caused by certain drugs and foodstuffs including most notably (albeit rarely) peanuts. Avoidance and drugs are effective in controlling the hypersensitivity responses but these disorders remain a significant healthcare issue. Drugs are often targeted at the effects of IgE-induced mast cell degranulation which is central to the pathogenesis of type I hypersensitivity reactions. Allergy to proteins in latex gloves is not at all uncommon and will clearly affect the dental team as well as patients; assessment and avoidance are important as mild localized

Table 6.12 Hypersensitivity reactions and their pathogenesis.

Hypersensitivity	Pathogenesis	Examples	Abnormality
Type I (immediate)	Innocuous antigen (e.g. pollen) recognized by IgE antibodies triggering mast cell degranulation in skin or mucosal surfaces	Allergic rhinitis	Acute effects including mucosal oedema (nasal and conjunctival) and sneezing
		Allergic asthma	Acute effects including bronchial constriction and inflammation
		Atopic eczema	Chronic inflammation of skin (rash)
		Systemic anaphylaxis	Acute effects including oedema, increased vascular permeability, circulatory collapse, death
Type II (antibody-mediated)	IgG antibody recognition of cell surface (and cell matrix) antigen leading to cell destruction (by ADCC, complement-induced lysis or phagocytosis)	Haemolytic disease of the newborn	Anaemia in rhesus-positive newborn with rhesus-negative mother
		Penicillin allergy	Antibodies to penicillin-coated red blood cells lead to complement-mediated lysis
Type III (immune complex-mediated)	Complexes of antibodies and antigens deposited in tissues and organs leading to immune-mediated tissue injury	Serum sickness after injection of antiserum or therapeutic antibodies	Tissue inflammation and damage evidenced by rash, arthritis, glomerulonephritis
Type IV (cell-mediated, delayed-type)	Inappropriate activation of T-cells	Graft-versus-host disease (cytotoxic T-cells), contact dermatitis, tuberculosis (T_H1 cell activation of macrophages), chronic asthma (T_H2-induced mast cell activation)	Chronic and persistent inflammation, tissues damage and loss of function

hypersensitivity response may progress to systemic anaphylaxis is some individuals. **Type IV hypersensitivity** has a distinct pathogenesis: it has a 'chronic' pathogenesis, is mediated by T-cells and is precipitated only days after exposure (hence, the name 'delayed-type'); this is precisely the type of inappropriate and excessive immune response seen in mycobacterial exposure (e.g. in the early stages of tuberculosis).

Vaccination

Vaccination against microbial pathogens is a practical application of immunology that, along with effective sanitation and the development of antibiotics, has had the most beneficial effects on human health in modern times. Vaccination involves active provision of effective immunity against disease (Tables 6.13 and 6.14). Vaccination

Table 6.13 UK vaccination programme for all.

Vaccine	Disease	Causative agent	Vaccination schedule
5-in-1 (DTaP/IPV/Hib)	Diphtheria	Diptheria toxin	2, 3 and 4 months, 12 months (Hib only, given in combination with meningitis C booster), 40 months (all except Hib in a '4-in-1' vaccine),
	Tetanus	Tetanus toxin	
	Whooping cough	Pertussis toxin	
	Polio	Polio virus	
	Pneumonia	*Haemophilus influenzae* type b	
	Meningitis	*Haemophilus influenzae* type b	
4-in-1 (DtaP/IPV) booster	Tetanus/diphtheria/ polio/whooping cough	As above	40 months
3-in-1 (Td/IPV) booster	Tetanus/diphtheria/polio	As above	13–18 years
Pneumococcal conjugate vaccine (PCV)	Pneumococcal pneumonia and pneumococcal meningitis	*Streptococcus pneumoniae*	2 months
Pneumococcal polysaccharide vaccine (PPV)	Pneumococcal pneumonia and pneumococcal meningitis	*Streptococcus pneumoniae*	Over 65 s
Rotavirus	Diarrheal disease	Rotavirus	2 and 3 months
Meningitis C	Meningitis, septicaemia	Meningococcal group C bacteria	3 and 12 months, 13–14 years
MMR	Measles		3 months, 40 months
	Mumps		
	Rubella		

exploits the principle of **immunological memory** whereby initial encounter with microbial antigens leads not only to the production of effector lymphocytes but also the development of long-lived quiescent lymphocytes in the lymph nodes (so-called memory B- and T-cells) which are primed and ready to respond quicker and more vigorously to secondary encounters with antigens. We know from studies of the population vaccinated many years earlier for smallpox that effective immunity is long-lasting and that immunological memory remains effective for many years even in the absence of antigen (smallpox was eradicated in 1980). The effectiveness of a vaccine depends on the manufacturing method, the use of adjuvants (substances added to the vaccine formulation to enhance immune responses), the route of immunization and the nature of the immune responses elicited. Vaccination is not just important for individual health but is a critical public health measure to protect populations against outbreaks of infectious diseases. Thus, if the majority of a community have protective immunity then the susceptible minority will be protected as the microorganism has a low probability of finding a non-immune host and the chain of infection cannot be created. The corollary of this is that the more non-immune people in the community then the greater the likelihood of disease outbreaks and

Table 6.14 Vaccinations for special groups.

Vaccine	Disease	Causative organism	Vaccination schedule
Shingles	Shingles	Herpes zoster virus (human herpes virus 3)	70–79 years
Human papilloma virus (HPV)	Genital warts, cervical cancer	HPV types 6, 11, 16 and 18	Girls aged 12–13 years (three injections)
Influenza	Influenza	Influenza virus	Over 65 s, pregnant women, immunocompromised children and adults, people with chronic heart and respiratory disease
Hepatitis B vaccine	Hepatitis, liver cancer	Hepatitis B virus	Individuals in contact with potentially infected bodily fluids (e.g. doctors, dentists, lab workers, children of infected mothers, etc.)
Tuberculosis (TB) vaccine	Tuberculosis, meningitis	*Mycobacterum tuberculosis*	Children in contact with infected individuals or recently arrived for countries with high levels of tuberculosis
Chicken pox vaccination	Chicken pox	Herpes zoster virus (human herpes virus 3)	Pregnant women, immunocompromised individuals
Travel vaccines	Available against numerous diseases including hepatitis A, yellow fever, typhoid, etc. Dependent on location and purpose of travel.		

epidemics. Maintaining this '**herd immunity**' is a major healthcare challenge. Some individuals in a community are particularly at risk from certain infections; an example of this is healthcare and laboratory workers routinely exposed to sources of blood-borne viruses and who are required to have hepatitis B vaccination (Table 6.14).

7

Oral Microbiology

Angela H. Nobbs

Bristol Dental School, University of Bristol, Bristol, UK

Learning Objectives

- To be able to list the constituents and communities that make up the oral microbiota.
- To be able to describe the formation and constituents of dental plaque biofilm.
- To understand the role that microorganisms play in the pathogenesis of caries and periodontal disease.
- To be able to list the common fungi, bacteria and viruses that cause oral infections.

Clinical Relevance

The oral cavity is host to a huge number and variety of microorganisms and dental plaque is an example of a mixed-species microbial biofilm. While only a small proportion of these microorganisms are responsible for infections they play a crucial role in the most common dental diseases such as caries and periodontal disease. The mechanism by which microorganisms can be transferred from one individual to another is central to cross-infection control and instrument sterilization strategies. Antimicrobials will be commonly prescribed by dentists and knowledge of the specific organisms they target as well as the mode of action is crucial to patient care. Oral microbiology is a very active area of dental research and new strategies for treating and avoiding infections are always being developed, especially those that will discourage further spread of antimicrobial resistance.

Introduction

The oral cavity is home to one of the most complex microbial ecosystems found in the human body. According to the Human Oral Microbiome database almost 700 bacterial taxa have been identified in the mouth to date. Of these, approximately 50% have been named, 17% are unnamed but cultivated and 34% are only known as uncultivated phylotypes. These bacteria are then joined by approximately 20–30 species of fungi and several viruses belonging to four major families. This complexity reflects the diverse microenvironments found in the oral cavity, with hard and soft tissues each providing

Basic Sciences for Dental Students, First Edition. Edited by Simon A. Whawell and Daniel W. Lambert.
© 2018 John Wiley & Sons Ltd. Published 2018 by John Wiley & Sons Ltd.
Companion website: www.wiley.com/go/whawell/basic_sciences_for_dental_students

unique habitats that promote the growth of distinct microbial communities. In a healthy individual, the oral microbial population, or **resident oral microbiome** (Table 7.1), can protect the host from invading pathogens via a biological exclusion phenomenon known as **colonization resistance**. Microbial colonization is also kept in check by the mouth's own battery of antimicrobial mechanisms. The resident microbiome and host defences thus work in partnership to promote a healthy oral cavity. However, problems can arise when this delicate equilibrium is disrupted, with initiation of disease.

Oral Microbiota

Gram-Positive Bacteria

Two genera of Gram-positive bacteria predominate in the oral cavity. The first is *Streptococcus* (Figure 7.1a). Streptococci are ubiquitous in the mouth and can comprise up to 80% of early dental plaque. Oral species can be classified into four main taxonomic groups based upon their 16S rRNA gene sequence: mitis, mutans, salivarius, anginosus (Table 7.2). However, they are often collectively cited as **viridans-group streptococci** because colonies cause greening of blood agar due to partial lysis of red blood cells (*viridis* is Greek for 'green'). This is referred to as alpha haemolysis and is indicative of hydrogen peroxide production. Mitis-group streptococci comprise a number of species that can be isolated from sites throughout the oral cavity and nasopharynx. Member species include *S. pneumoniae*, a major pathogen associated with otitis media, bronchitis, meningitis and pneumonia, while several other species (e.g. *S. gordonii*), although predominantly **commensals** in the mouth, have been associated with systemic infections such as infective endocarditis (Feature box 7.1). Similarly, anginosus-group streptococci colonize both soft and hard substrata in the mouth and are frequently isolated from abscesses, both dental and at extra-oral sites. Mutans-group streptococci primarily colonize hard surfaces within the mouth and are strongly associated with dental caries (tooth decay), while salivarius-group streptococci preferentially target the tongue and other mucosal surfaces.

The second major genus of Gram-positive bacteria is *Actinomyces*. These rod-shaped bacteria (Figure 7.1b) are common components of dental plaque but, as opportunistic pathogens, are also associated with root-surface caries and abscess formation. Two species predominate in the human mouth: *A. naeslundii* and *A. oris*. A third species, *A. israelii*, is recognized as the major causative agent of actinomycosis, a chronic inflammatory disease that primarily targets the oral mucosae (Feature box 7.2, Figure 7.2).

Several other Gram-positive bacteria have been slow to identify due to fastidious growth requirements that have hindered cultivation. These include major plaque constituent *Granulicatella adiacens*, and several anaerobic species associated with periodontal or endodontic infections, such as *Parvimonas micra*, *Peptostreptococcus stomatis*, *Finegoldia magna* and *Filifactor alocis*. Several *Lactobacillus* species are also common isolates from the mouth. These are typically found in relatively low abundance, but elevated levels can be indicative of a high carbohydrate diet.

Gram-Negative Bacteria

Knowledge of the Gram-negative component of the resident oral microbiome has been significantly improved by the introduction of molecular-based identification approaches. This is because many Gram-negative species have strict growth and/or nutritional requirements, making cultivation difficult. *Veillonella* species are **obligate anaerobes** and unable to metabolize carbohydrates directly. These bacteria are therefore reliant upon uptake of intermediary metabolites released by other plaque microbes as an energy source. Similarly, *Porphyromonas gingivalis* utilizes peptides rather than sugars for growth and is unable to

Table 7.1 Predominant microbial genera found within the oral cavity.

Genus/Family	Classification/morphology	Preferred site(s)
Bacteria		
Actinomyces	Gram-positive rods/filaments	Plaque, mucosae, tongue
Aggregatibacter	Gram-negative rods	Subgingival pockets
Bifidobacterium	Gram-positive rods	Plaque
Corynebacterium	Gram-positive rods/filaments	Plaque
Eikenella	Gram-negative rods	Subgingival pockets
Eubacterium	Gram-positive rods/filaments	Subgingival pockets
Filifactor	Gram-positive rods	Subgingival pockets
Finegoldia	Gram-positive cocci	Subgingival pockets
Fusobacterium	Gram-negative rods	Plaque
Gemella	Gram-positive cocci	Mucosae
Granulicatella	Gram-positive cocci	Plaque, mucosae
Lactobacillus	Gram-positive rods	Plaque, tongue
Neisseria	Gram-negative cocci	Teeth, mucosae, tongue
Parvimonas	Gram-positive cocci	Subgingival pockets
Peptostreptococcus	Gram-positive cocci	Subgingival pockets
Porphyromonas	Gram-negative rods	Subgingival pockets
Prevotella	Gram-negative rods	Subgingival pockets
Propionibacterium	Gram-positive rods	Subgingival pockets
Rothia	Gram-positive rods (variable)	Plaque, tongue
Streptococcus	Gram-positive cocci	Plaque, mucosae, tongue
Tannerella	Gram-negative rods	Subgingival pockets
Treponema	Gram-negative spirochaetes	Subgingival pockets
Veillonella	Gram-negative cocci	Plaque, mucosae, tongue
Fungi		
Aspergillus	Mould	Tongue
Aureobasidium	Yeast	Tongue
Candida	Yeast	Tongue, appliances
Cladosporium	Mould	Tongue
Cryptococcus	Yeast	Tongue
Fusarium	Mould	Tongue
Saccharomyces	Yeast	Tongue
Viruses		
Herpesviridae	Double-stranded DNA virus	Mucosae
Papillomaviridae	Double-stranded DNA virus	Mucosae
Picornaviridae	Single-stranded RNA virus	Mucosae
Retroviridae	Single-stranded RNA virus	Mucosae

(a)　　　　　　　　　　　　　　　　　　(b)

(c)　　　　　　　　　　　　　　　　　　(d)

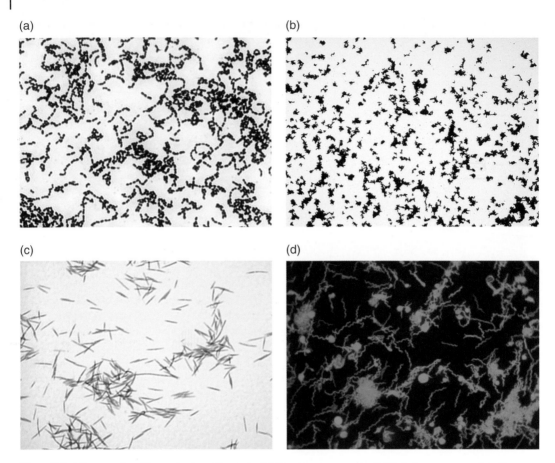

Figure 7.1 Micrographs of important oral bacteria. (a) *Streptococcus gordonii*, (b) *Actinomyces naeslundii*, (c) *Fusobacterium nucleatum*, (d) *Treponema denticola*.

tolerate oxygen. This bacterium is typically located below the gum line and is strongly associated with periodontal disease, as well as severe systemic diseases such as atherosclerosis (Feature box 7.1). Other periodontopathogens include *Prevotella intermedia*, which is an obligate anaerobe but can ferment carbohydrates, and *Aggregatibacter actinomycetemcomitans*, which is a **capnophilic** bacterium particularly associated with aggressive periodontitis.

One of the most abundant Gram-negative obligate anaerobes is *Fusobacterium nucleatum* (Figure 7.1c). This bacterium forms characteristically long filaments and is considered crucial to the accretion of dental plaque due, in part, to its promiscuous coaggregation capabilities with other members of the oral

microbiota. Recently it has also been associated with systemic conditions including pregnancy complications and bowel cancer. Other striking morphologies include those of *Treponema*, such as *T. denticola*, and of TM7. As spirochaetes, *Treponema* species exhibit a corkscrew-like morphology (Figure 7.1d), whereas TM7 can form filaments up to 40 μm in length. Treponemes can be cultured *in vitro*, albeit with difficulty, but successful cultivation of TM7 remains elusive.

It should be noted that not all Gram-negative oral microbes are intolerant of oxygen. Both *Neisseria* species and *Eikenella corrodens* are **facultatively anaerobic**. Accordingly, many of these bacteria can be found at sites throughout the oral cavity. *Neisseria* species play an important role in

Table 7.2 Oral streptococci.

Group	Species	Preferred site(s)
Mitis	S. mitis	Teeth, dental appliances, mucosal tissues
	S. oralis	
	S. pneumoniae	
	S. gordonii	
	S. sanguinis	
	S. parasanguinis	
	S. cristatus	
	S. infantis	
	S. oligofermentans	
	S. australis	
	S. peroris	
Anginosus	S. anginosus	Teeth, dental appliances, mucosal tissues
	S. constellatus	
	S. intermedius	
Mutans	S. downei	Teeth, dental appliances
	S. mutans	
	S. sobrinus	
Salivarius	S. salivarius	Tongue and other mucosal tissues
	S. vestibularis	

early plaque formation, while *Eikenella corrodens* is primarily associated with periodontal disease.

Fungi

While less abundant than bacteria, fungal species are consistently found as members of the resident oral microbiome. Both **unicellular yeasts** and **multicellular moulds** have been found in the oral cavity. By far the most common genus is *Candida* and, in particular, *Candida albicans*, with a carriage frequency of up to 40% (Figure 7.3). Other common genera include *Cladosporium*, *Aureobasidium* and *Saccharomyces*. Fungi are most frequently isolated from the dorsum of the tongue, but also readily colonize materials such as acrylic from which dental appliances

are constructed. Consequently, individuals who wear dentures are likely to harbour a greater fungal burden (predominantly *C. albicans*) within their mouths than those individuals who are appliance-free. The clinical relevance of a diverse population of fungal species in the oral cavity remains relatively unknown. Nonetheless, it is well recognized that oral fungal colonization and subsequent disease is particularly problematic among the immunocompromised.

Viruses

As for other microorganisms, the advent of molecular-based identification techniques has transformed understanding of the viral component of the oral microbiome. Approximately 90% of adults harbour viruses and those most frequently found within the oral cavity belong to four major families: *Herpesviridae*, *Papillomaviridae*, *Picornaviridae* and *Retroviridae*. Furthermore, both herpes viruses and papilloma viruses are able to enter periods of **latency** and persist for the lifetime of the host once acquired. Such latency makes it difficult to determine the influence of viral colonization on health and disease. Nonetheless, within the oral cavity viruses have been associated with the development of ulcers, tumours, autoimmune diseases and periodontitis.

Microbial Communities in the Mouth

Oral Microenvironments

Redox potential, pH and **nutrient availability** at any given site within the mouth will dictate which microorganisms can grow, while **receptor availability** underpins sites of microbial colonization (**tissue tropism**). The anatomy of the oral cavity therefore presents microbes with unique habitats that favour the accumulation of distinct microbial communities. Epithelia of the hard and soft palates, buccal mucosa and gingivae

---

Feature box 7.1 Oral bacteria and systemic disease

There is growing evidence that periodon-topathogens may be linked with severe systemic conditions. Atherosclerosis is associated with inflammatory plaque accumulation in blood vessels of the cardiac system. Proinflammatory cytokines, periodontal pathogens or their antigens may therefore initiate or exacerbate these effects following entry into the bloodstream from sites of periodontal disease, particularly as the inflammation and tissue destruction at these sites increases the likelihood of bacteraemia. Indeed, DNA from bacteria such as *P. gingivalis*, *F. nucleatum* and *A. actinomycetemcomitans* has been detected in atherosclerotic plaques. There is also an association between periodontitis and adverse pregnancy outcomes such as preterm birth. Since successful pregnancy is reliant upon a delicate balance of hormones, cytokines and proteases, disruption of this balance by periodontopathogens could mediate adverse effects. Again, in support of this, both *P. gingivalis* and *F. nucleatum* have been isolated from amniotic fluid and have been shown to induce preterm birth in animals. Systemic effects are not, however, restricted to periodontopathogens, and associations are also seen with members of the commensal microbiota. This may relate to the fact that even daily practices such as toothbrushing or eating hard foodstuffs have been shown to induce a transient bacteraemia. A classic example is infective endocarditis, a relatively rare but often fatal infection of the heart valves. Viridans streptococci are responsible for approximately 50% of infective endocarditis cases in the Western world. Underpinning this association is the capacity for these streptococci to colonize heart valves and promote thrombosis through interactions with host platelets, leading to formation of the infective vegetation.

Feature box 7.2 Cervicofacial actinomycosis

Cervicofacial actinomycosis is an infection affecting the lower jaw caused by members of the *Actinomyces* genus, with *A. israelii* responsible for over 90% of cases. An infected root canal, tooth extraction or other form of trauma enables these bacteria to infect submandibular tissues, with resultant swelling. The swelling may be localized or diffuse, and sinus tracts develop within the swollen tissues from which a thick, yellow exudate is expressed. This pus contains characteristic aggregates of calcified *Actinomyces* filaments, known as 'sulphur granules'.

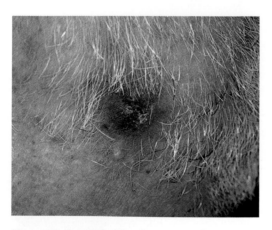

Figure 7.2 Cervicofacial actinomycosis. Source: Courtesy of T. Brooke.

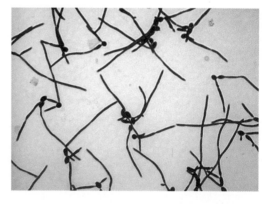

Figure 7.3 Gram stain of *Candida albicans* showing filamentous growth (true hyphae and pseudohyphae) arising from mother cells (blastospores).

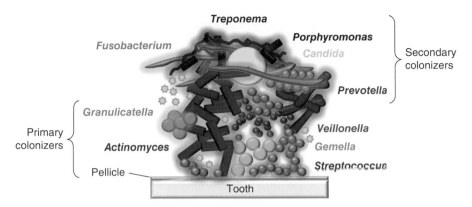

Figure 7.4 Spatiotemporal model of plaque accretion. Primary colonizers associate with components of the acquired pellicle on the tooth surface and with each other via coadhesion/coaggregation. This generates a substratum with which incoming secondary colonizers can then associate. As the plaque matures, production of extracellular polymeric substance provides structural integrity and a conduit for the exchange of molecules. Nutritional adaptation, intermicrobial signalling (yellow stars) and beneficial/antagonistic interactions lead to the formation of distinct microbial societies within the plaque community that provide optimal metabolic networks and protection. Ultimately a climax community is formed that, in times of health, exists in equilibrium with its host.

are exposed to the external environment and thus are primarily colonized by aerobic or facultatively anaerobic microbes. The principal exception to this is with the dorsum of the tongue, where the highly papillated surface can generate anoxic areas and thus support complex communities incorporating anaerobic microorganisms. Desquamation of soft tissues does, however, serve to minimize overall microbial burden at these sites. By contrast, non-shedding surfaces such as teeth or dental appliances are more stable substrata, with tooth pits and fissures and interproximal sites offering added protection from shear forces. These hard surfaces thus have capacity to support much larger and more diverse microbial populations.

Dental Plaque Formation

Successful colonization of the oral cavity is driven by one fundamental concept: stick or be swallowed. Flushing activities of saliva are highly effective, with millions of microbes swallowed every day. Therefore it is critical that microbes entering the mouth are able to rapidly attach to a surface. Nonetheless, acquisition of the oral microbiome is not a random process, but rather follows a general spatiotemporal model. This is exemplified by dental plaque formation on teeth (Figure 7.4). Colonization of the tooth begins with attachment of **pioneer** (or **primary**) **colonizers** to specific receptors within the acquired salivary pellicle, the precise composition of which is host-dependent (Feature box 7.3). These pioneer colonizers are predominantly streptococci, together with *Actinomyces* and *Veillonella* species, and express surface molecules (**adhesins**) that mediate attachment to salivary components such as mucins, agglutinins, proline-rich proteins and α-amylase. This layer of early colonizers then serves as a substratum for further incoming microbes, known as **secondary colonizers**, thereby facilitating accretion and diversification of the microbial community as plaque matures. For example, both streptococci and actinomycetes can bind to each other and also to *P. gingivalis*. Such physical interactions occur via specific receptor–ligand partnerships in a process known as **coaggregation** (when both partner microbes are in suspension) or **coadhesion** (when one partner microbe is already immobilized). *F. nucleatum* can bind the most diverse range of partner microbes identified to date, including both early colonizers (forming so-called 'corncob' structures with streptococci) and secondary colonizers. This species is therefore considered a critical 'bridging' microorganism within plaque.

Interbacterial interactions have not evolved to exclusively facilitate physical attachment, and **mutualistic relationships** based upon compatible metabolic or nutritional requirements also influence plaque community development. For example, as plaque matures, facultative anaerobes (e.g. streptococci) deplete oxygen within the local environment, generating anoxic pockets in which anaerobic secondary colonizers (e.g. *T. denticola*, *P. gingivalis*) can grow. Streptococci also excrete lactate as a waste product of glycolysis. Lactate is then utilized as an energy source by *Veillonella* species, which are unable to perform glycolysis themselves. In kind, uptake of lactate by *Veillonella* increases the flux of glucose to lactate, thereby promoting streptococcal growth. This reciprocal relationship is one of the reasons why streptococci and *Veillonella* occur together within early plaque, and such **nutritional co-dependencies** may explain why many members of the oral microbiome have yet to be cultivated independently. The goal of all oral microorganisms is, however, to ensure their survival and consequently some interbacterial interactions are **antagonistic**. Those species that occupy the same micro-environment are often in competition for available binding sites or nutrients. Some bacteria have therefore evolved strategies to enhance their competitive advantage. Many oral streptococci secrete hydrogen peroxide, which can damage and kill other microbes through the generation of oxidizing free radicals. Other bacteria secrete peptides, known as **bacteriocins**, which specifically inhibit the growth of closely related species. Examples include mutacins produced by *S. mutans* that target other oral streptococci, and actinobacillin produced by *A. oris*, which is toxic to both streptococci and other actinomycetes.

Intermicrobial Signals

An additional factor that influences overall plaque development is **intermicrobial signalling**. Many oral microbes release **diffusible signalling molecules**. These can be detected by other members of the microbiota, who may respond by modulating gene expression or metabolic activity. For example, *Veillonella atypica* secretes a short-range signalling molecule that is detected by *S. gordonii*. In response, *S. gordonii* upregulates expression of enzyme α-amylase and so the breakdown of intracellular carbohydrate reserves, ultimately excreting additional lactate for utilization by *V. atypica*. Often signalling mechanisms are regulated according to population density, with gene modulation only occurring once a critical threshold concentration of signalling molecule has been reached. This is known as **quorum sensing**. A key quorum sensing molecule implicated in dental plaque formation is autoinducer-2 (AI-2). This is synthesized by enzyme LuxS, and carriage of the *luxS* gene is highly conserved among Gram-negative and Gram-positive bacteria. Several species can respond to AI-2, regardless of its origin, and thus AI-2 is known as a 'universal' signalling molecule. While relatively little is understood about its detection, AI-2 is required for cooperative growth between *S. gordonii* and *P. gingivalis*, *A. oris* or *C. albicans*.

Extracellular Matrix

As the plaque community expands, production of **extracellular polymeric substance** (**EPS**) leads to the establishment of a protective matrix in which the plaque microorganisms become embedded. Thus dental plaque is an archetypal **biofilm**. The principal function of the matrix is to provide structural integrity to the biofilm, but can also act as a conduit for the exchange of molecules among the microbial community. Matrix components are either actively secreted or are released following cell lysis. Polysaccharides are present in the greatest abundance and include **insoluble glucans** (glucose polymers) synthesized by oral streptococci from dietary sucrose. More recently, **extracellular DNA** (eDNA) has also been shown to be an integral matrix constituent. Growth as a biofilm confers significant benefits upon the plaque microbiota, such as increased resistance to removal by shear forces and to host antimicrobial defences. Furthermore, inter-microbial communication results in coordinated, optimized gene expression, so that the collective metabolic efficiency and survival of the biofilm community is greater than the sum of its parts.

Climax Community

The plaque community will continue to develop until shear forces limit any further expansion, but its overall architecture and organization undergo continuous reorganization. Plaque composition changes significantly from initial microbial acquisition at birth through to adulthood, and across different sites of the tooth, in response to varying environmental conditions. Nonetheless, microbial succession ultimately results in a plaque community within each niche that is in equilibrium with its host and so remains fairly stable. This is known as a **climax community**. Microbial homeostasis underpins the colonization-resistance capabilities of the resident plaque microbiome and helps to maintain overall oral health. However, disruption of the host-microbe equilibrium in response to a change in local environmental conditions can shift the climax community composition, enabling outgrowth of pathogenic microorganisms and subsequent oral disease. This forms the basis of the **ecological plaque hypothesis**.

Microbiology of Caries

Disease

Dental caries is one of the most ubiquitous bacterial infections of humans, with a global prevalence of approximately 35%. Dental caries can be defined as an infection of bacterial origin that causes **demineralization** of hard tissues and destruction of the organic matter of the tooth. Demineralization occurs as a result of **acid production** (predominantly lactate) by bacteria fermenting carbohydrates, and causes formation of a **carious lesion** within the tooth. The initial lesion is sub-surface due to acid diffusion, but can progress to a clinically detectable primary lesion known as a 'white spot'. At this stage, caries can be reversed by remineralization and regrowth of hydroxyapatite crystals. If this does not occur, the lesion progresses, leading to collapse of the tooth surface above the lesion and formation of a small **cavity**. With advanced caries this cavity can then progress to the dentine and into the pulp chamber, ultimately resulting in pulp necrosis and formation of periapical abscesses. While its pathogenesis remains the same, dental caries can be classified according to lesion location, rate of progression and the tissues affected (Table 7.3).

Table 7.3 Types of dental caries.

Type	Features
Enamel smooth surface	Relatively rare due to ease with which surfaces can be cleaned
Enamel pit and fissure	Occlusal surfaces particularly prone to lesions
Approximal	Common due to ease with which bacteria/food become trapped
Root	Associated more with elderly due to gingival recession
Recurrent	Occurs around existing restorations
Rampant	Widespread severe lesions Primarily in individuals with a reduced salivary flow rate
Early childhood	Caries of primary dentition
Severe early childhood (nursing-bottle)	Rampant caries of primary dentition Associated with prolonged use of bottles/pacifiers containing concentrated fermentable carbohydrates

S. mutans was isolated from a human carious lesion by Clarke in 1924, but it was not until studies performed by Keyes and Fitzgerald with hamsters in the 1950s that the role of bacteria in dental caries was recognized. These experiments showed that golden hamsters developed tooth decay when fed a high-sugar diet, whereas albino hamsters fed the same diet remained caries-free. However, when albino hamsters were caged with or fed the faecal pellets from golden hamsters, these animals then became caries-active. This demonstrated that golden hamsters harboured a transmissible agent responsible for caries. A *Streptococcus* was subsequently isolated from hamster carious lesions and shown to satisfy Koch's postulates of infectious disease. Nonetheless, it was not until 1968 that this bacterium was accepted as the *S. mutans* originally identified by Clarke.

Aetiology

Given the mechanism of caries progression, the bacteria associated with disease are those that are effective acid producers (**acidogenic**) and/or are tolerant of highly acidic and thus low-pH conditions (**aciduric**). The predominant **cariogenic bacteria** associated with all forms of the disease are the mutans-group streptococci and, specifically relating to human disease, *S. mutans* serotypes c, e and f, and *S. sobrinus* serotypes d and g. Using *S. mutans* as a model, a number of virulence attributes have been identified that contribute to the cariogenicity of these bacteria (Figure 7.5). The first is ability to **bind to the tooth surface** and in *S. mutans* this is principally mediated by a protein adhesin on the cell surface known as SpaP or P1. This adhesin belongs to the AgI/II family of polypeptides that is conserved across virtually all oral streptococci, and promotes strong attachment to acquired pellicle constituent glycoprotein 340 (gp340; otherwise known as salivary agglutinin (SAG)). *S. mutans* is also a prolific producer of **matrix polysaccharides** that promote its retention within plaque. This results from activities of three glucosyltransferases (GtfB–D) and one fructosyltransferase (Ftf), which synthesize glucan or fructan polymers respectively from fermentable carbohydrate (sucrose). Insoluble glucans are particularly effective for retention, as they are bound by four glucan-binding proteins on the *S. mutans* cell surface (GbpA–D), thereby strengthening overall structural integrity of the plaque biofilm. Polysaccharide synthesis also relates to the highly acidogenic nature of this bacterium. *S. mutans* can metabolize dietary carbohydrate to produce a variety of acids, including lactate. Furthermore, glucans, fructans and intracellular polysaccharide stores made by *S. mutans* can be metabolized once dietary sources of carbohydrate are unavailable. This prolongs the duration of acid release and thus the time period over which the tooth is exposed to a pH that triggers demineralization

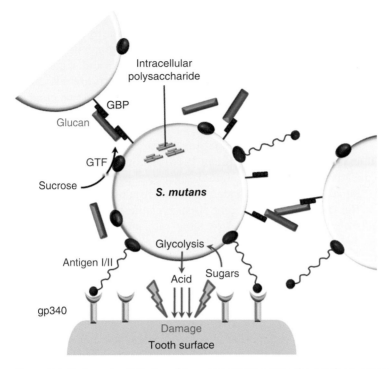

Figure 7.5 Cariogenic attributes of *S. mutans*. Antigen I/II polypeptides promote attachment to gp340 within the acquired pellicle on the tooth surface, while glucosyltransferases (GTFs) synthesize glucans from fermentable carbohydrate. Glucans in turn are bound by glucan-binding proteins (GBPs), providing additional structural stability to the plaque biofilm. Glucans, together with intracellular polysaccharide stores, can be broken down via glycolysis to yield energy, with lactic acid released as a waste product. This causes a drop in pH in the local environment. If this reaches pH 5.5 or lower, demineralization of the tooth surface occurs, leading to formation of a carious lesion.

(below pH 5.5). *S. mutans* is also highly aciduric and thus able to thrive under low pH conditions, unlike many other members of the oral microbiota.

Like mutans streptococci, lactobacilli are efficient producers of lactic acid and able to withstand low-pH conditions. However, they lack the specialized colonization attributes seen with *S. mutans* that promote strong attachment to the tooth surface. As such, while isolated from all forms of carious lesion, lactobacilli are not thought to initiate smooth surface caries. Rather, other bacteria (e.g. *Streptococcus*, *Bifidobacterium*) trigger early smooth surface lesions, and the resulting acidic conditions then promote outgrowth of the aciduric lactobacilli. Acid production by lactobacilli then further exacerbates lesion progression. Lactobacilli may,

however, have capacity to initiate pit/fissure or approximal caries if they become physically trapped within these sites.

Actinomyces species are less prolific acid producers than mutans streptococci or lactobacilli. However, these bacteria are frequently isolated from root surface carious lesions. At these sites, cementum rather than enamel forms the outermost layer. Cementum has a lower mineral content and is therefore more readily dissolved than enamel, making roots susceptible to acid attack by *Actinomyces*.

Traditionally these cariogenic bacteria were identified by isolation from lesions and subsequent cultivation. However, with the advent of culture-independent identification techniques, it is now recognized that the spectrum of cariogenic microbes is much wider and the pathogenesis of disease more complex. Species of *Veillonella*, *Bifidobacterium* and *Propionibacterium* are now considered important in the progression of caries. *Rothia dentocariosa* and *Propionibacterium* species have been found to have a strong association with carious lesions that form within dentine, and *Scardovia wiggsiae* is an emerging pathogen associated with severe forms of early childhood caries. Thus, rather than caries arising from the actions of a single causative bacterium, it is more likely that a change in ecological conditions disrupts the resident microbiome so that the effects of a collective of cariogenic microbes predominate (i.e. ecological plaque hypothesis). Host and environmental factors are therefore also critical in influencing overall caries risk. The flow rate and buffering capacity of an individual's saliva affects how effectively acid can be removed or neutralized to minimize demineralization, while diets with a high intake of fermentable carbohydrate (quantity and frequency) will promote conditions that favour growth of cariogenic microorganisms.

Microbiology of Periodontal Diseases

Classification

The term **periodontal disease** encompasses a range of conditions that target the supporting structures of the teeth. These diseases are widespread in both developed and developing countries, and affect an estimated 50% of adults over 30 years of age in the USA. Periodontal diseases typically result from a combination of bacterial factors and the host immune response, and are associated with polymicrobial infections rather than a single causative agent. The development of periodontal disease is characterized by the loss of junctional epithelium from the base of the gingival crevice along the root of the tooth, forming a **periodontal pocket**. The mildest form of periodontal disease is **gingivitis**,

which manifests as inflammation of the gingival tissues in response to plaque accumulation. Not all cases of gingivitis progress to more severe periodontitis and, if good oral hygiene is restored, the effects are reversible. However, it is widely recognized that gingivitis usually precedes onset of periodontitis. **Periodontitis** is distinguished from gingivitis by the progressive and irreversible loss of attachment between the tooth and gingivae, periodontal ligament and alveolar bone, ultimately resulting in tooth loss (Figure 7.6). Different disease manifestations vary according to locality, rate and severity of tissue destruction, and can be strongly influenced by host and environmental factors. Given the spectrum of conditions, classification of periodontal diseases has proven challenging, but they are currently divided across eight main categories (Table 7.4). An emerging form of periodontitis associated with dental implants is **peri-implantitis**. This results from microbial infection of the soft and hard tissues surrounding an implant. Such infections are often acute and highly destructive, resulting in significant bone loss and implant failure.

Host Factors

Plaque accumulation triggers **host innate and adaptive immune defences** in the surrounding soft tissues. Minor inflammation of gingival tissues may occur, but usually the microbial challenge will be successfully contained. Neutrophils play a critical role at this stage, which is why neutrophil abnormalities are strongly associated with periodontitis. However, if the immune response is ineffective, environmental conditions generated by the **inflammation** will instead promote outgrowth of microorganisms that dysregulate the host inflammatory response further, resulting in tissue and bone destruction. Bacterial antigens induce humoral responses and the generation of antibodies. These trigger inflammation and release of **prostaglandins** via the complement cascade, which then stimulate bone resorption. Cell-mediated immunity also responds to

Figure 7.6 Effects of periodontitis. Healthy periodontal tissue (left) contains connective tissue and alveolar bone, which support the tooth root. In addition, the oral epithelium covers this supporting tissue, and a specialized junctional epithelium connects it to the tooth surface. The space between the epithelial surface and the tooth is named the sulcus and is filled with gingival crevicular fluid. In cases of periodontitis (right), a dental plaque biofilm accumulates on the surface of the tooth and tooth root and causes the destruction of periodontal connective tissue and alveolar bone. Source: Darveau 2010. Reproduced with permission of *Nature Reviews Microbiology*.

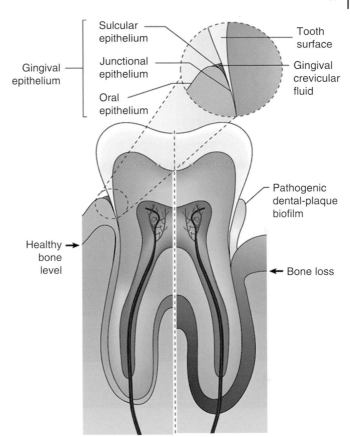

microbial challenge through **T- and B-cell activation** and **polymorphonuclear leukocyte (PMN)/monocyte recruitment**. This results in the release of **proinflammatory mediators**, such as TNF-α and IL-1, ultimately leading to bone resorption following osteoclast activation, and to loss of connective tissue following release and activation of proteolytic enzymes including **matrix metalloproteinases (MMPs)**.

Bacterial Factors

While the aetiology of periodontal disease is complex, involving consortia of microbes rather than individual species, collectively **periodontopathogens** possess a number of virulence attributes. First is the capacity to **colonize subgingival sites**. Many periodontopathogens are secondary colonizers and so their attachment is mediated by coadhesion to antecedent primary colonizers. Alternatively, some bacteria can bind directly to receptors expressed on the surface of gingival epithelial cells or to components of the extracellular matrix (ECM). Periodontopathogens also employ a number of strategies for **evading or disrupting host immune defences** and so promoting their persistence at subgingival sites. Bacteria such as *P. gingivalis* or *A. actinomycetemcomitans* can induce their uptake into epithelial cells following attachment, the intracellular environment providing protection from external immune defences. In addition, these bacteria can target PMNs. *P. gingivalis* expresses a polysaccharide capsule that is anti-phagocytic, and can modulate host expression of proinflammatory mediators such as IL-8, thereby impairing phagocyte recruitment. *A. actinomycetemcomitans* produces a potent exotoxin known

Table 7.4 Classification of periodontal diseases.

Type	Features
Gingival diseases	Plaque-induced or non-plaque-induced forms Reversible inflammation of the gingival margins Can be exacerbated by systemic factors (e.g. pregnancy, HIV or HSV-1 immunosuppression)
Chronic periodontitis	Localized or generalized forms Most common form of periodontitis Severity correlates with plaque/calculus burden Slow/moderate progression Can be modified by systemic (e.g. diabetes, HIV) or environmental (e.g. smoking) factors
Aggressive periodontitis	Localized or generalized forms Rare and usually occurs in adolescents Severity does not correlate with plaque/calculus burden Rapid tissue destruction Commonly associated with neutrophil dysfunction Strong genetic component implicated due to familial clustering
Periodontitis as a manifestation of systemic disease	Systemic disease induces onset of periodontitis Systemic diseases include haematological and genetic disorders that often cause neutrophil abnormalities
Necrotizing periodontal diseases	Painful necrosis (death) of gingival tissues, periodontal ligament and alveolar bone Common predisposing factors include smoking, stress and HIV infection
Abscesses of the periodontium	Often result from acute exacerbation of pre-existing periodontal pockets
Periodontitis associated with endodontic lesions	Endodontic lesion is draining through a pre-existing periodontal pocket
Developmental or acquired deformities and conditions	Tooth-related and mucogingival factors that may modify or predispose to periodontitis, including occlusal trauma and gingival recession

as leukotoxin, which specifically lyses neutrophils, monocytes and a lymphocyte subpopulation. Several periodontopathogens are **asaccharolytic**, meaning that they obtain their energy from catabolism of amino acids rather than sugars. These bacteria therefore express a multitude of **proteolytic enzymes** to break down tissue components into growth nutrients. However, in the pursuit of obtaining nutrients, the actions of these proteases can also disrupt host immunity by degrading antibodies, antimicrobial peptides, cytokines and components of the complement cascade.

Another key feature of periodontopathogens is their capacity to **induce or exacerbate the tissue destruction** associated with periodontal disease and again, many of these effects are mediated by **bacterial proteases**. Classic examples are RgpA and Kgp, two major proteases of *P. gingivalis* that are collectively known as **gingipains**. Gingipains can disrupt ECM by breaking down collagens, fibronectin and laminin, and can also activate host MMPs, which in turn cause further damage to ECM and the periodontium. Other subgingival bacterial hydrolases cause similar damage by targeting hyaluronic acid or chondroitin sulphate. Once epithelial barriers have been breached these tissues are then susceptible to further damage from **cytotoxic metabolites** released by some periodontopathogens. These metabolites include volatile fatty acids such as butyric acid, indole, ammonia and volatile sulphur compounds such as hydrogen sulphide or methyl mercaptan. In addition to tissue damage, **lipopolysaccharide** (**LPS**) of both *P. gingivalis* and *A. actinomycetemcomitans* has been shown to activate osteoclasts and so promote alveolar bone resorption.

Aetiology

Determination of the causative agents of periodontal disease remains an ongoing challenge. Identification of microorganisms within periodontal pockets does not implicate specific species, but rather **complex communities** of microorganisms, the composition of which shifts with disease severity. Species of *Porphyromonas*, *Treponema*, *Tannerella*, *Prevotella* and *Aggregatibacter* have all been strongly associated with periodontal disease. These putative periodontopathogens have been identified on the basis of a number of criteria, including greater abundance in diseased versus healthy sites, induction of responses within the host associated with disease and expression of relevant virulence factors. It should be noted, however, that the spectrum of periodontopathogens is likely even greater still. Evidence for this comes from the recent application of metagenomics to identification of the subgingival microbiome. This has revealed a large number of novel phylotypes, several of which are not yet able to be cultivated or are difficult to grow, such as TM7 or *F. alocis*. Further research is now required to determine the contribution of such microbes to progression of periodontal disease. It should also be noted that, given their capacity to modulate host immune responses, it is thought that herpes viruses might work in synergy with bacteria to contribute to the progression of periodontal disease.

Many putative periodontopathogens can be found in healthy individuals, albeit in relatively low abundance. This highlights the concept of periodontal disease as an **opportunistic infection**. The resident microbiome normally serves to maintain numbers of pathogenic microbes at levels below clinical significance but if this is disrupted periodontal disease can arise. This usually correlates with a transition from the predominantly Gram-positive bacteria associated with health to consortia with an abundance of Gram-negative obligate anaerobes. The trigger for this shift is the host mounting an inflammatory response against accumulated plaque, which results in an increased influx of **gingival crevicular fluid** (GCF) into the gingival crevice. GCF is rich in proteinaceous components, thereby providing nutrients for the asaccharolytic subgingival bacteria. As these bacteria grow, so their collective metabolic activity results in a rise in local pH and a fall in redox potential. These conditions further promote outgrowth of anaerobic periodontopathogens, with the concomitant increase in their metabolic products, proteolytic enzymes and other virulence factors contributing to overall tissue destruction.

Other Oral Infections

Endodontic Infections

Infections of the tooth pulp, root canals or root apex are collectively known as **endodontic infections**. These sites are typically sterile, but microorganisms can gain access via cracks or microfractures following placement of restorations or other trauma, or via areas of exposed dentine. Several oral streptococci are able to penetrate **dentinal tubules** and while these bacteria might not be the causative agents of disease *per se*, other pathogens such as *P. gingivalis* have been shown to 'piggy back' on streptococci and so be transported within these sites. Such mechanisms may explain why the most prevalent genus found in infected root canals is *Streptococcus*, while the overall microbiota is dominated by anaerobic bacteria, including species of *Porphyromonas*, *Dialister*, *Treponema*, *Olsenella* and *F. alocis*. **Pulpal infection** triggers host inflammatory responses that in turn cause tissue destruction and the onset of clinical symptoms, exacerbated by microbial factors. This host–microbe–environment

---

Feature box 7.4 Ludwig's angina

If not effectively treated, a dentoalveolar infection may spread through the soft tissues of the neck and floor of the mouth, causing painful swelling of the submental, sublingual and submandibular spaces. This condition is known as Ludwig's angina, in recognition of the physician who first described it. Inflammation of the submental and sublingual spaces raises the floor of the mouth, with elevation and displacement of the tongue, while swelling of the submandibular space can restrict the airway. As a result, individuals develop difficulties with swallowing and breathing and, if not adequately managed, airway compromise can result in death. Bacteria most commonly associated with this condition include species of *Prevotella*, *Porphyromonas*, *Fusobacterium* and viridans streptococci.

---

interplay is thus very like periodontal disease. Where **pulp necrosis** occurs, infection may progress to the periapical region of the root, with continued dysregulation of host inflammatory responses resulting in periapical alveolar bone resorption and formation of a **periapical** (or **dentoalveolar**) **abscess**. Acute dentoalveolar abscess is the most common orofacial bacterial infection and, if inadequately treated, may progress to a condition known as Ludwig's angina (Feature box 7.4).

Bone Infections

In addition to affecting soft tissues, dentoalveolar infections may progress to the bone, causing a condition known as **osteomyelitis**. This manifests as inflammation of the medullary bone within the maxilla or mandible, the latter being more susceptible due to a relatively poor blood supply. Infections may be acute or chronic, with the swelling causing severe pain and difficulty with jaw movements. Microbiota associated with this condition are similar to those for periodontal and endodontic infections, typically comprising polymicrobial infections of viridans streptococci and anaerobes such as *Parvimonas*, *Prevotella* or *Fusobacterium*. Individuals receiving bisphosphonate drugs for the treatment of osteoporosis or breast cancer are particularly susceptible to this condition.

Perhaps unsurprisingly, bone infections can also occur following a tooth extraction, a classic example being **dry socket** (Figure 7.7).

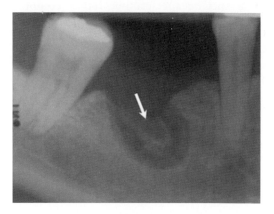

Figure 7.7 Radiograph showing dry socket (arrow), 3 months post-extraction. Source: Courtesy of T. Brooke.

This condition occurs after 0.5–5% of routine extractions and 25–30% of surgical extractions. It is characterized by the absence of a blot clot within the socket, and inflammation (**alveolar osteitis**) of the exposed alveolar bone. These sites are associated with increased pain and prolonged healing. Microbial infection has not been definitively proven as the cause of this condition, but its association with pronounced **halitosis** (oral malodour) implies the presence of volatile sulphur compounds and thus obligate anaerobes.

Fungal Infections

Candida albicans is responsible for more than 90% of oral fungal infections, with other *Candida* species such as *C. glabrata* and *C. dubliniensis* contributing the remaining 10%.

Although harboured in the mouths of approximately 40% of the healthy adult population, *C. albicans* is usually maintained at numbers below clinically significant levels by the resident microbiome. *C. albicans* is therefore an **opportunistic pathogen**, requiring a shift in local conditions to generate an environment in which it can proliferate and cause disease. Consequently, candidal infections occur in individuals who have some form of cellular immune deficiency, are immunosuppressed or who experience some form of disruption to their commensal oral microbiota. These infections may be **superficial** (cutaneous or mucocutaneous) or **invasive**. Invasive candidal infections have a high mortality rate and are becoming increasingly problematic among older people and in the hospital environment.

C. albicans has a number of virulence attributes that contribute to its pathogenicity. *C. albicans* is **pleomorphic** (i.e. has several morphological forms), and typically grows as spherical blastospores or as filamentous forms known as pseudohyphae or true hyphae (Figure 7.3). Each morphological form has a distinct profile of surface molecules and so by frequently switching morphologies, *C. albicans* is able to evade components of the host immune response. **True hyphae** are particularly associated

with virulence. This is due to the presence of hyphae-specific adhesins that are critical for effective colonization and biofilm formation, particularly on epithelial tissues or prosthetic devices. Furthermore, hyphae are able to penetrate epithelial layers to access deeper tissues, and are anti-phagocytic, both mechanisms serving to promote candidal persistence. *C. albicans* also expresses a number of **hydrolytic enzymes** that can promote localized tissue damage. These include secreted aspartyl proteases (SAPs) that can degrade host ECM, and phospholipases, which can degrade phospholipids and thus host cell membranes.

Superficial *Candida* infections of the oral cavity are collectively known as **oral candidosis** (or **candidiasis**), but can be further divided into four primary infections based upon their clinical presentation (Table 7.5). Of these infections, chronic erythematous candidosis (otherwise known as ***Candida-associated denture stomatitis***) is the most common (Figure 7.8). As the name implies, this infection is associated with dentures, with approximately 65% of denture wearers presenting with clinical symptoms. The majority of infections involve upper dentures, as here the close-fitting device restricts salivary flow across the palate, generating conditions in which *Candida* can proliferate.

Table 7.5 Types of oral candidosis.

Infection	Features	Predisposing factors
Pseudomembranous	'Oral thrush' Acute (although chronic variant associated with HIV/AIDS) Easily removed, white, plaque-like lesions on mucosae with underlying erythema	Age extremes Immunosuppression Steroid inhaler use
Acute erythematous	Painful, red patches on dorsum of tongue	Use of broad-spectrum antibiotics
Chronic hyperplastic	Typically asymptomatic White, plaque-like lesions on mucosa at corners of the mouth that difficult to remove Lesion sites may become malignant (5–10%)	Middle-aged, male smokers
Chronic erythematous	Typically asymptomatic Inflammation of palatal mucosa under denture	Poorly fitting dentures with or without poor oral hygiene

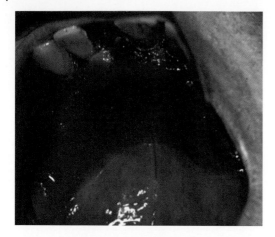

Figure 7.8 *Candida*-associated denture stomatitis. Source: Courtesy of T. Brooke.

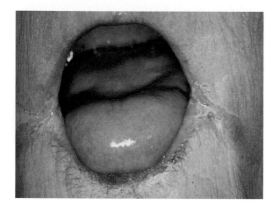

Figure 7.9 Angular cheilitis. Source: Courtesy of T. Brooke.

Upon removal of the device, evidence of candidal growth between the denture and palate can be clearly seen, with the resulting host immune response causing the palate to become red and inflamed. It is common for bacteria to also be present on the device, such as oral streptococci or *Staphylococcus aureus*. These bacteria are thought to both exacerbate the host immune response and to promote candidal colonization through formation of a **polymicrobial biofilm**. *Candida* is also found in conjunction with bacteria for a condition known as **angular cheilitis** (Figure 7.9). This commonly occurs in conjunction with denture stomatitis as a result of leakage of *Candida*-containing saliva at the corners of the mouth. This triggers a host inflammatory response, causing erythema and the formation of lesions. Bacteria such as *S. aureus* and oral streptococci are often found alongside *Candida* within these lesions and likely contribute to their persistence.

Viral Infections

As mentioned, most adults will harbour viruses, often acquiring them early in childhood. However, many of these viruses exhibit periods of latency. As such, following resolution of the (often symptomatic) **primary infection** associated with initial acquisition, a virus can be carried for the remainder of its host's lifetime. This carriage may be asymptomatic, or disruption to the host immune system may allow virus **reactivation** and onset of symptomatic **secondary infections**. Many viruses can be transmitted by aerosols. The oral cavity can therefore serve as a portal for viruses to enter the body, and saliva can provide a vehicle for virus transmission. Once inside the host, viruses can disseminate and cause disease at sites throughout the body. This section will focus on those viruses for which the orofacial tissues are a predominant site of infection.

Of the almost 300 types of herpes virus identified to date, eight are known to infect humans. All eight have been detected in saliva and are associated with a variety of disease manifestations. Human herpesvirus-1 (otherwise known as **herpes simplex virus 1 (HSV-1)**) is the most abundant of the herpes viruses, infecting 80–90% of adults in developed countries. Acquisition usually occurs in early childhood, typically causing a mild **herpetic gingivostomatitis** that is often mistaken for 'teething'. Within 10 days, symptoms resolve and HSV-1 becomes latent. Approximately 40% of infected individuals will suffer recurrent secondary infections triggered by factors such as stress or immunosuppression. These infections characteristically present as cold sores around the lips (**herpes labialis**) (Figure 7.10), but can also cause intraoral ulceration of the hard palate.

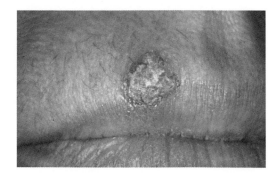

Figure 7.10 Herpes labialis (cold sore) caused by reactivation of HSV 1. Source: Courtesy of T. Brooke.

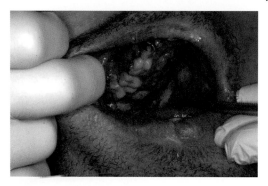

Figure 7.11 Burkitt's lymphoma caused by EBV. Source: Courtesy of T. Brooke.

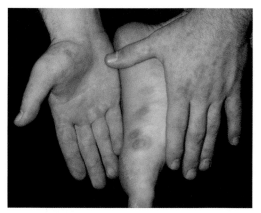

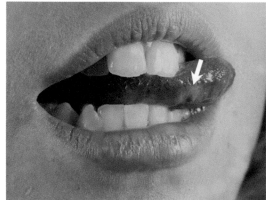

Figure 7.12 Hand, foot and mouth disease. Arrow indicates tongue lesion. Source: Courtesy of T. Brooke.

Another common herpesvirus is human herpesvirus-4 (otherwise known as **Epstein– Barr virus (EBV)**), occurring in 70% of adults. Again, acquisition in early childhood usually leads to an asymptomatic primary infection but if acquired in adulthood, EBV can cause **infectious mononucleosis** (otherwise known as glandular fever or 'kissing disease' due to its most common mode of transmission). Individuals present with fever, swollen adenoid glands (lymphadenopathy), fatigue and small haemorrhages on the palate, but the condition is self-limiting. Another oral manifestation of EBV is **hairy leukoplakia**. This is characterized by formation of a white lesion on the side of the tongue with vertical corrugations that give it a 'hairy' appearance, and is indicative of HIV infection/AIDS or other severe immunosuppression.

Due to its capacity to replicate within and transform B-cells, EBV is also associated with B-cell lymphomas, including **Burkitt's lymphoma**, an aggressive tumour of the jaws (Figure 7.11). In addition, transformation of oral epithelial cells by EBV has been linked with **nasopharyngeal carcinoma**. **Human herpesvirus-8** is another well-recognized oncogenic virus and is the likely causative agent of **Kaposi's sarcoma**. This is a lymphoid vascular tumour typically found in HIV-infected individuals, with lesions often forming in the mouth.

Belonging to the family *Picornaviridae*, **coxsackieviruses** and particularly serotype A16 are causative agents of '**hand, foot and mouth' disease** (Figure 7.12). Primarily affecting young children, this is a common, typically mild condition whose name derives from the sites in which lesions develop. Within the mouth, these include the tongue, soft palate and pharyngeal mucosa. Coxsackieviruses can also cause a childhood condition known as **herpangina**. This is an acute, febrile illness of sudden onset that is characterized by the presence of vesicular lesions on the oral and pharyngeal mucosae.

Alongside EBV, members of the *Papillomaviridae* family are associated with cancer at various sites within the host, including the oral cavity. Such conditions include **oral squamous cell carcinoma**, with which **human papillomavirus-16** is particularly associated, and focal epithelial hyperplasia (or **Heck's disease**). This latter condition presents as papules on the lower lip, buccal mucosa and tongue, with a high prevalence of **human papillomavirus-13**. However, not all growths caused by papillomaviruses are malignant, and these viruses are also common causes of mucosal warts (**verruca vulgaris**). Within the mouth these are typically found on the labial and lingual mucosae, with transmission arising from warts on the hands or orogenital contact (Figure 7.13). Interestingly, there is growing evidence that oral bacteria such a *P. gingivalis* may be involved in oral carcinoma, potentially indicating additional examples of bacterial–viral synergy in oral disease.

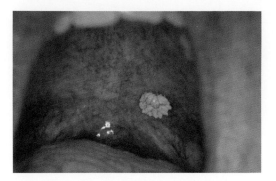

Figure 7.13 Verruca vulgaris (wart) caused by human papillomavirus. Source: Courtesy of T. Brooke.

Summary

Oral microbiology has advanced significantly over the past few decades. In its infancy, interest was sparked by just one or two microorganisms associated with disease. However, today there is a growing appreciation for the vast complexity of the oral microbiome, comprising a multitude of bacteria, fungi and viruses. These complex communities are in constant dialogue with each other and with their host, sensing and responding to changes in ecological conditions to perpetuate their own survival. For the vast majority of us, this resident microbiome exists in harmony with our body, even affording protection from assaults by more pathogenic microorganisms. However, when this delicate equilibrium is disrupted, pathogenic cohorts can proliferate and initiate a spectrum of oral infections. The polymicrobial nature of these infections complicates their treatment. Identification of vaccine candidates that are effective against communities of microorganisms is probably not feasible, while the rapid spread of antibiotic resistance is already driving the need to devise alternative antimicrobial therapies. Unpicking the oral microbiome to understand the delicate interplay between its members and their host is thus essential for development of novel strategies to control these polymicrobial diseases.

8

Introduction to Pathology

Paula M. Farthing

School of Clinical Dentistry, University of Sheffield, Sheffield, UK

Learning Objectives

- To be able to list the aetiology (causes) of human disease including environmental and genetic factors.
- To be able to describe the mechanisms of cellular responses to cell injury.
- To list the differences between necrosis and apoptosis.
- To be able to describe the basic processes of neoplasia, healing and repair.
- To be able to describe the histological features and processes that mediate acute and chronic inflammation.

Clinical Relevance

An understanding of the causes and mechanism of disease is central to clinical practice. The oral cavity may be affected by a number of diseases, some specific to this region and others similar to elsewhere in the body. Occasionally systemic (body-wide) conditions manifest themselves in the mouth and thus the dentist may be the first to recognize abnormalities that indicate the presence of disease. Microscopic examination of the pathological changes that occur in tissues is a key tool in the diagnosis and treatment planning of a number of oral diseases and explaining the clinical manifestations of the disease (see Feature box 8.1). As with a number of other chapters this information is also crucial to understanding the scientific basis of treatment strategies.

Introduction

Pathology is the scientific study of disease in all its aspects. It covers the causes (aetiology) and the pathogenic mechanisms of disease; that is, the series of events that takes place during the development of disease. In addition, pathology covers the changes that take place in the tissue as a result of the disease process (histopathological changes), the resulting clinical changes that may be observed as well as how the disease progresses and what will happen to the individual as a result of the disease. As you can see pathology is very broad and it forms the basis of clinical practice. A thorough

---

Basic Sciences for Dental Students, First Edition. Edited by Simon A. Whawell and Daniel W. Lambert.
© 2018 John Wiley & Sons Ltd. Published 2018 by John Wiley & Sons Ltd.
Companion website: www.wiley.com/go/whawell/basic_sciences_for_dental_students

---

Feature box 8.1 Role of the oral pathologist

Oral pathology is the study of diseases of the oral and maxillofacial complex including the salivary glands, teeth, oral mucosa, lips and jaws. It is a specialty of dentistry and oral pathologists diagnose oral disease from oral biopsies by studying the changes that have taken place in the tissues (i.e. the histopathological changes). A biopsy is removal of tissue from a patient and it may be either incisional where a small part of the lesion is taken away to make the diagnosis or it may be excisional where the entire lesion is removed. An oral pathologist provides a written report to the clinicians detailing the changes they can see and coming to a diagnosis. This is important to plan the future management of the patient. Many oral cancers are treated by excisional biopsies and the oral pathologist will comment on whether the cancer is completely excised and also provide an idea of the prognosis (outcome) for the patient. Many oral pathologists who work in dental schools undertake research on the pathogenesis of oral diseases in collaboration with scientists and other oral clinicians. In addition they teach undergraduate dental students and other oral health care professionals.

---

understanding of the causes of disease, the changes that are taking place in the body and the clinical manifestations of that disease are essential for accurate diagnosis and appropriate patient management.

Aetiology of Disease

The causes of disease may be divided into two main groups: environmental factors and genetic causes.

Environmental Causes of Disease

There are many environmental causes of disease but most fall into the groups shown in Table 8.1.

Infectious agents are an important cause of oral disease. Periodontal disease is caused by the build-up of bacteria known as microbial plaque on the teeth. In certain people this leads to loss of the alveolar bone which surrounds and supports the teeth. Teeth become mobile and may eventually be lost.

Viruses also cause disease and there are a number which specifically affect the oral cavity. One of these is herpes simplex type 1. The virus is ubiquitous and almost everyone is exposed to it early on in life. The initial or primary infection only produces symptoms in a few people, who suffer from blisters on their gums and palate. These rupture to form ulcers (a break in the lining mucosa), which are painful. In addition the patient feels unwell and has a temperature. The disease

Table 8.1 Environmental causes of disease.

Category	Cause
Infectious agents	Bacteria, viruses, fungi, prions, protozoa
Physical agents	Trauma, radiation, extremes of temperature
Chemical agents	Strong acids and alkalis, chemical carcinogens, therapeutic and non-therapeutic agents or drugs
Nutritional deficiency/excess	For example starvation, excess sugar
Abnormal immunological reactions	For example pemphigus vulgaris
Hypoxia: lack of oxygen to the tissues	For example anaemia, problems with heart or lungs, arterial blockage

lasts for 10–14 days. In some patients the virus is not eliminated from the body by the normal immune response and lies dormant in the nervous system. Under times of stress and in sunlight the virus reappears on the lips and forms cold sores.

Fungal infections are also common in the oral cavity and most are caused by *Candida albicans*. This fungus is a weak pathogen: it does not cause disease easily and usually only does so if there is a defect in the ability of the individual to combat it. One such cause is wearing dentures continually and not taking them out even at night. *Candida* can grow on the surface of the denture because it is not exposed to saliva, which under normal circumstances would keep it under control.

Protozoa are rare in the UK and do not usually cause oral disease. However, examples are amoebic dysentery and trypanosomes which cause sleeping sickness. Prions are also a rare cause of disease but in recent years much interest has focused on human bovine encephalopathy (Creutzfeldt–Jakob disease). This disease takes years to develop and affects the brain. There is no cure. The relevance to dentistry is that it may be transmitted through dental instruments if they are not sterilized properly.

Physical agents are a common cause of oral disease as the mouth is subjected to significant trauma. Causes of trauma include teeth, dentures and orthodontic appliances. Almost everyone has bitten their tongue at some point. Further causes of trauma are extreme hot and cold. The mouth is resilient but a very hot pizza or boiling hot tea or coffee can cause burns. However, these burns heal very quickly compared to similar lesions on the skin.

Chemical agents are an important cause of disease. Strong acids and alkali will cause damage to the oral cavity and internal organs if swallowed, but this is rare. Chemicals known as carcinogens which work over a long period of time may cause cancer; for example, tobacco in various forms is associated with oral cancer. Drugs may also cause disease: most drugs are used therapeutically but almost all have side

effects and a few may cause damage which can be life threatening. The decision whether to use a drug to treat a particular disease is a balance between the therapeutic value of that drug and the side effects of using it. In contrast, many drugs are used non-therapeutically: alcohol is an example.

Nutritional excess is a relatively common cause of disease. Excess sugar is an important cause of dental caries and overeating of fatty and sugary foods leads to weight gain and obesity. This itself is associated with a number of diseases such as type 2 diabetes, high blood pressure and heart disease. Nutritional deficiency is also relatively common not only in poorer countries where people do not have enough to eat or may be restricted in what they can eat, but also in the Western world. Poor diet or lifestyle mean that some people do not have sufficient nutrients, including vitamins. In other patients their body is unable to absorb nutrients even though they may be present in the diet.

The immune response is normally protective but occasionally may be the cause of problems. For example, some diseases are the result of the body mounting an immune response against itself. One example that affects the oral cavity and/or skin is pemphigus vulgaris. The body makes antibodies against desmosomes which hold the epithelial cells together. When the antibody binds the cells separate and form blisters which then burst, leaving ulcers.

Hypoxia or lack of oxygen to the tissues may be caused by one of three mechanisms:

1) a reduction in the ability of the blood to carry oxygen: this occurs in anaemia and sometimes in carbon monoxide poisoning;
2) a reduction in perfusion of the tissues caused by problems with the lungs and/or heart;
3) lack of perfusion of the tissues caused by blockage of arteries.

All these may cause tissue damage which may have serious consequences. For example, strokes and heart attacks may be caused by blockage of arteries.

Psychological factors are important in disease and sometimes interact with other causes. For example, psychological factors are important in addiction to alcohol, which is consumed in excess. They may also influence symptoms of a disease and how a patient perceives their illness.

Genetic Factors in Disease

Genetic factors play an important role in disease although the extent to which this is true varies between diseases and individuals. Normal single genes or groups of genes may increase an individual's susceptibility to disease or conversely their resistance to disease. A good example is in the development of lip and skin cancer, both of which are caused by damaging effects of ultraviolet light. In Australia the indigenous aboriginal population are dark-skinned and the melanin is able to counteract the ultraviolet (UV) light. In contrast, white-skinned Australians have arrived relatively recently in Australia and are biologically adapted to living in more temperate northern climates where there is relatively little sunlight. They do not have sufficient melanin in their skin to counteract the effects of UV light and are particularly prone to lip and skin cancer.

Another important area where normal genes may play an important role in the development of disease are the genes that control the immune response. These are known as the human leukocyte antigen genes (HLA genes) in humans but in animals they are referred to as the major histocompatibility complex or MHC. There are very many variants or polymorphisms of these genes and they are classified into different HLA types. An individual's HLA phenotype will determine their susceptibility to a number of diseases including infections and autoimmune disease such pemphigus vulgaris referred to earlier.

Abnormal genes or groups of genes may also play a role in disease. An example of where a defect in a single gene causes disease is in Huntington's disease. The affected gene is on chromosome 4 and it shows an autosomal dominant pattern of inheritance. If either one of the parents have the gene then the offspring have a 50:50 chance of inheriting it. The gene codes for a protein called huntingtin which affects the functions of neurones. The symptoms do not become apparent until between the ages of 25 and 50 years and include physical and mental changes.

Abnormalities in chromosomes may also cause disease. For example, Down's syndrome patients have an extra copy of chromosome 21 which means that every cell has three instead of two copies. This is known as trisomy and patients suffer from delayed development and have characteristic facial features. In addition, about half of all patients have congenital heart and other defects.

Although some diseases are caused by gene or chromosome abnormalities most diseases are multifactorial and are caused by a combination of environmental factors interacting with the combined activity of several normal genes. This presents problems in trying to work out the aetiology of the disease and why only some people are affected. For example, it is well known that smoking is strongly correlated with lung cancer and that people who smoke have an increased risk of developing lung cancer. However, some people who do not smoke still get lung cancer whereas others smoke their entire lives and do not get the disease. This difference is likely to be the result of genetic factors and individual susceptibility to the disease.

Mechanisms of Disease

The aetiological agents described cause disease by affecting the activity of individual cells. This in turn can lead to changes in the tissues which may affect the function of that tissue and may be obvious clinically. The cell damage may be reversible in which case the cell will return to normal once the aetiological agent is removed or it may be irreversible and the cell may die. In some cases the injury may be irreversible but sub-lethal and the cell

Figure 8.1 Cell responses to injury.

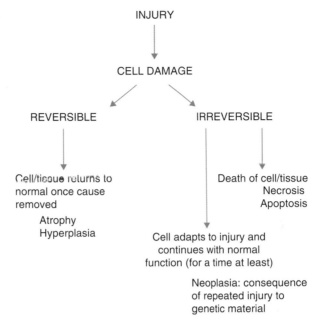

will survive. Alternatively, the cell may be able to adapt to the injury and continue with its normal function (Figure 8.1).

Irreversible Cell Injury

When the effects of the damage are so severe that the cell is no longer able to survive it is said to be **necrotic**. A necrotic cell shows specific structural or morphological changes which can be recognized histopathologically. The cytoplasm of such a cell is usually pink (eosinophilic) and glassy on staining with haematoxylin and eosin. Changes also occur in the nucleus which may be small and darkly staining (pyknosis), fragmented into pieces (karyohexis) or pale staining and faint (karyolysis) (Figure 8.2).

Necrosis

When many cells in an organ or tissue die then an area of necrosis is present (see Feature box 8.2). The two main changes that take place are that the cell proteins are denatured and enzymes destroy the rest of the cell. These enzymes may come from the necrotic cells in which case the process is termed **autolysis** or they may come from

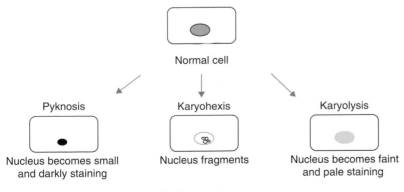

Figure 8.2 Nuclear changes in cellular necrosis.

Feature box 8.2 Pulpal necrosis

The pulp lies in the centre of the tooth and unlike the rest is composed of soft tissue. It contains vessels and nerves which provide the blood supply and sensation to the tooth. The vessels and nerves enter the tooth through the apical foramen- a small opening at the apex of the root. In response to destruction of the enamel and dentine usually by dental caries, the pulp becomes damaged and inflamed. This results in the formation of oedema, which is a special type of tissue fluid known as an inflammatory exudate (see section on inflammation). Because the pulp is surrounded by dentine the tissue pressure rises rapidly and this may be so great it presses on the vessels entering through the root apex and causes them to collapse. As a result the blood supply to the pulp ceases and the pulp dies and becomes necrotic. The patient will experience pain when the tissue pressure rises and this may be very severe. However, once the pulp has become necrotic the pain disappears. A tooth with a necrotic pulp is sometimes referred to as dead or non-vital and may appear grey in colour. Although a dead tooth may no longer be painful, the inflammation may spread from the pulp and reach the periodontal ligament and bone surrounding the root apex, resulting in periapical infection which itself may cause problems. Once a pulp becomes necrotic it is necessary to carry out an endodontic or root treatment to remove all the necrotic pulp and prevent periapical infection occurring.

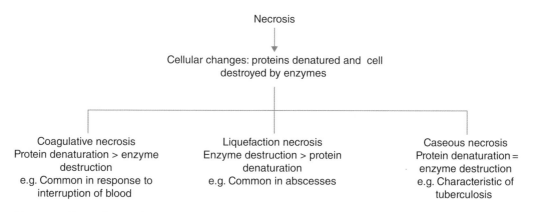

Figure 8.3 Types of necrosis.

infiltrating leucocytes, which is **heterolysis**. Macroscopically several different types of necrosis are recognized depending on the balance between protein denaturation and enzymatic destruction. Coagulative necrosis usually occurs in response to interruption of blood supply and is characterized predominantly by protein denaturation. The outline of the cells in the tissue can still be seen but they are eosinophilic and the nuclei show karyolysis and karyohexis. With time autolysis will occur. Liquefaction (or colliquative) necrosis occurs when enzymatic destruction is marked and the necrotic tissue becomes liquefied. This type of necrosis is common in abscesses. Caseous necrosis occurs when there is both protein denaturation and enzymatic digestion and the tissue takes on a 'cheesy', eosinophilic appearance. This type of necrosis is seen in tuberculosis (Figure 8.3).

Apoptosis

A specific type of cell necrosis called **apoptosis** occurs during normal development and is important in the formation of tissues and organs. It is sometimes referred to as programmed cell death as it occurs naturally and not in response to injury. Individual cells die but they are surrounded by normal healthy cells. Apoptosis also occurs in adults as part of normal tissue turnover but it is also used by cytotoxic T-lymphocytes as part of their killing mechanism. The initial changes occur in the nucleus which fragments and then the cell degrades itself from within using enzymes. In neoplasms the balance between apoptosis and cell division is disturbed either as a result of inhibition of apoptosis or increase in cell division or a combination of both and the number of cells in the tissue increases.

Neoplasia

Neoplasia means new growth and it is a term that refers to the excessive and irreversible growth of cells. There is an accumulation of genetic changes due to various types of sublethal but irreversible injury which includes viruses and chemical carcinogens. Initially these genetic changes may not affect the function of cells but with time and successive injury the normal genetic mechanisms which control growth of the cells is lost and they proliferate out of control. It is important to distinguish neoplasia, which is irreversible proliferation, from hyperplasia, which is reversible (see later in this chapter).

The genes which are damaged are of two types: tumour-suppressor genes and oncogenes. Tumour-suppressor genes prevent cell division and if they are damaged may not function properly and proliferation increases. Conversely oncogenes promote cell division and may be activated continuously without the normal control mechanisms that supress their activity. Many neoplasms occur because of genetic changes in both tumour-suppressor genes and oncogenes (Figure 8.4). Exactly which tumour-suppressor genes and oncogenes are damaged varies not only between different tumour types but also sometimes between tumours of the same type from different patients. This variability means that treatments targeting specific genetic changes often do not work for all patients.

Neoplasms are divided broadly into two types: benign and malignant (Table 8.2) The major difference between the two is that benign neoplasms remain localized and do not spread from their tissue of origin. In contrast malignant neoplasms do not remain localized but spread via the bloodstream or the lymphatic vessels to distant organs and tissues.

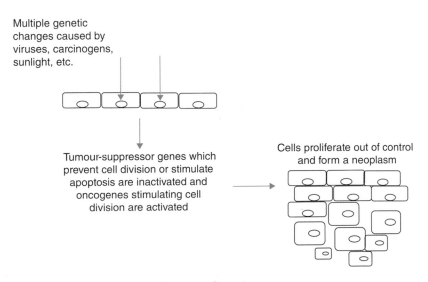

Figure 8.4 Mechanism of neoplastic transformation.

Table 8.2 Characteristics of different types of neoplasm.

Benign	Malignant
Resemble the tissue of origin	Less likely to resemble tissue of origin
Remain localized and do not spread to other sites in the body	Do not remain localized but spread to other sites in the body (metastasize)
Grow by expansion and are well circumscribed	Infiltrate and invade surrounding tissues

They then start to grow at these new sites. The process by which the cells spread is called metastasis. Other differences between the two types is that the margins of benign neoplasms tend to be well defined and they are often surrounded by a capsule made of connective tissue. This makes their surgical removal relatively easy. In contrast malignant neoplasms infiltrate and destroy the tissue in which they arise and may also infiltrate adjacent tissues and organs. This together with their tendency to metastasize means they are more difficult to treat.

Reversible Cell Injury

In this type of injury the cell will return to normal once the cause is eliminated. In some cases few changes are apparent but in some hydropic swelling is seen. Cells take in water, appear cloudy and contain vacuoles. In other cases fat accumulates within cells and tissues. This may occur following ingestion of poisons or in metabolic diseases such as diabetes.

Atrophy

Cells may also respond to certain types of injury by becoming smaller: **atrophic**. The change is referred to as atrophy and may affect whole tissues and organs. In these cases a reduction in the number of cells in the tissue or organ may also occur. Atrophy is common following a reduction in blood supply but may also be seen following a reduction in functional activity: a muscle will become smaller if it is not used because of a bone fracture or following interruption of the nerve supply. Atrophy is also seen in endocrine organs following a reduction in the stimulating hormone and is part of the normal ageing process. In the oral cavity the oral mucosa may become atrophic in response to certain inflammatory diseases (for example, lichen planus) or in response to iron-deficiency anaemia. However, in this case the mucosa is atrophic because there is a reduction in the number of epithelial cells rather than a decrease in the size of individual epithelial cells.

Hypertrophy

Cells may also respond to injury by becoming **hypertrophic**; that is, larger than normal. Often, however, hypertrophy is physiological and is part of the normal response to increased functional demands. A good example is the hypertrophy of skeletal muscle which follows extensive gym work and training. Pathological hypertrophy may occur is response to abnormal functional demands. This may be seen in cardiac muscle if a patient has high systemic blood pressure or chronic lung disease. The heart muscle becomes hypertrophic in an effort to pump blood round the body against the raised blood pressure but eventually the blood supply to the heart becomes insufficient to maintain the hypertrophic muscle and the heart no longer pumps efficiently. Blood remains in the ventricles at the end of each beat which dilates the heart muscle and further decreases its ability to pump efficiently.

Often hypertrophy is associated with **hyperplasia** which is an increase in the number of cells in a tissue or organ. This may be physiological or pathological in origin. Physiological hyperplasia of the endometrial lining of the womb occurs as part of the normal menstrual cycle in females and once hormone levels drop the lining is shed. Pathological hyperplasia occurs in the oral

---

Feature box 8.3 Metaplasia

Squamous metaplasia occurs when one type of specialized epithelial cell such as respiratory ciliated epithelial cells change to stratified squamous epithelium. The nasal cavity and the antral sinuses are lined by columnar respiratory epithelium. The cilia on the surfaces of these cells perform a specific function in that they move in synchrony with each other and are able to move the surface layer of mucous towards the back of the nose to be swallowed. Microorganisms in the nose and sinuses become trapped by the mucous and they are destroyed by the acid in the stomach when the mucous is swallowed. Squamous metaplasia may occur following repeated infection, particularly in the sinuses. This means the sinuses are lined by stratified squamous epithelium rather than ciliated epithelium and the mucous which traps the microorganisms does not move but stays in the sinuses. The microorganisms are able to grow in the mucous and this contributes to repeated chronic infection or chronic sinusitis.

---

cavity in response to ill-fitting dentures; the connective tissue component of the mucosa overgrows to form a nodule. Occasionally the epithelial component of the mucosa is hyperplastic in response to human papilloma virus and forms a squamous cell papilloma.

Cells may also respond to injury by undergoing **metaplasia**. This is a reversible change where one cell type changes into another (see Feature box 8.3). A common example is when ciliated respiratory epithelium changes to stratified squamous epithelium in response to chronic trauma. In the nasal cavity and in the antral sinus this may cause functional problems. Other examples of metaplasia occur in connective tissues and in the oral cavity fibroblasts which normally form collagen change into osteoblasts and form bone. This is common fibrous hyperplasia in response to irritation by dentures: often these overgrowths contain bone.

Inflammation

All vascular tissues in the body respond to injury by mounting an inflammatory response. This is protective and its purpose is to either destroy, dilute or wall off the damaged area and cause of injury and to initiate repair. It is important to realize that the tissue has to be vascular because without a blood supply an inflammatory response is not possible. Enamel is one example of an avascular tissue and another is the cornea.

Two Types of Inflammation are Recognized: Acute and Chronic

Acute inflammation is a short-lived process (hours or days) which usually develops in response to a single episode of injury, for example in response to a wound or a tooth extraction. In contrast **chronic inflammation** is more prolonged and may last weeks, months or years. It usually occurs in response to continuous or multiple episodes of injury. Periodontal disease and rheumatoid arthritis are examples. However, it is important to realize that the boundaries between acute and chronic inflammation are indistinct and in practice they may form a continuum. In addition they may coexist and in chronic inflammation there may be an acute episode.

Acute Inflammation

A tissue that is acutely inflamed is red, warm, swollen and painful and is usually associated with loss of function. These changes occur very quickly following injury

Event	Effect	
Vasoconstriction of arterioles	Affected area becomes white	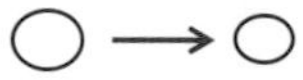
Arteriolar, capillary and venule dilation	Affected area red and warm	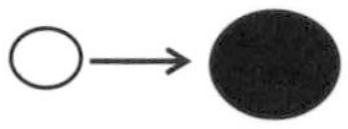
Increased vascular permeability	Swelling due to oedema	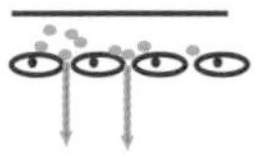
Vascular stasis	Loss of fluid slows blood flow	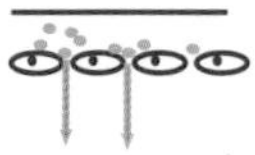

Figure 8.5 Vascular events.

and are mediated by changes in the blood supply to the tissues. Later, after a number of hours, inflammatory cells become important.

Vascular Events
See Figure 8.5.

1) **Transient vasoconstriction** (reduction in the diameter) of the arterioles. This is caused by a local axon reflex and the affected area becomes white. It may only last a few seconds. You will be able to see it if you draw your finger nail firmly across your skin.
2) **Arteriolar, capillary and venule dilation**. Inflammatory mediators which are released following tissue damage all act to relax the vascular smooth muscle and blood flow to the area increases. The affected area becomes warm and red.
3) **Increased vascular permeability**. The blood vessels become more permeable due to the action of inflammatory mediators which increase the spaces between endothelial cells lining the blood vessels. This results in leakage of fluid and plasma proteins (inflammatory exudate) into the damaged area. The inflammatory exudate is called oedema and the area becomes swollen.
4) **Vascular stasis**. Loss of fluid from the blood into the tissues results in slowing of blood flow.

Explanation of Vascular Events
Vasodilation is mediated principally by histamine, serotonin, nitric oxide (NO) and prostaglandins. Histamine and serotonin are synthesized and stored in mast cells (found in tissues) and platelets (in blood) respectively and can be released immediately they are required. Mast cells release histamine in response to many stimuli including physical trauma, neuropeptides (substance P), components of the complement system (C3a and C5a) and cytokines (e.g. IL-1). Serotonin is released in response to platelet aggregation.

NO is a gas which is synthesized rapidly by endothelial cells and macrophages in response to cytokines and other stimuli. Prostaglandins are one of the metabolic products of arachidonic acid which is formed by the action of phospholipases on phospholipids in the cell membrane. They are synthesized by the action of the enzyme cyclooxygenase and several different types exist including prostaglandin G2, F2 and E2 (Figure 8.6). The anti-inflammatory agents aspirin and indomethacin inhibit prostaglandin production which in part explains their anti-inflammatory properties.

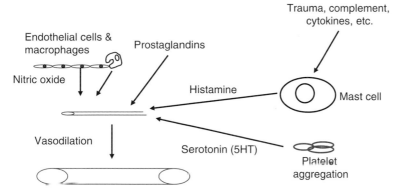

Figure 8.6 Explanation of vascular events: vasodilation.

Increased Vascular Permeability and Formation of Oedema

This is mediated predominately by histamine in the early stages which increases the inter-cellular gaps between endothelial cells and makes the vessels more 'leaky'. Complement components C3a and C5a have a similar effect as do cytokines such as IL-1 and TNF, although these tend to act in the later stages of inflammation. Leukotrienes which are also metabolites of arachidonic acid (see earlier) may also play a role.

In health the hydrostatic pressure of the blood at the beginning of the capillary bed tends to force fluid from the blood into the tis-sues but the plasma proteins remain in the circulation. This loss of fluid means that the plasma proteins are more concentrated and so the osmotic pressure of the blood increases during blood flow through the capillaries. At the end of the capillary bed the osmotic pressure exerted by the plasma pro-teins draws fluid back into the circulation and the result is that the amount of fluid that leaves at the beginning of the capillary bed equals the amount of fluid that enters at the end.

During inflammation there is a large increase in hydrostatic pressure due to the increased blood flow and this results in an increase in fluid entering the tissues at the beginning of the capillary bed. However, because of the increased permeability of the vessels the plasma proteins also enter the tissues and this results in decreased osmotic pressure of the blood and increases the osmotic pressure of the tissue. No osmotic gradient exists at the end of the capillary bed to draw fluid back into the blood and it remains in the tissues as oedema. This is an example of an inflammatory exudate (Figure 8.7).

Role of Oedema

The two most important functions of oedema are to dilute bacterial or other toxins and to deliver the components of the blood to the tissues to activate the inflammatory response. The most important components are as follows.

Complement Complement is a cascade of proteins which are present in an inactive form in the blood. They are activated by reactions of antibody with antigen (classical pathway) or by interactions with microbial agents or other agents (alternative path-way) and the resulting cascade of nine pro-teins (C1–C9) plays an important role in inflammation.

C3a and C5a are known as anaphylotoxins and they cause inflammatory vascular changes, stimulate histamine release and promote the formation of other inflamma-tory mediators such as leukotrienes and prostaglandins. C5a also attracts phagocytic cells to the inflamed area (see later) and C3b aids phagocytosis by sticking to the surface of microorganisms (opsonization).

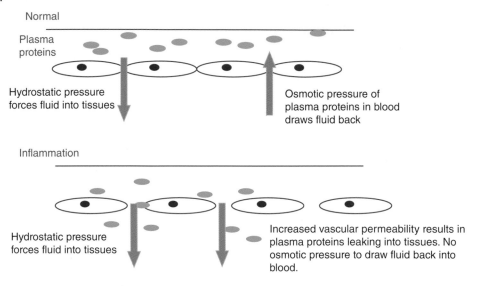

Figure 8.7 Formation of oedema.

The terminal C9 component is also known as the membrane attack complex and is able to destroy microorganisms.

Clotting Cascade   The clotting cascade, similar to complement, is a cascade of proteins which results in the formation of a fibrinous clot. Clotting is initiated by activated platelets or tissue damage and undergoes an amplification phase which includes a number of factors such as Factor VIII. It is a deficiency of the later which results in the bleeding disorder haemophilia. The end result of the clotting cascade is that prothrombin is converted to thrombin and thrombin converts fibrinogen to fibrin which forms a meshwork. This together with embedded platelets forms a plug and not only stops bleeding but may help form a barrier to the spread of infection. Many of the clotting factors such as thrombin and the Hageman factor also stimulate responses which promote the inflammatory response (see later).

Kininogens and Kinins   Kininogens are plasma proteins that are converted into kinins by the action of proteases (e.g. thrombin). One of the most important kinins is bradykinin which has similar inflammatory effects to histamine.

Antibodies

Antibodies may be present and if they encounter their specific microorganism will bind to its surface. This process is called opsonization and it aids phagocytosis of the microorganism by macrophages and neutrophils.

Cellular Events

The two principle leukocytes or inflammatory cells which play an important role in the acute inflammatory response are neutrophils and macrophages. (In certain types of inflammation basophils and eosinophils may be important.) Neutrophils and monocytes (which are macrophage precursors) are present in blood and in health are present in the centre of the vessels. In order to enter the tissues they undergo the following:

1) **margination**: movement to periphery of the bloodstream,
2) **pavementation**: adhesion to endothelium,
3) **emigration**: through blood vessel wall.

See Figures 8.8 and 8.9.

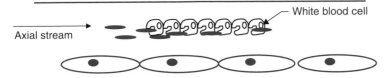

Figure 8.8 White cell distribution in the vessels of normal tissue. In normal blood flow, white and red blood cells are present in the centre of the vessel surrounded by the liquid part of the blood.

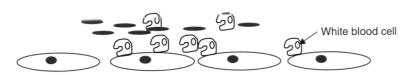

Figure 8.9 White cell distribution in inflammation. (1) In inflammation the white blood cells move to the edges of the vessel. This is called margination and is due to vascular stasis. (2) They then adhere to the endothelial cells. This is known as pavementation. (3) White blood cells emigrate between endothelial cells and into the tissues, attracted by chemokines.

Once in the tissue the cells:

1) **aggregate** around inflammatory sites,
2) **phagocytose** and **kill** microorganisms and cellular debris.

Explanation of Cellular Events
Margination of cells from the centre to the periphery of the blood vessels is the passive result of vascular stasis.

Pavementation Once the cells contact the endothelium they bind weakly by adhesion molecules known as selectins and roll along the surface of the endothelial cells due to blood flow. Cytokines and chemokines (small polypeptide chemical messengers) produced by endothelial cells activate cell adhesion molecules on both the leukocytes as well as the endothelial cells themselves, so the cells bind together firmly. These cell adhesion molecules are usually members of the integrin family (e.g. LFA-1) on the leukocyte surface and the immunoglobulin superfamily of adhesion molecules such as ICAM-1 on the endothelial cell surface. They are upregulated by inflammatory cytokines such as IL-1, TNF-α and chemokines.

Emigration and Aggregation Leukocytes push their way through the intercellular spaces between endothelial cells and migrate towards the site of inflammation. They are attracted into the tissues by chemokines such as IL-8, leukotrienes and C5a, and also by the products of some microorganisms. The movement of cells up a concentration gradient is known as chemotaxis and the agents that cause this migration are chemo-attractants.

Phagocytosis Neutrophils and macrophages are able to engulf and destroy microorganisms and necrotic tissue. This process is known as phagocytosis. In the initial phase the phagocyte sends out a number of extensions (pseudopodia) to completely surround the microorganism which becomes internalized in a phagosome. It is then destroyed in a phagolysosome by enzymes and an oxygen-dependent mechanism. During this process some of the lysomomal enzymes may be released into the tissues, resulting in damage.

Phagocytosis is promoted when the phagocyte is able to bind to the microorganisms or dead cells and often binding is promoted by opsonins. These are proteins which bind to the surface of both microorganisms and phagocytes, forming a bridge or bond between the two. Good examples are IgG antibodies and the complement component C3b.

Neutrophils arrive first at sites of acute inflammation. They are able to engulf debris and microorganisms but they have a very short life span and die after phagocytosis, spilling their proteolytic enzymes and causing tissue damage. In certain circumstances neutrophils may kill microorganisms by throwing out neutrophil extracellular traps (NETs). These surround and kill the microorganisms. They are composed of antimicrobial peptides derived from the nuclear contents of the neutrophil which undergoes a special form of cell death known as NETosis.

If many neutrophils are attracted into the tissue pus may form. This is a dense accumulation of neutrophils and dead or necrotic tissue and clinically is known as an abscess. It is described in greater detail later.

Macrophages arrive later, have a relatively long life span, can phagocytose many times and grow to a large size. They engulf dead neutrophils, red blood cells, microorganisms and necrotic tissue. They also release inflammatory mediators, which can thus promote healing (Figure 8.10).

Pain

Inflamed tissue may be painful for a number for reasons:

- increase in tissue pressure due to oedema or pus,
- release of inflammatory mediators which stimulate pain fibres; for example, bradykinin, prostaglandins. These agents may also cause fever.

Outcome of Acute Inflammation
Complete Resolution

This occurs when the injury is short-lived and there is little destruction of tissue. The vascular permeability returns to normal and the oedema drains away in the lymphatic vessels. Necrotic cells and microorganisms are removed by macrophages and there is regeneration of the normal tissues and complete return to normal function without scarring. Complete resolution is relatively common in the oral cavity in response to trauma.

Healing by fibrosis

If tissue damage is very severe and the cells destroyed are unable to regenerate then healing by fibrosis may occur. The necrotic debris is removed by macrophages and replaced by **granulation tissue** (Figure 8.11). This is composed of fibroblasts which lay down

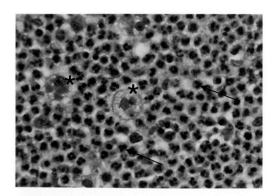

Figure 8.10 Histological appearance of pus: dense accumulations of neutrophils which have multilobed nuclei (arrows). Macrophages are larger and engulf necrotic tissue and dead neutrophils (*).

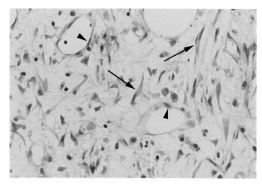

Figure 8.11 Histological section of granulation tissue from a healing wound. Fibroblasts are indicated by arrows and endothelial cells lining the blood vessels by arrowheads. The large round cells containing brown pigment are macrophages which have engulfed red blood cells.

(a)

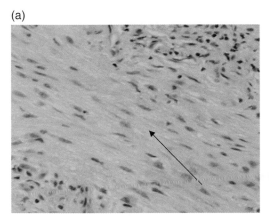

(b)

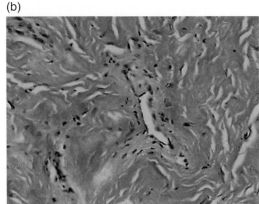

Figure 8.12 Maturation of granulation tissue. (a) Fibroblasts lay down collagen (arrow) and the tissue becomes less cellular and vascular. (b) Scar tissue composed of dense collagen may form.

collagen, and endothelial cells which form new blood vessels. With time the granulation tissues matures, becomes less vascular and forms dense fibrous (scar) tissue (Figure 8.12). **Scar formation** occurs quite commonly on the skin in response to traumatic injury and may also occur in specialized tissues such as heart, liver and brain. Scarring is uncommon in the oral cavity.

Formation of an abscess may also lead to scarring. An abscess forms when there is massive accumulation of neutrophils which cause substantial tissue damage. The abscess becomes walled off by granulation tissue but sometimes it may drain and discharge on the surface. This promotes healing as much of the necrotic tissue is removed. If this does not happen then the necrotic tissue is resorbed by macrophages and replaced by granulation tissue which eventually form a scar.

Progression to chronic inflammation

Progression to chronic inflammation may occur when the acute inflammatory response fails to get rid of the injurious agent or when there is interference with the normal processes of healing. This is described in greater detail below.

Chronic Inflammation

Chronic inflammation is sometimes referred to as frustrated healing. This is because inflammation, repair and continued tissue destruction occur simultaneously. It may last for weeks, months or years.

Causes of Chronic Inflammation

The first possible cause is as a result of previous acute inflammation that has failed to resolve. This may be due to:

- foreign material such as grit or retained sutures;
- the cause has not been eliminated. A good example occurs in the bone at the apex of a non-vital (i.e. necrotic) tooth. An acute inflammatory reaction will not result in healing because the cause of the inflammation (i.e. the non-vital tooth containing microorganisms and necrotic tissue) is still present;
- poor healing due to inadequate blood supply.

The second cause is that inflammation may be chronic and low grade from onset. This usually occurs in response to a chronic low-grade stimulus:

- certain microorganisms, for example *Mycobacterium*, which causes tuberculosis;
- prolonged exposure to low-grade toxins: these may be exogenous (e.g. silica which causes silicosis) or endogenous (e.g. toxic lipids in plasma associated with atherosclerosis);

- autoimmune disease: the body mounts an immune reaction against a component of self (e.g. rheumatoid arthritis).

Features of Chronic Inflammation

Chronic inflammation, like acute inflammation, is characterized by both vascular and cellular changes but the cellular changes are more marked. Vascular changes are minimal with some increase in blood flow, formation of limited amounts of oedema and vascular stasis.

Cellular Changes

The inflammatory cells of chronic inflammation are macrophages, lymphocytes and plasma cells. In certain cases eosinophils and basophils may be present and sometimes scattered neutrophils may be seen. Repair in the form of vascular granulation tissue composed of fibroblasts and endothelial cells is also present, which may mature to form scar tissue. Superimposed on these cells is continued tissue destruction which may be caused by the aetiological agent or by the host response (inflammatory cells).

Cells in Chronic Inflammation

Macrophages

Macrophages are derived from blood monocytes and are attracted into the tissues by the mechanisms described in the section on acute inflammation. Once in the tissue they become activated by cytokines, for example IFN-γ produced by activated T-cells, or by certain bacterial products including endotoxin. Macrophages play a pivotal role in chronic inflammation (Figure 8.13).

Their four main functions are:

1) phagocytosis: removal of microorganisms, necrotic tissue and cells, cellular debris, etc.;
2) production of cytokines (e.g. IL-1, TNF) and chemokines; these play an important role in attracting other inflammatory cells such as lymphocytes to the site and also in regulating the immune response;
3) presentation of antigen to T-cells, which stimulates the immune response;
4) stimulation of repair by producing growth factors which initiate fibroblast proliferation, collagen deposition and angiogenesis (formation of new blood vessels).

Unfortunately the products secreted by macrophages can also cause tissue damage. Reactive oxygen species which are used to destroy microorganisms can also destroy host cells and proteases released by macrophages may degrade the extracellular matrix and damage cells.

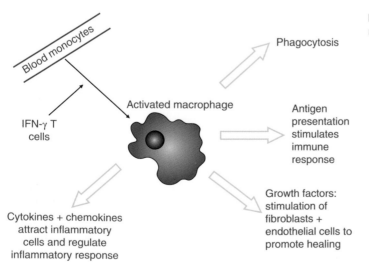

Figure 8.13 Activation of macrophages.

Blood monocytes

IFN-γ T cells

Activated macrophage

Phagocytosis

Antigen presentation stimulates immune response

Cytokines + chemokines attract inflammatory cells and regulate inflammatory response

Growth factors: stimulation of fibroblasts + endothelial cells to promote healing

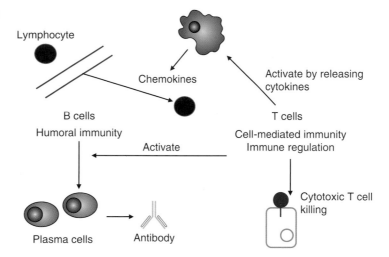

Figure 8.14 Activation of lymphocytes.

Lymphocytes

Both T- and B-lymphocytes may be present in chronic inflammation and they enter from peripheral blood by the same mechanisms as neutrophils and macrophages. B-cells are important in humoral immunity and if activated will differentiate into plasma cells and produce antibodies. The latter are effective against foreign antigens on microorganisms and occasionally in certain autoimmune diseases will react against the host. T-cells are important in cell-mediated immune reactions against virally infected cells, neoplasms and bacteria, which survive within cells. Cytotoxic T-cells are able to kill such cells and other types of T-cell such as T helper cells are able to regulate the immune response and activate B-cells and macrophages (Figure 8.14).

Repair

The body attempts to repair itself by forming granulation tissue: immature fibrous tissue composed of fibroblasts and endothelial cells. Fibroblasts produce collagen and endothelial cells form blood vessels. Granulation tissue is very vascular and is stimulated by growth factors released by macrophages. With time granulation tissue matures to form scar tissue. The number of blood vessels and fibroblasts decrease and the amount of collagen increases. Scar tissue is relatively avascular. Chronic inflammation may be characterized by both granulation tissue and scarring.

Tissue Destruction

Continued tissue destruction is one of the hallmarks of chronic inflammation and the precise cause varies with the type of disease. Some destruction is caused by products of microorganisms; for example, dental caries is caused by acid produced by bacteria in microbial plaque. In other diseases it is the host response that causes the destruction. It has already been mentioned that macrophages produce free oxygen and proteases which damage cells and the extracellular matrix but neutrophils also release enzymes that cause damage. Necrotic tissue releases damaging mediators that perpetuate the inflammatory response and cytotoxic T-cells also kill host cells if recognized as foreign or if they are virally infected.

Granulomatous Inflammation

This is a distinctive pattern of inflammation that is characterized by the formation of 'granuloma'. A granuloma is composed of:

- macrophages that resemble epithelial cells: epithelioid macrophages,
- lymphocytes,
- multinucleate giant cells (see Figure 8.15).

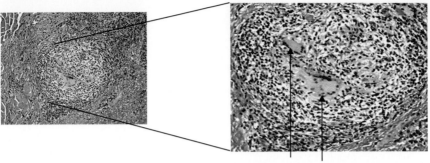

Multinucleate giant cells (arrows), lymphocytes and
epithelioid macrophages

Figure 8.15 Granulomatous inflammation.

Note: a granuloma is *not* the same as granulation tissue.

Granulomas form in response to a number of different stimuli. These include:

- infection: tuberculosis, syphilis, leprosy,
- certain immune reactions (e.g. Crohn's disease, sarcoidosis),
- foreign material (e.g. sutures, talc).

Tuberculosis is a good example of granulomatous inflammation and it is caused by the organism *Mycobacterium tuberculosis*. Unlike the majority of bacteria, mycobacteria are able to survive within cells and when engulfed by macrophages are able to proliferate inside them. The host resists the mycobacteria by mounting a cell-mediated immune response (T_H1 response) which boosts the ability of the macrophage to kill the bacteria. However, mycobacteria have waxy cell walls and complete destruction of the organisms is very difficult even if the macrophages are activated. As a result even if the bacterium is killed parts of the wall remain and continue to stimulate the cell-mediated immune response. This is now a hypersensitivity response and results in the formation of a granuloma. Monocytes are attracted from peripheral blood and differentiate into epithelioid macrophages. Some monocytes fuse to form giant cells which may be of the Langhans (nuclei in horseshoe arrangement)

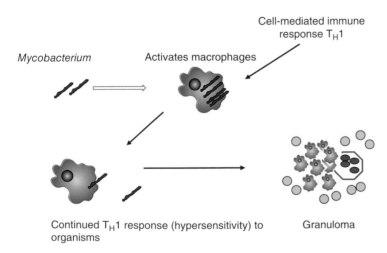

Figure 8.16 Tuberculosis.

or foreign body type (scattered arrangement of nuclei). Activated T-cells are attracted. In addition, the immune response causes caseous necrosis which can be quite marked. Thus the cell-mediated immune response protects the host against the *Mycobacterium* but also causes tissue destruction. It is a paradox that patients with the most efficient host response against the mycobacteria suffer most damage whereas those patients who do not mount much of a response suffer very little damage (Figure 8.16).

Granuloma also form in other diseases such as Crohn's disease and sarcoidosis and although it is likely that there is a T_H1 cell-mediated immune reaction, what initiates it is less clear. Foreign material may also stimulate a similar response but in such cases the cause is usually obvious.

Summary

In summary, chronic inflammation occurs either when an acute inflammatory reaction fails to get rid of the cause or in response to a chronic low-grade infection/aetiology. It is characterized by repair and destruction occurring simultaneously and by the presence of chronic inflammatory cells: macrophages, lymphocytes and plasma cells. Macrophages in particular are important in controlling the inflammatory response and in addition to phagocytosis they stimulate repair as well as causing tissue damage. A special type of chronic inflammation called granulomatous inflammation occurs in response to foreign bodies such as sutures and certain microorganisms; for example, tuberculosis as well as in immune conditions such as sarcoidosis.

9

Head and Neck Anatomy
Stuart Hunt

School of Clinical Dentistry, University of Sheffield, Sheffield, UK

Learning Objectives

- To be able to list the cranial nerves and the structures they innervate.
- To be able to describe the skeletal, muscular and vascular features of the face and neck.
- To able to describe the features of the temporomandibular joint and how the muscles function in mastication.
- To be able to describe the anatomical features of the oral cavity, pharynx, larynx, orbit and paranasal sinuses.

Clinical Relevance

All dentists must have a detailed knowledge of head and neck anatomy. It is essential to understand the complex 3D structure of the orofacial tissues and their relationship to each other during dental procedures so that specific structures can be located and undesirable damage to normal tissue avoided. For example, nerves need to be located to administer local anaesthetic but nerve damage must be avoided during third molar surgery. Anatomical knowledge is essential to interpret medical images of the head and neck region. Specialist anatomical terminology must be used to accurately record clinical procedures and findings.

The Cranial Nerves

The cranial nerves underpin the functions of the head and neck, and so are highly relevant to dental practice. When viewing the base of the brain it is possible to see the 12 pairs of cranial nerves that are part of the peripheral nervous system (the other part consisting of the 31 pairs of spinal nerves). These cranial nerves, except for the accessory nerve (XI), originate from the brain or brainstem and exit the cranium through the foramina or fissures. The cranial nerves contain neurones of distinct types that have a variety of functions and are essential for the head and neck to operate normally. Some functions are the same as **spinal nerves** (general), whereas other functions are specific to **cranial nerves** (special). These can be further divided into **somatic** (related to the body) and **visceral**

Basic Sciences for Dental Students, First Edition. Edited by Simon A. Whawell and Daniel W. Lambert.
© 2018 John Wiley & Sons Ltd. Published 2018 by John Wiley & Sons Ltd.
Companion website: www.wiley.com/go/whawell/basic_sciences_for_dental_students

(related to organs) classifications. Finally, function can be divided into **afferent** (sensory) or **efferent** (motor) categories.

The Olfactory Nerves (CN I)

Special visceral afferent neurones convey the sense of smell from the nose to the brain. Olfactory nerves originate in the olfactory epithelium in the roof of the nasal cavity and pass through perforations in the cribriform plate of the ethmoid bone to terminate by synapsing with secondary neurones in the olfactory bulbs (Figure 9.1b). These fibres project posteriorly as the olfactory tracts, running along the underside of the frontal lobes, which in turn synapse in the olfactory areas of the brain.

(a)

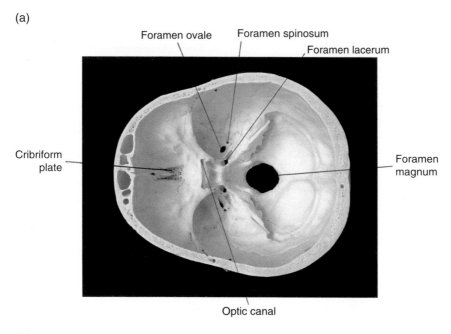

(b)

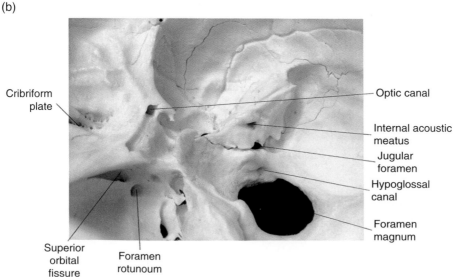

Figure 9.1 The foremen of the skull.

The Optic Nerves (CN II)

The optic nerves are the largest of the cranial nerves and contain special sensory afferent neurones for vision and are the axons of cells that connect indirectly with the photoreceptors (rods and cones) in the retina at the back of each eye. The optic nerves exit the orbits via the optic canals and soon after unite to form the optic chiasma, where nasal retinal axons cross to the opposite side and temporal retinal axons remain on the same side. The axons then divide again and continue as the optic tracts, which terminate in the lateral geniculate nucleus of the thalamus. Postsynaptic fibres from the lateral geniculate nucleus synapse in the visual cortex of the occipital lobe of the brain.

The Oculomotor (CN III), Trochlear (CN IV) and Abducens (CN VI) Nerves

Cranial nerves III, IV and VI can be conveniently grouped together as they are all general somatic efferent nerves that control movement of the eyeball via the extraocular muscles. They all enter the corresponding orbit via the superior orbital fissure (Figure 9.1b).

The **oculomotor nerves** innervate the majority of the extraocular eye muscles including the superior, inferior and medial rectus muscles, and the inferior oblique muscle. In addition they control elevation of the upper eyelid by innervation of the levator palpebrae superioris muscle. The oculomotor nerves also contain a general visceral efferent component that consists of preganglionic parasympathetic axons destined to innervate the intrinsic muscles of the eye.

The **trochlear nerves** innervate the superior olique muscle of the corresponding orbit and are the only cranial nerves that originate from the posterior surface of the brainstem.

The **abducens nerves** innervate the lateral rectus muscle of the corresponding orbit.

The Trigeminal Nerves (CN V)

The trigeminal nerves are the second largest cranial nerves and are mostly composed of general somatic afferent fibres, but also contain a minor special visceral efferent component that supplies motor innervation to the muscles of mastication. They are the most relevant cranial nerves for dental practice as they are the major sensory nerves for the head, supplying cutaneous innervation to the face and also deeper structures such as the paranasal sinuses and most importantly the mucous membranes of the oral cavity, the upper and lower dentition, and their supporting structures. As the name suggests (*tri*geminal) each of the two trigeminal nerves divides into three major branches (before leaving the cranium): the ophthalmic (V_1), maxillary (V_2) and mandibular divisions (V_3). Of these branches, only the mandibular division contains motor axons; the other two branches are purely sensory. Due to supplying distinct areas of the head, each branch leaves the cranium via a specific fissure/foramen. The ophthalmic branch leaves the cranium through the superior orbital fissure, while the maxillary and mandibular branches leave via the foramen rotundum and foramen ovale, respectively. The ophthalmic branch carries sensory innervation from the skin of the anterior part of the scalp, forehead, upper eyelid and the dorsum of the nose. The maxillary branch receives sensory information from the skin covering the side of the nose, lower eyelid, cheek and upper lip. The mandibular branch supplies the skin covering the mandible, including the lower lip and chin. By remembering this cutaneous pattern of innervation it is possible to determine which branch of the trigeminal nerve supplies the deeper structures, as the branch supplying these structures will be the same branch supplying the overlying skin.

The Facial Nerves (CN VII)

The facial nerves facilitate a number of different functions and therefore contain several types of nerve fibre. Their major function, and neurone component, as their name suggests, is to supply motor innervation to the muscles of facial expression via special visceral efferent fibres. The facial nerve emerges from the brain as a large motor root and a smaller sensory root (nervus intermedius). Both roots enter the facial canal via the internal acoustic meatus and fuse together. In the middle ear, the facial nerve gives off the greater petrosal nerve, which carries general visceral efferent fibres to the lacrimal gland and mucous glands of the nose, maxillary sinus and palate. The facial nerve continues through the bony canal, where the remaining general visceral efferent and special visceral afferent fibres branch off forming the chorda tympani nerve. This nerve passes through the squamotympanic fissure and carries taste sensation from the anterior two-thirds of the tongue and provides preganglionic parasympathetic fibres that are destined to stimulate secretomotor function in the submandibular and sublingual salivary glands. The main part of the facial nerve, now consisting of purely motor fibres, exits through the stylomastoid foramen, giving off branches to the posterior belly of digastric and stylohyoid muscles, *en route* to supply the muscles of facial expression. The nerve passes through the parotid salivary gland and divides into five branches (temporal, zygomatic, buccal, mandibular and cervical) that supply the muscles of facial expression.

The Vestibulocochlear Nerves (CN VIII)

These nerves contain special somatic afferent fibres and are responsible for conveying the special senses of hearing and balance via the vestibular and cochlear components, respectively. Like the facial nerve, the vestibucochlear nerve also passes through the internal acoustic meatus.

The Glossopharyngeal Nerves (CN IX)

The glossopharyngeal nerves contain a variety of nerve fibre types. They convey general sensation from the posterior one-third of the tongue, palatine tonsils and oropharynx via general somatic afferent fibres and also carry the sense of taste from the posterior one-third of the tongue via special visceral afferent fibres. In addition, general visceral afferent fibres receive information from the chemoreceptors of the carotid body and baroreceptors of the carotid sinus. The general visceral efferent component supplies preganglionic parasympathetic nerves that are involved in stimulating secretomotor function in the parotid salivary gland. Finally, the remaining special visceral efferent fibres supply motor innervation to the stylopharyngeus muscles. The glossopharyngeal nerves arise from the brain as a collection of rootlets that fuse together soon after passing through the jugular foramen.

The Vagus Nerves (X)

The vagus nerves have an extensive course through the body and contain a variety of neuronal fibre types. General somatic afferent fibres carry sensory information from the larynx, laryngopharynx and the skin of the external ear. Special visceral afferent fibres carry taste sensation from the epiglottis and pharynx. Special visceral efferent fibres innervate one extrinsic muscle of the tongue (palatoglossus), the muscles of the soft palate (except tensor veli palatine), pharynx (apart from stylopharyngeus) and larynx. The general visceral efferent fibres innervate smooth muscle and glands in the pharynx, larynx, thoracic viscera and abdominal viscera. General visceral afferent fibres carry information from the thorax and abdomen. They start their long journey as they exit the cranial cavity through the jugular foramen and travel through the neck inside the carotid sheath, between the carotid artery and internal jugular vein.

The Accessory Nerves (CN XI)

The accessory nerves are the only cranial nerves that enter the cranial cavity and exit again. The spinal part of the nerve originates from the upper five cervical segments of the spinal cord and enters the cranium through the foramen magnum. This part of the nerve contains general somatic efferent fibres that supply motor innervation to the sternocleidomastoid and trapezius muscles. Before the nerve leaves the cranium it is joined by fibres from the vagus nerve. These cranial roots then join with the vagus nerve as they leave the cranium through the jugular foramen.

The Hypoglossal Nerves (CN XII)

These nerves contain general somatic efferent fibres that supply motor innervation to all intrinsic and extrinsic (except for palatoglossus) muscles of the tongue. They exit the cranial cavity through the hypoglossal canals, which are either side of the foramen magnum.

Clinical tests for nerve function are shown in Table 9.1.

The Face and Neck

The Skeletal Components of the Neck

The skeletal components of the neck are comprised of the seven cervical vertebrae, the hyoid bone (that does not directly articulate with any other bones) and the laryngeal cartilages. The cervical vertebrae are structurally distinct from thoracic vertebrae, having a small body, a bifid spinous process and also transverse foramina (for the transmission of blood vessels and nerves). C7 is intermediary in structure, having a long slender spinous process that can be felt through the skin at the base of the neck. The first two cervical vertebrae are specialized: C1 (also known as the atlas) has no body and articulates with the occipital condyles on the base of the skull, allowing nodding movements of

Table 9.1 Clinical tests for cranial nerve function.

Cranial nerve number	Cranial nerve name	Clinical test
I	Olfactory	Ask patient to identify characteristic smells such as coffee, peppermint, etc.
II	Optic	Test visual acuity (Snellen chart).
III	Oculomotor	Ask the patient to track the movement of a pen torch across all visual fields and check for full range of eye movement.
IV	Trochlear	As for III.
V	Trigeminal	Use the sharp blunt test across all regions of the face to test for sensation carried by V_1, V_2 and V_3.
VI	Abducens	As for III.
VII	Facial	Inspect for facial symmetry. Ask the patient to make exaggerated facial expressions.
VIII	Vestibulocochlear	Test hearing with a tuning fork. Place the vibrating tuning fork near the external entrance of the ear. To test for sensineural hearing loss, place the base of the vibrating tuning fork on the mastoid process.
IX	Glossopharyngeal	Test for gag reflex by touching the pharyngeal wall.
X	Vagus	Ask the patient to open their mouth and say 'Ahh'. Check for symmetrical elevation of the soft palate.
XI	Accessory	Ask the patient to turn their head and shrug their shoulders against resistance provided by your hand.
XII	Hypoglossal	Ask the patient to protrude their tongue. The tongue will deviate to the affected side.

the head. C2 (the axis) has a process, called the dens, that projects upwards from its body. The dens is formed from the body of C1 that has fused with the body of C2 during development. The anterior surface of the dens articulates with posterior surface of the arch of the atlas and allows shaking movements of the head.

Muscles of the Neck

The most relevant muscle groups in the neck are the superficial, suprahyoid and infrahyoids.

Platysma is the most superficial muscle of this group and lies just below the surface of the skin of the neck. It originates from the fascia covering the pectoralis muscles and forms a flat broad sheet that attaches to the inferior border of the mandible and the muscles around the mouth. Platysma is technically a muscle of facial expression and in innervated by the cervical branches of the facial nerve. It acts to tighten the skin of the neck and also depress the corners of the mouth. **Sternocleidomastoid** is a paired strap-like muscle that is an important landmark of the neck. It originates from the medial third of the clavicle and also the manubrium. The two heads join and attach to the mastoid process and lateral part of the superior nuchal line. If one muscle contracts the head and neck bend to the ipsilateral (same) side, which results in the face tilting upwards and turning to the contralateral (opposite) side. If both muscles contract the neck is flexed and the head extended. **Trapezius** is a paired triangular muscle that originates from the superior nuchal line, external occipital protuberance and the spinous processes of the cervical and thoracic vertebrae. It inserts on the lateral third of the clavicle and parts of the scapula. Trapezius is used to shrug the shoulders as it raises the scapula. Both the sternocleidomastoid and trapezius are innervated by the **spinal accessory nerve** (CN XI). The suprahyoid and infrahyoid muscles are described in a later section.

The Skeletal Components of the Head and Face

The skull is made of 22 bones, eight of which form the cranium: frontal, temporal (two), sphenoid, ethmoid, parietal (two) and occipital bones. Fourteen bones are associated with the face: maxilla (two), nasal (two), palatine (two), zygomatic (two), lacrimal (two), vomer, inferior nasal concha (two) and the mandible (Figure 9.2). Apart from the articulation between the mandible and the temporal bone, contacts between the bones of the skull are non-mobile and are known as sutures.

Muscles of Facial Expression

The muscles of facial expression are responsible for creasing the skin of the face (i.e. facial expressions) but they are also involved in closing the orifices (i.e. eye and mouth) that they surround. The most relevant muscles to learn about are those that surround the eye and the mouth. **Occipitofrontalis** has two bellies separated by an aponeurosis. The occipital belly originates from the superior nuchal line and inserts into the aponeurosis. The frontal belly originates from the aponeurosis and inserts into the skin of the eyebrows and the orbicularis oculi muscle. When contraction of the occipital belly fixes the aponeurosis in place the frontal belly can contract to raise the eyebrows. The **orbicularis oculi** originates from the orbital rim and encircles the orbit. This muscle can be used to screw up the eyes tightly. The **orbicularis oris** surrounds the mouth and can control the shape and size of the orifice. There are a number of muscles that elevate the upper lip: **levator labii superioris**, **levator anguli oris**, **zygomaticus major** and **minor**. The muscles responsible for depressing the lower lip are depressor **labii inferioris** and **depresser anguli oris**. The **buccinator** forms the lateral wall of the oral cavity and helps to push food back into the oral cavity proper during mastication. It originates from the alveolar processes of the maxilla and

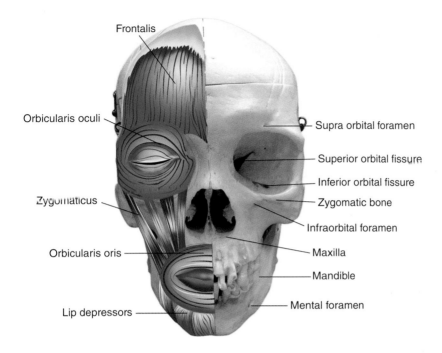

Frontalis

Orbicularis oculi

Zygomaticus

Orbicularis oris

Lip depressors

Supra orbital foramen

Superior orbital fissure

Inferior orbital fissure

Zygomatic bone

Infraorbital foramen

Maxilla

Mandible

Mental foramen

Figure 9.2 The face.

mandible, as well as the pterygomandibular raphe. The muscle fibres converge at the corner of the mouth, blending with orbicularis oris and other dilators of the mouth to form the **modiolus**.

Facial Nerve

The muscles of facial expression receive motor innervation from the facial nerve (CN VII). The facial nerve emerges from the stylomastoid foramen, giving off branches to the occipital belly of occipitofrontalis, posterior belly of digastric and stylohyoid muscles before entering the parotid salivary gland. Before leaving the gland the facial nerve branches into five main divisions: temporal (supplying frontalis), zygomatic (supplying orbicularis oculi), buccal (supplying buccinator and muscles that elevate the upper lip) mandibular (supplying muscles that depress the lower lip) and cervical (supplying platysma).

Cutaneous Innervation

The head and neck receive cutaneous innervation from a number of different nerves and their branches. In particular, the skin of the face and anterolateral scalp receives sensory innervation from the terminal branches of the trigeminal nerve. The terminal branch of the ophthalmic branch of trigeminal is the supraorbital nerve that supplies the skin of the forehead, upper eyelid and a central strip of the nose. The skin of the lower eyelid down to and including the upper lip receives sensory innervation from the terminal branch of the maxillary branch of trigeminal, the infraorbital nerve, which emerges from the infraorbital foramen. It also supplies the skin of the medial side of the cheek, the lateral aspect of the nose and the corresponding oral mucosa in the mouth. Branches of the mandibular division of trigeminal supply the skin of the lower lip, chin, skin over the ramus of the mandible, lateral cheek and part of the temple. The auriculotemporal nerve supplies sensory innervation to the temple and external ear. The buccal nerve pierces buccinator to supply the skin overlying and the corresponding oral mucosa of the cheek adjacent to the lower molar teeth. The mental nerve, which branches from the inferior alveolar nerve, emerges from the mental foramen to supply the skin of the chin and lower lip, labial mucosa and gingivae of mandibular teeth. The remaining cutaneous innervation of the face and neck is derived from the cervical plexus and the first four cervical spinal nerves.

Blood Vessels of the Head and Neck

The main arteries supplying the head and neck branch from the common carotid and subclavian arteries.

The common carotid arteries bifurcate in the neck to produce the external and internal carotid arteries. The internal carotid has no branches in the neck and travels, adjacent to the internal jugular vein within the carotid sheath, towards the cranium to supply the brain. The external carotid artery is **external** to the carotid sheath and provides many branches that supply the tissues of the head and neck, including the oral cavity. The **superior thyroid artery** is the first branch from the external carotid artery supplying structures below the hyoid bone including the infrahyoid muscles, sternocleidomastoid, muscles of the larynx and the thyroid gland. The **ascending pharyngeal artery** supplies the pharyngeal walls and also a branch that supplies the palatine tonsil. The lingual artery supplies the tongue, the floor of the mouth and the suprahyoids. The **facial artery** arises superior to the lingual artery (or may branch from a common trunk) and emerges onto the face at the inferior border of the mandible, anterior to the masseter muscle. It then travels diagonally across the face to the medial corner of the eye. The skin of the posterior neck and scalp, and behind the ears, is supplied by the **occipital and posterior auricular arteries**, respectively. The two terminal branches of the external carotid artery arise within the parotid salivary gland. The smaller of the two is the **superficial temporal artery**, which branches to supply the skin of the scalp. The larger terminal branch is the **maxillary artery**, which gives off a number of important branches. The **middle meningeal artery** passes through foramen spinosum to supply the dura and the skull. The **inferior alveolar artery** enters the mandibular canal to supply the mandibular dentition.

The subclavian artery gives rise to branches that supply the structures of the head and neck. The **inferior thyroid artery** branches from the thyrocervical trunk to supply the thyroid gland, larynx and trachea. The **vertebral artery** also branches from the subclavian artery. It travels up through the neck via the transverse foramina of the cervical vertebrae and enters the cranium via foramen magnum to supply the brain.

The venous drainage of the head and neck is via the internal and external jugular veins. The internal jugular vein is responsible for draining the brain and other deeper structures of the head and neck, whereas the external jugular vein drains the more superficial extracranial structures. The internal jugular vein leaves the cranium through the jugular foramen and travels inferiorly within the carotid sheath, alongside the internal carotid artery and vagus nerve, which is deep to sternocleidomastoid, before emptying into the subclavian vein. Along its course the internal jugular vein receives a number of tributaries including the facial, lingual, pharyngeal and superior thyroid veins. The external jugular vein is formed by the merger of the posterior division of the retromandibular vein and the posterior auricular vein. It travels superficial to sternocleidomastoid before emptying into the subclavian vein.

Lymphatic Drainage of the Head and Neck

The lymphatic system is a network of vessels that begin in peripheral tissues and eventually connect with veins. Lymphatic capillaries combine to former larger vessels that feed into collecting ducts which empty into the venous system to return fluids and solutes from peripheral tissues to the general circulation. The larger vessels are interrupted by lymph nodes, which are important organs in the production of lymphocytes. Understanding the lymphatic system is important for monitoring spread of infection, which can cause swollen lymph nodes (lymphadenopathy) and also for understanding how some tumours, including oral cancer, spread. There are clusters of lymph nodes that are responsible for regional drainage of lymphatic fluid. The submental nodes drain the central lower lip, the chin, floor of the mouth, tip of the tongue and the incisor teeth. They drain into the jugulo-omohyoid node of the deep cervical chain and the submandibular nodes. The submandibular nodes drain the face, gingivae and teeth, floor of the mouth, and the tongue. They also drain into the deep cervical chain via the jugulo-omohyoid node. The preauricular (parotid) nodes drain lymphatic fluid from the anterolateral scalp, eyelids and external ear into the deep cervical chain. The postauricular (mastoid) nodes drain the posterolateral scalp into the deep cervical nodes. Lymph from the posterior scalp and upper neck drains into the deep cervical nodes via the occipital nodes. The superficial cervical nodes are responsible for monitoring lymph from the superficial structures of the neck.

The Temporomandibular Joint

The temporomandibular joint (TMJ) is formed by the underside of the **temporal bone** and the head of the **mandibular condyle** (Figure 9.3a). The articulating surface of the temporal bone includes the convex articular eminence and the concave glenoid fossa. The head of the mandibular condyle is convex and so is most stable when in the glenoid fossa. The joint is most unstable when the condyle is aligned with the articular eminence. The right and left TMJs are connected by the mandible and so one joint cannot move without there being some

movement in the other. These joints allow for movement of the mandible during speech and mastication.

The articulating surfaces are covered in fibrocartilage and the joint is separated into two compartments by a fibrocartilagenous disc. The disc is continuous with the upper head of the lateral pterygoid muscle and connects the muscle to the posterior aspect of the joint. It is pulled forward by the lateral pterygoid to stabilize the joint when the head of the condyle moves anteriorly out of the glenoid fossa and onto the articular eminence.

The TMJ is enclosed by the fibrous joint capsule. The synovial membrane that lines the joint capsule secretes synovial fluid that lubricates the joint and fills the joint compartments. There are three paired ligaments that attach the mandible to the cranium: **temporomandibular**, **stylomandibular** and **sphenomandibular**. The temporomandibular ligament is essentially a thickening of the joint capsule and is considered the major joint ligament as it prevents excessive posterior movement of the mandible. The remaining two minor ligaments are classed as minor ligaments, which connect the mandible to the cranium. The sphenomandibular ligament is relevant for dental practice as it attaches to the lingula, covering the opening of the mandibular foramen. The sphenomandibular ligament may therefore act as a physical barrier to local anaesthesia of the inferior alveolar nerve. The capsule and ligaments provide proprioceptive information on joint position via sensory nerves from branches of the mandibular division of the trigeminal nerve (auriculotemporal and masseteric nerves). See Feature box 9.1.

Muscles of Mastication

The muscles of mastication are comprised of four pairs of muscles attached to the mandible: masseter, temporalis, medial pterygoid and lateral pterygoid (Figure 9.3b). These muscles function with the TMJ to allow

(a)

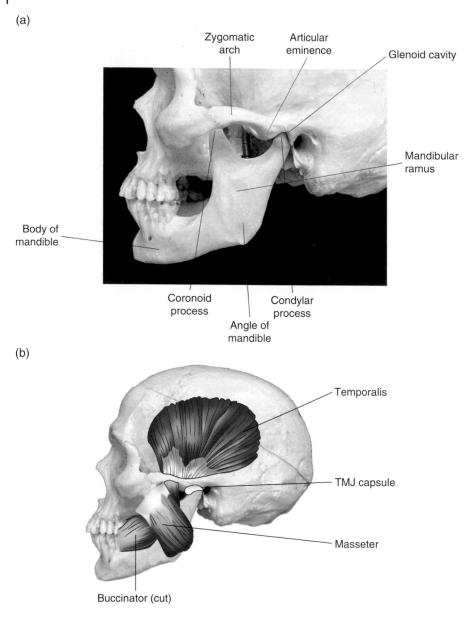

(b)

Figure 9.3 (a) The TMJ and (b) muscles of mastication.

Feature box 9.1 Dislocation of the TMJ

Trauma to the mandible or even opening your mouth too wide can lead to dislocation of the TMJ. The TMJ can only dislocate anteriorly because its movement is restricted medially and posteriorly by bone. The mandibular condyle overrides the articular eminence resulting in the mouth being fixed in an open position. The dislocation should be reduced immediately. If this does not

happen the muscles of mastication may go into spasm, which 'locks' the dislocated joint in position. In this case, muscle relaxants may be prescribed to reduce the spasm and allow manual reduction. Dislocation of the TMJ will lead to stretching of the associated ligaments and joint capsule, which means that repeated dislocation is more likely in the future.

movement of the mandible. They are all innervated by the mandibular division of the trigeminal nerve.

The masseter originates from the zygomatic arch, inserts onto the external surface of the mandible and is a powerful elevator of the mandible.

The temporalis is a broad, fan-shaped muscle that originates from the temporal fossa and inserts onto the apex, anterior and posterior borders, and medial surface of the coronoid process via a tendon. This extends on the anteromedial border of the ramus as far down as the retromolar fossa, which is important when designing lower dentures. The anterior, vertical muscle fibres elevate the mandible, whereas the posterior, more horizontal muscle fibres retract the mandible.

The medial pterygoid is divided into deep and superficial heads, and elevates the mandible. The deep head originates from the medial surface of the lateral pterygoid plate, whereas the superficial head originates from the pyramidal process of the palatine bone and maxillary tuberosity of the maxilla. Both heads insert onto the medial surface of the ramus and angle of the mandible.

The lateral pterygoid is involved in protrusion of the mandible and is divided into upper and lower heads. The upper head originates from the infratemporal surface of the greater wing of the sphenoid bone and inserts on the anterior aspect of the articular disc and capsule. The lower head originates from the lateral surface of the lateral pterygoid plate and inserts into the anterior surface of the neck of the mandible at the pterygoid fovea.

Movement of the mandible during speech or mastication is facilitated by the TMJ and the associated muscles. Two types of movement are permitted at the joint: rotational and sliding. Rotation of the head of the condyle allows slight depression of the mandible, but continued opening requires the condyle (and articular disc) to slide forwards and downwards onto the articular eminence, which happens with bilateral contraction of the lateral pterygoid muscles. The mouth is opened further still by the action of the digastric and other suprahyoid muscles, which depress the mandible. This can only happen if the hyoid bone is fixed by simultaneous contraction of the infrahyoid muscles. Bilateral contraction of masseter, temporalis and medial pterygoids will serve to elevate the mandible and close the mouth.

During mastication a special movement is required, called lateral excursion, to bring the teeth on one side into occlusal contact. The lateral pterygoid on the protruding side contracts, moving the condyle forward onto the articular eminence. The contralateral condyle remains in the glenoid fossa, held in place by the posterior fibres of temporalis, but rotates about a vertical axis. This results in a lateral deviation of the mandible, called Bennett movement, to the side of the condyle that is still in the glenoid fossa. When the left lateral pterygoid contracts the mandible will deviate to the right side and vice versa. The mandible deviates to the working side where the teeth are brought in maximal occlusal contact for mastication, whereas the other side is known as the balancing side. The process alternates resulting in a side-to-side movement of the mandible.

The Oral Cavity

The mouth can be divided into two main regions: the **vestibule** (sulci between the cheeks or lips and the teeth) and the **oral cavity** proper (the space inside and including the teeth).

The upper and lower furrows of oral mucosa between the cheeks and the alveolar processes are called the buccal sulci. Those between the lips and alveolar processes are called the labial sulci. The upper and lower lips are connected to the corresponding alveolar ridge by the upper and lower labial frenulum, respectively. The opening of the parotid duct can be found opposite the maxillary second molar.

The roof of the oral cavity is formed anteriorly by the bony hard palate and posteriorly by the muscular soft palate. Behind the anterior teeth is the incisive papilla and posterior to this are ridges of tissue called the palatine rugae. Attached to the posterior border of the hard palate is the soft palate. Hanging from the posterior border of the soft palate is a muscular structure called the uvula.

The soft palate is highly mobile and consists of four paired muscles: palatoglossus, palatopharyngeus, tensor veli palatini and levator veli palatini. Palatoglossus extends from the median palatine raphe and inserts into the lateral surface of the tongue, forming the palatoglossal arch (anterior pillar of fauces). When these muscles contract they depress the soft palate and elevate the posterior tongue to form a sphincter separating the oral cavity from the pharynx. Palatopharyngeus originates in the soft palate and inserts into the inferior pharyngeal constrictor muscle and the thyroid cartilage, forming the palatopharyngeal arch (posterior pillar of fauces). Contraction of these will depress the soft palate or elevate the larynx and pharynx. Between these arches you will find the palatine tonsil.

As the name suggests, levator veli palatini elevates the soft palate. Originating from the inferior aspect of the petrous temporal bone and the medial side of the cartilaginous part of the auditory tube, the muscle inserts into the median palatine raphe.

The tensor veli palatini originates from the scaphoid fossa and the lateral aspect of the cartilaginous part of the auditory tube. The muscle forms a tendon which turns medially around the pterygoid hamulus and inserts into the median palatine raphe. Contraction of tensor veli palatini tenses the soft palate and also opens the auditory tube to allow air flow between the middle ear and the pharynx.

These muscles are innervated by the pharyngeal plexus except for tensor veli palatini, which is innervated by a division of the mandibular branch of trigeminal.

The tongue occupies a large area of the oral cavity and is used during mastication, swallowing and speech. It is the anterior two-thirds of the tongue that is clearly visible, whereas the posterior one-third of the tongue extends into the throat. The anterior dorsal surface of the tongue is covered with tiny projections called filiform papillae that give the tongue its velvety appearance. These contain no taste buds, but are thought to allow the tongue to grip food. The other dorsal papillae, fungiform and circumvallate papillae, contain many taste buds (there are also taste buds in the foliate papillae on the posterolateral surface of the tongue). A V-shaped groove called the sulcus terminalis demarcates the division of the tongue into anterior two-thirds and posterior one-third. The posterior one-third of the tongue contains a mass of lymphoid tissue call the lingual tonsil, where papillae are absent. The ventral (underside) surface of the tongue has a different appearance due to the thin smooth lining mucosa, through which the large deep lingual veins are visible. The lingual frenulum, a band of tissue in the midline, connects the ventral surface of the tongue to the floor of the mouth.

The tongue is made up of striated (voluntary) muscle, which can be divided into two groups: intrinsic and extrinsic. The tongue is divided longitudinally in the midline by the fibrous median septum (see Feature box 9.2). Intrinsic muscles have both attachments within the tongue itself, whereas extrinsic muscles have one attachment within the tongue and one external to the tongue.

There are four groups of **intrinsic muscles** in the tongue. The **superior longitudinal** muscles run directly below the dorsal mucosa and from the base of the tongue to the apex. These fibres shorten the tongue and turn the apex upwards. The **inferior longitudinal** muscles are near the ventral surface of the tongue. They too shorten the tongue, but curl the apex downwards. The **transverse** muscle fibres run from the median septum passing to the lateral aspects of the tongue. Contraction of these fibres will narrow and lengthen the tongue. The **vertical** muscle fibres run between the dorsal and ventral

Feature box 9.2 Lymphatic drainage of the tongue

The tongue is divided longitudinally in the midline by the fibrous median septum, which forms a barrier to the movement of lymphatic fluid. However, this barrier is incomplete at the tip and posterior regions of the tongue, which allows bilateral drainage of lymphatic fluid. Thus, an oral squamous cell carcinoma (OSCC) at the tip or base of the tongue is likely to spread bilaterally to regional lymph nodes (to lymph nodes on both sides). In contrast, an OSCC located adjacent to the median septum is more likely to spread unilaterally (to lymph nodes on only one side), limiting its spread.

surfaces of the tongue. Contraction of these fibres will flatten and broaden the tongue.

There are four pairs of **extrinsic** muscles of the tongue. The **genioglossus** muscles are large fan-shaped muscles that are separated in the midline by the median septum. They originate from the upper genial tubercles on the medial surface of the body of the mandible. Contraction of these muscles produces a range of movements including protrusion and flattening of the tongue. Each **styloglossus** originates from the respective styloid process of the temporal bone and inserts into the lateral aspect of the tongue. The action of these muscles is to retract the tongue. The **hyoglossus** muscles originate from the body and greater cornu of the hyoid bone, inserting into the lateral surface of the tongue. These muscles depress the tongue. **Palatoglossus** has already been described in the muscles of the soft palate.

All of the intrinsic and extrinsic muscles (except for palatoglossus) receive their motor innervation from cranial nerve XII, the hypoglossal nerve.

The floor of the mouth bears a number of characteristic features due to the salivary glands that open there. The submandibular salivary glands have a large lobe that is superficial to the mylohyoid muscle and a small lobe that is deep to mylohyoid and lies in the floor of the mouth. The submandibular duct runs from the superficial lobe, hooking around the posterior free border of mylohyoid and through the deep lobe. It opens into the floor of the mouth through the sublingual papilla, which are found on either side of the lingual frenulum. The sublingual salivary glands lies entirely in the floor of the mouth, with their upper surface being directly below the lining mucosa. These glands open through numerous small openings along the sublingual folds.

The physical floor of the mouth is a muscular sling formed by the mylohyoid muscles. They are attached along the mylohyoid line on the medial aspect of the mandible and unite in a midline raphe. There are free posterolateral borders as the medial posterior fibres insert into the anterior body of the hyoid bone. Mylohyoid is innervated by the mylohyoid nerve, a branch of the inferior alveolar nerve before it enters the mandibular foramen. Mylohyoid, along with geniohyoid, stylohyoid and digastric muscles belong to the family of suprahyoid muscles. Deep to the mylohyoid muscles are the geniohyoid muscles, which originate from the inferior genial tubercles and insert on the body of the hyoid bone. Geniohyoid receives motor innervation from C1 via the hypoglossal nerve.

Superficial to mylohyoid lies the anterior belly of digastric, a muscle with two separate bellies. The anterior belly originates from the intermediate tendon and inserts at the digsatric fossa on the lower surface of the body of the mandible. The posterior belly originates at the mastoid notch and inserts at the intermediate tendon. Due to different embryological origins each belly has a different innervation. The anterior belly is innervated by the mylohyoid nerve (mandibular division of trigeminal) and the posterior belly receives innervation from a branch of the facial nerve. The stylohyoid originates from the styloid process and inserts on the body of the hyoid bone. It is innervated by a branch of the facial nerve. The suprahyoid muscles can elevate the hyoid bone and larynx during swallowing. If the hyoid bone is fixed in place by simultaneous contraction of infra- and suprahyoids, the suprahyoids can then depress the mandible.

Sensory Innervation of the Oral Cavity

Tongue and Floor of Mouth

The lingual nerve is a branch of mandibular division of the trigeminal nerve (Figure 9.4). It also contains a chorda tympani component which carries taste sensation from the anterior two-thirds of the tongue and preganglionic parasympathetic fibres to the submandibular and sublingual salivary glands. The lingual nerve carries somatic sensation from the anterior two-thirds of the tongue, the mucosa covering the floor of the mouth and the lingual gingivae of the mandibular dentition. The nerve is susceptible to damage in the oral cavity by dental procedures as it lies close to the roots of the third molar tooth and is only covered by a thin layer of mucosa. The posterior one-third of the tongue receives sensory, taste and secretomotor innervation from the glossopharyngeal nerve.

Maxillary Dentition, Hard and Soft Palate

The maxillary division of the trigeminal nerve supplies the maxillary dentition, the gingivae and supporting structures. The maxillary nerve passes through the pterygopalatine fossa on its course to the floor of the orbit. The nerve passes through the infraorbital canal, and is known as the infraorbital nerve, before emerging into the face through the infraorbital foramen.

The greater and lesser palatine nerves branch from the maxillary nerve in the pterygopalatine fossa and travel through the pterygopalatine canal to reach the palatine bone. The greater palatine nerve passes through the greater palatine foramen and passes anteriorly, between the mucoperiosteum and bone, as far as the canine tooth. The greater palatine nerve supplies sensory innervation to the mucosa of the hard palate and the palatal gingivae. The lesser palatine nerve passes through the lesser palatine

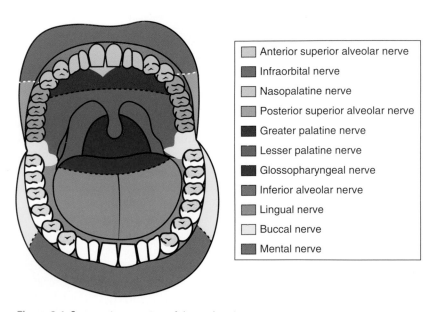

Legend:
- Anterior superior alveolar nerve
- Infraorbital nerve
- Nasopalatine nerve
- Posterior superior alveolar nerve
- Greater palatine nerve
- Lesser palatine nerve
- Glossopharyngeal nerve
- Inferior alveolar nerve
- Lingual nerve
- Buccal nerve
- Mental nerve

Figure 9.4 Sensory innervation of the oral cavity.

foramen to supply sensory innervation to the soft palate and palatine tonsils.

The posterior superior alveolar nerve arises from the maxillary nerve in the pterygopalatine fossa and passes through the pterygopalatine fossa before entering bone through the posterior alveolar foramina and passing through bony canals to supply the maxillary molar teeth. The nerve also provides sensory innervation for the mucous membrane lining the maxillary sinus.

The anterior superior alveolar nerves branch from the infraorbital nerve and travel down through the anterior wall of the maxillary sinus to supply the maxillary central incisors, lateral incisors, canine and supporting tissue. When present, the middle superior alveolar nerve usually branches from the infraorbital nerve and travels through the lateral wall of the maxillary sinus to supply the maxillary premolar teeth.

Mandibular Dentition

The mandibular dentition and periodontal tissues receive sensory innervation from the inferior alveolar nerves. The nerve is a branch of the mandibular division of trigeminal that enters the bone of the mandible via the mandibular foramen. The nerve travels in the mandibular canal as far as the mental foramen. The canine and incisor teeth are supplied by the incisive nerve, which is a continuation of the inferior alveolar nerve. The mental nerve exits the mandible through the mental foramen to innervate the skin of the lower lip and chin, the labial mucosa and gingivae of the anterior teeth.

The Pharynx and Larynx

The Pharynx

The pharynx is a muscular tube that acts as a conduit for air and food passing to the larynx and oesophagus, respectively. It can be divided into discrete anatomical regions: **nasopharynx** (behind the nasal cavity), **oropharynx** (behind the oral cavity) and **laryngopharynx** (behind the larynx). The lateral and posterior walls of the pharynx are formed by the pharyngeal constrictor muscles. There are three pairs of constrictor muscles: **superior**, **middle** and **inferior**. Each constrictor muscle has a different origin, but they all insert posteriorly into the median pharyngeal raphe (a fibrous band of tissue that is attached to the pharyngeal tubercle on the base of the skull). The superior constrictor fibres originate from the pterygoid hamulus, mandible and pterygomandibular raphe. The middle constrictor originates from the hyoid bone and stylohyoid ligament. The inferior constrictor muscle originates from the thyroid and cricoid cartilages. These muscles contract peristaltically to move food into the oesophagus during swallowing. The pharyngeal constrictors are innervated by the pharyngeal plexus, which contains a sensory component from the glossopharyngeal nerve and a motor component from the vagus nerve.

The Larynx

The larynx is part of the respiratory tract and is therefore reinforced by cartilage. However, laryngeal cartilages articulate with each other at synovial joints to allow precision movement. The primary function of the larynx is to close the trachea and protect the lower respiratory tract from inhalation of food or liquids during swallowing or vomiting. Its secondary function is the generation of noise by vibration of the vocal folds (**phonation**).

Laryngeal Cartilages

The five cartilages that form the larynx are suspended from the hyoid bone. The largest of these is the thyroid cartilage that is composed of two laminae that are fused anteriorly. The thyroid cartilage and hyoid bone are connected by the thyrohyoid membrane. The cricoid cartilage is shaped like a signet ring and is the only complete ring of cartilage in the respiratory tract. It has a backwards

---

Feature box 9.3 Making an emergency airway

Understanding the anatomy of the larynx is important in an emergency situation. If you suspect that a patient's larynx (or anyone else's for that matter) is obstructed, preventing passage of air, you may need to create an emergency airway. The patient should be laid flat on their back with their neck fully extended. You should palpate the laryngeal cartilages, identifying the cricothyroid membrane between the cricoid and thyroid cartilages. In a clinical setting, an incision should be made in the cricothyoid membrane with a scalpel and a tracheotomy tube inserted to keep the emergency airway open. In a non-clinical setting the hole could be made with any sharp implement and the hole kept open with the plastic tube from a ballpoint pen.

---

facing broad lamina and a narrow band anteriorly. The cricoid cartilage and thyroid cartilage articulate at the cricothyroid joints. The inferior border of the thyroid cartilage is joined to the cricoid cartilage by the cricothyroid membrane, an important site for the creation of an emergency airway (see Feature box 9.3). The cricoid cartilage also articulates with the paired arytenoid cartilages that sit on the superiolateral border of the cricoid lamina. They articulate at the cricoarytenoid joints. The epiglottis is a leaf-shaped cartilage with the stem attached to the inner aspect of the thyroid laminae. During swallowing the larynx is elevated and the epiglottis folds to help prevent food entering the trachea.

Vocal Folds

The vocal folds are paired folds in the mucous membrane lining the inside of the larynx, which are bulked out by underlying muscle. They are usually open except during swallowing and speech. During swallowing the vocal folds are forcefully closed (adducted) to prevent food entering the lower respiratory tract. However, speech requires adduction, tension and fine adjustment to allow the vocal folds to vibrate and phonate. The vocal ligament and vocalis muscle attach to the vocal process of the arytenoid cartilages posteriorly and the inner aspect of the thyroid cartilage anteriorly. Above the true vocal folds are a pair of vestibular folds, which contain mucous

glands to produce lubrication. The vocal aperture or rima glottis is formed anteriorly by the vocal folds and posteriorly by the vocal processes of the arytenoid cartilages.

Movement of the Vocal Folds

The cartilages that form the larynx articulate by synovial joints to allow changes in tension and position of the vocal folds. When the hyoid bone is fixed in position, due to the action of the infrahyoid muscles, the cricoid cartilage can pivot at the cricothyroid joint, bringing the anterior band towards the inferior aspect of the thyroid cartilage. This also results in movement of the superior surface of the lamina, and hence the arytenoid cartilages sitting on top, backwards. This will increase the length and tension of the vocal folds.

Three types of movement are possible at the cricoarytenoid joints: *sliding* apart or together, *rotation* about a vertical axis and *tilting* forwards or backwards. When the arytenoids slide medially this will adduct (close) the vocal folds, whereas sliding laterally with abduct (open) the vocal folds. If they rotate inwards the vocal folds will be adducted (closed) and vice versa. Tilting backwards will increase the length and tension, but decrease thickness. The opposite is also true.

Laryngeal Muscles

A number of muscles are responsible for the movement of the vocal folds: The **posterior cricoarytenoids** are the only abductors (openers) of the vocal folds. They are attached to the posterolateral aspect of the cricoid cartilage and the muscular process of the corresponding arytenoid cartilage. They rotate the arytenoid cartilages outwards and so open the vocal folds. The **transverse interarytenoid** is an unpaired muscle. The muscle is attached to the muscular process of each arytenoid cartilage and acts to slide them medially (together) to adduct the vocal folds. The **oblique interarytenoids** form a cross shape as each muscle passes from the muscular process of one arytenoid cartilage to the apex of the opposite arytenoid cartilage. Each muscle is continuous with the **aryepiglottic muscle** of the aryepiglottic fold. Together the oblique interarytenoids and the aryepiglottic muscles help to narrow the laryngeal opening. The **thyroarytenoid** arises from the inferior, inner aspect of the thyroid cartilage and inserts into the antero-lateral surface of the arytenoid cartilage. The **lateral cricoarytenoid** originate from lateral aspect of the cricoid band and attach to the muscular process of the arytenoid. Both the thyroarytenoid and the lateral cricoarytenoid muscles act to adduct the vocal folds by rotating the arytenoid cartilages inwards. The **vocalis** muscle is formed by the lower, deeper fibres of thyroarytenid and it runs parallel to the vocal ligament. Vocalis tilts the arytenoids forwards towards the thyroid cartilage. Its action therefore shortens the vocal folds, which increases thickness, decreases tension and lowers vocal pitch. The remaining laryngeal muscle is **cricothyroid**, which originates at the anterolateral surface of the cricoid band and attaches to the inferior cornu and lamina of the thyroid cartilage. The cricothyoid causes movement at the cricothyroid joint (discussed earlier) that results in increased tension in the vocal folds and a higher vocal pitch.

Innervation of the Larynx

The superior laryngeal nerves, which are branches of the right and left vagus nerves, divide into internal and external branches. The internal laryngeal nerve provides sensory innervation to the mucosa above the vocal folds. The external laryngeal nerve supplies motor innervation to the cricothyroid muscle. All other laryngeal muscles are innervated by the recurrent laryngeal nerves (also branches of the vagus nerves). In addition, they also supply sensory innervation to the mucosa below the vocal folds.

Thyroid Gland

The thyroid gland is inferior to the thyroid cartilage and is made of two lobes connected by the isthmus. There is sometimes a third lobe called the pyramidal lobe that projects upwards from the isthmus. The gland is encased in a fibrous sheath. Four small parathyroid glands are usually present adjacent to or embedded within the posterior to the thyroid gland. The thyroid receives arterial blood from the superior (branch of the external carotid) and inferior (branch of the thyrocervical trunk) thyroid arteries. Superior and inferior thyroid veins drain venous blood into the internal jugular and brachiocephalic veins, respectively.

The Orbit

The orbit is the cavity in the skull that houses the globe (eyeball), associated muscles, nerves and blood vessels (Figure 9.5). The walls of the orbit are made by contributions from seven different bones. The roof of the orbit is formed by the orbital plate of the frontal bone and the lesser wing of the sphenoid bone. The floor is composed of the orbital plate of the maxilla, the orbital surface of the zygomatic bone and the small orbital plate of the palatine bone. The medial wall is formed by the frontal process of the maxilla, lacrimal, ethmoid and body of the sphenoid bone. The bones forming the lateral wall are the orbital surface of the zygomatic bone and the greater wing of the sphenoid. The orbit contains a number of

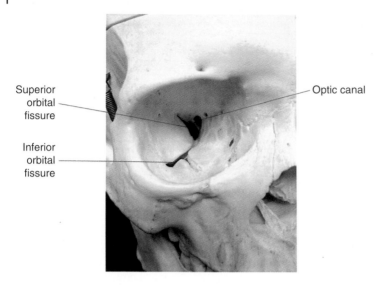

Superior orbital fissure

Inferior orbital fissure

Optic canal

Figure 9.5 The orbit.

spaces or foramina for the passage of nerves and blood vessels. The optic canal passes through the lesser wing of the sphenoid bone acting as a conduit for the optic nerve and the ophthalmic artery. The greater and lesser wings of the sphenoid bone are separated by the superior orbital fissure, which allows passage of the oculomotor, trochlear and abducens nerves and the superior ophthalmic vein. The inferior ophthalmic vein and maxillary branch of trigeminal pass through the inferior orbital fissure.

Extraocular Muscles and their Innervation

The extraocular muscles are responsible for the movement of the eyeball and also the upper eyelid (Figure 9.6). Movement of the upper eyelid is controlled by the levator palpebrae superioris muscle, the uppermost muscle in the orbit. It originates from the lesser wing of the sphenoid at the apex of the orbit and inserts into the tarsal plate of the upper eyelid. It is innervates by the superior branch of the oculomotor nerve.

There are four rectus muscles attached to each eye. They originate from the common tendinous ring that is attached to the bone around the opening of the optic canal. The muscles project forwards, forming a cone of muscle around the optic nerve, and insert onto the sclera of the eyeball, in front of the coronal equator. The superior rectus lies deep to levator palpebrae superioris and acts primarily to elevate the eyeball, but also contributes to adduction and intorsion of the eye. Superior rectus is innervated by the superior branch of the oculomotor nerve. The inferior rectus depresses, adducts and extorts the eyeball. The medial rectus moves the eye medially (adducts). The inferior and medial recti are innervated by the inferior branch of the oculomotor nerve. The lateral rectus muscle moves the eye laterally (abducts) and is supplied by the abducens nerve.

The oblique muscles do not originate from the tendinous ring. The superior oblique originates from the body of the sphenoid bone, medial to the opening of the optic canal. The muscle passes forward above the medial rectus and anteriorly becomes tendinous. The tendon loops through the trochlear and passes beneath the superior rectus to attach to the eyeball behind the coronal equator. The superior oblique acts to depress,

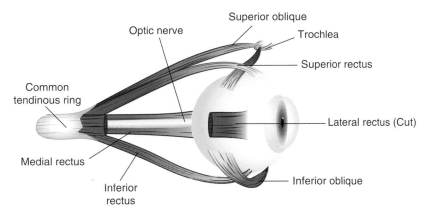

Figure 9.6 Schematic of eye with muscles.

abduct and intort the globe. It is supplied by the trochlear nerve. The inferior oblique is the only extraocular muscle to arise from the front (floor) of the orbit. It attaches to the lateral surface of the eye, behind the coronal equator. The inferior oblique is supplied by the inferior branch of the oculomotor nerve and acts to elevate, abduct and extort the globe.

The Paranasal Air Sinuses

Although the nasal cavity is not highly relevant for dental practice, the paranasal air sinuses are very important. The sinuses are air-filled spaces within the frontal, sphenoid, maxillary and ethmoid bones that communicate with the nasal cavity. The sinuses are lined with respiratory epithelium that can be inflamed as a result of infection. The most relevant to dental practice are the maxillary and frontal air sinuses.

Maxillary Air Sinus

The floor of the sinus is in intimate contact with the roots of the premolar and molar teeth. The lining mucosa of the sinus receives sensory innervation from the superior alveolar nerves, which is clinically relevant due to the phenomenon of referred pain: infection of the maxillary sinus may manifest as toothache. Infection in the maxillary sinus is common due to the drainage opening being two-thirds up the medial wall of the sinus. The opening is situated in the hiatus semilunaris in the middle meatus of the nasal cavity.

Frontal Air Sinus

The frontal air sinus is not highly relevant apart from the fact that it also opens into the hiatus semilunaris. It is possible for infection to travel from the frontal sinus and into the maxillary sinus by running along the hiatus semilunaris.

10

Tooth Development, Tooth Morphology and Tooth-Supporting Structures

Alistair J. Sloan

School of Dentistry, University of Cardiff, Cardiff, UK

Learning Objectives

- To be able to describe the mechanisms and stages of tooth development.
- To understand the processes of dentinogenesis and mineralization, and the control of root formation.
- To be able to accurately describe the morphological features of individual teeth.
- To understand the processes of amelogenesis and enamel mineralization.
- To be able to describe the features and roles of periodontal ligament, junctional epithelium and alveolar bone.

Clinical Relevance

Detailed knowledge of tooth anatomy is absolutely essential for all dental care professionals to enable them to identify, chart and record patient dentition and any procedures that have been or will be carried out on them. An understanding of tooth development enables the clinician to recognize the mixed dentition in children and appreciate the underlying basis of dental anomalies. The tooth-supporting structures are key to tooth stability and physiology but are also specifically targeted by some oral conditions such as periodontal disease.

Introduction

Tooth development or, to give it its correct term, **odontogenesis** consists of a complex series of reciprocal cellular interactions, leading to the formation of the dentition from epithelial and mesenchymal cells in the stomatodeum. Enamel, dentine, cementum and the periodontal tissues all develop during the appropriate stages of embryonic development, with formation of the tooth-supporting tissues (cementum, periodontal ligament and alveolar bone) lagging behind that of the tooth crown. Primary teeth begin at around the sixth to eighth weeks of intra-uterine life, and the permanent teeth begin to form in the twentieth week. It is the specific epithelial–mesenchymal interactions which dictate the

---

Basic Sciences for Dental Students, First Edition. Edited by Simon A. Whawell and Daniel W. Lambert.
© 2018 John Wiley & Sons Ltd. Published 2018 by John Wiley & Sons Ltd.
Companion website: www.wiley.com/go/whawell/basic_sciences_for_dental_students

correct formation of the tooth and help determine the formation of the specific teeth in the correct areas of the dental arch.

Early Tooth Development

The primitive oral cavity, the **stomatodeum**, is lined by a two- to three-cell thickness of epithelium. Beneath this is embryonic connective tissue, the ectomesenchyme (Figure 10.1). The initial observable stage of tooth development within the stomatodeum is a thickening of the epithelium. This thickening is called the **primary epithelial band** and forms at approximately 6 weeks of intrauterine life. This primary epithelial band rapidly divides into two structures termed the **dental lamina** and the **vestibular lamina**. Proliferation of vestibular lamina into the ectomesenchyme gives rise to the vestibule/sulcus. The vestibular lamina cells rapidly enlarge, then degenerate, leaving a cleft which becomes the vestibule.

The dental lamina is the structure from which the tooth germs develop. Proliferation of the dental lamina between 6 and 7 intrauterine weeks determines the positions of future deciduous teeth with a series (20) of epithelial ingrowths into ectomesenchyme (10 each in the developing jaw). This ingrowth of the epithelial dental lamina into the underlying mesenchyme leads to a bud of

cells at the distal aspect of the dental lamina and is called the **bud stage** of tooth development (Figure 10.2). Each bud is separated from the ectomesenchyme by a basement membrane. This incursion initiates condensation from the supporting ectomesenchyme which is observed as a cluster of ectomesenchymal cells closely packed beneath and around the epithelial bud. The remaining ectomesenchymal cells away from the bud are arranged with less regular order.

During tooth development two key processes are essential. The first is **morphodifferentiation**, which is the determination of the shape of the crown of the tooth through the shape of the amelodentinal junction of the forming tooth. The second process is

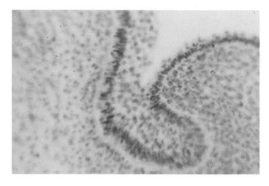

Figure 10.2 The bud stage of tooth development. The bud is formed from the invading epithelium and concurrent condensation of surrounding ectomesenchymal cells.

(a)

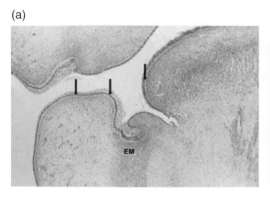

(b)

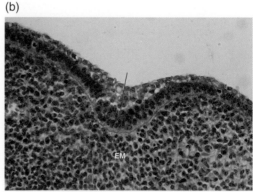

Figure 10.1 (a) The primitive oral cavity, the stomatodeum, with the ectomesenchyme (EM) lying beneath a lining of epithelium (arrows) and (b) the primary epithelial band (arrow).

histo-differentiation, where cells of the developing tooth differentiate into morphologically and functionally distinct groups of cells responsible for secretion of various dental tissues. Control and regulation of this differentiation is through specific and reciprocal cellular interactions between the epithelial and mesenchymal compartments.

The epithelial bud continues to proliferate into the ectomesenchyme and the first signs of an arrangement of cells in the tooth bud appear in the **cap stage**. A small group of ectomesenchymal cells stop producing extracellular substances and do not separate from each other, resulting in an aggregation (condensation) of these cells immediately adjacent to the epithelial bud. This is the developing **dental papilla**. During this transitional stage, the bud grows around the ectomesenchymal aggregation and has the appearance of a cap, becoming the **enamel** (or **dental**) **organ**. A condensation of ectomesenchymal cells called the **dental follicle** surrounds the enamel organ, limiting the dental papilla (Figure 10.3). These three structures (enamel organ, dental papilla, dental follicle) are the constituent elements of the **tooth germ**. It is the enamel organ that is responsible for the synthesis and secretion of the enamel whereas the dental papilla is responsible for the formation of the dentine and pulp.

The dental follicle will produce the supporting structures of a tooth. As the specific tooth tissues (enamel, dentine, pulp, periodontium) arise from specific embryological tissues it explains why enamel is epithelial in origin whereas dentine, pulp and periodontal tissues are mesenchymal in origin.

As tooth development progresses, there is a distinct histo- and morpho-differentiation of the enamel organ as it prepares for secretory function. Alongside this, there is an increase in size of the tooth germ. Both of these changes signify transition to the **early bell stage**. The enamel organ takes on a bell shape during this stage with continued cell proliferation. Histo-differentiation occurs of the enamel organ into four distinct cell layers within it (Figure 10.4). A single layer of cubiodal cells are observed at the periphery of the enamel organ and limit its size. This single layer of cells is known as the **outer enamel epithelium**. Conversely, the single cell layer adjacent to the dental papilla is known as **inner enamel epithelium** and it is these cells that differentiate into ameloblasts giving rise

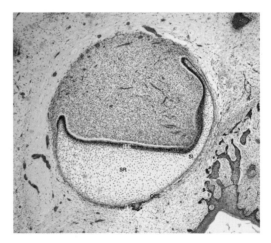

Figure 10.4 The enamel undergoes specific cellular changes in preparation for secretory function and four distinct cell layers are formed in this part of the tooth germ due to cellular proliferation and histo-differentiation. These four cell layers are the inner enamel epithelium (IEE), outer enamel epithelium (OEE), the stellate reticulum (SR) and the stratum intermedium (SI), which is a two- to three-cell-layer-thick area lying next to the inner enamel epithelium.

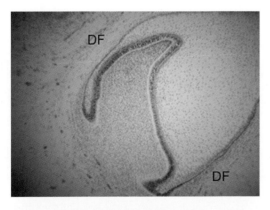

Figure 10.3 The dental follicle (DF) surrounds the enamel organ and limits the dental papilla. It is this structure that is responsible for formation of the supporting structures of the tooth.

to the secretion of enamel. Where these cells of the inner and outer enamel epithelium meet is an area termed the **cervical loop**. The majority of the cells situated between the outer and inner enamel epithelium are termed the **stellate reticulum**. These cells secrete hydrophilic glycosaminoglycans which increase the extracellular space and the cells interconnect through desmosomes giving them a stellate or star-shaped appearance. A two- to three-cell-thick layer of cells lying adjacent to inner enamel epithelium and with a flattened shape is the **stratum intermedium**.

To summarize, the layers of the enamel organ in order of innermost to outermost consist of inner enamel epithelium, stratum intermedium, stellate reticulum and outer enamel epithelium. During this stage of development, as it progresses from cap stage to early bell stage, a localized thickening of cells appears at the inner enamel epithelium around the cusp tip. This is known as the **enamel knot** and is a signalling centre within the developing tooth that provides positional information for tooth morphogenesis and regulates the growth of tooth cusps. The enamel knot produces a range of molecular signals, including fibroblast growth factors (FGFs), bone morphogenetic proteins (BMPs), Sonic Hedgehog (Shh) and Wnt signals. These molecular signals direct the growth of the surrounding epithelium and mesenchyme and have putative roles in signalling and regulation of crown development. The enamel knot is transitory and the primary enamel knot is removed by apoptosis. Secondary enamel knots may appear later during development that regulate the formation of the future cusps of the teeth.

Late Tooth Development

Continued epithelial–mesenchymal interactions signal further histo-differentiation of the four cell layers of the enamel organ as it prepares for amelogenesis. As tooth development progresses from early to late bell stage,

cell morphology in the enamel organ is directly related to function. The cells of the outer enamel epithelium are cuboidal with a high nucleus to cytoplasm ratio. These cells have a non-secretory protective role and will eventually become part of the dentogingival junction. The stellate reticulum cells sit within their extracellular matrix. The inner enamel epithelium cells appear as low/short columnar cells with a central nucleus and few organelles. These cells are beginning to differentiate into **pre-ameloblasts**.

Separating the inner enamel epithelial cells from the ectomesenchymal dental papillae is the **dental basement membrane**. The function of the basement membrane is to mediate the epithelial/mesenchymal compartments during development and odontoblast differentiation prior to dentine secretion. At this stage, the dental papillae consist of undifferentiated ectomesenchymal cells with relatively small amounts of extracellular matrix (apart from a few fine collagen fibrils) and these cells do not yet have a specialized secretory function.

Late bell stage is also known as the **crown stage** of tooth development and further cellular changes occur. In all prior stages of tooth development, all of the inner enamel epithelium cells were proliferating to contribute to the increase of the overall size of the tooth germ. However, during the crown stage, cell proliferation stops at the location corresponding to the sites of the future cusps of the teeth and the inner enamel epithelial cells change in shape from cuboidal to short columnar cells with nuclei polarized at the end of the cell away from the basement membrane.

The adjacent layer of cells on the periphery of the dental papilla increase in size, become columnar and their nuclei polarize away from the basement membrane. This change in cell morphology determines their differentiation into **odontoblasts**. The differentiation of ameloblasts from the cells of the inner enamel epithelium and the differentiation of odontoblasts form papillar cells at the periphery of the dental papilla are initiated at the site of the future cusp tips. The odonto-blasts secrete an organic collagen-rich matrix called **pre-dentine** towards the basement membrane. As the odontoblasts secrete pre-dentine they retreat and migrate towards the centre of the dental papilla. Cytoplasmic extensions are left behind as the odontoblasts move inward, creating a unique, tubular microscopic appearance of dentine as pre-dentine is secreted around these extensions.

As soon as dentine formation begins, the dental basement membrane degenerates and the short columnar cells of the inner enamel epithelium, the pre-ameloblasts, come into contact with the pre-dentine and terminally differentiate into **ameloblasts**, beginning to secrete an organic rich matrix against the dentine. This matrix is already partially mineralized and will mature to become the enamel. Whereas dentine formation proceeds in a pulpal direction, enamel formation moves outwards, adding new material to the outer surface of the developing tooth.

It is during this stage of tooth development that the tooth germ loses its attachment to the oral epithelium as it becomes encased in the newly formed bone of the developing jaw. The dental lamina disintegrates into discrete islands of cells known as the **glands of Serres**. Most of these degenerate but some remain quiescent in jaw bone and if stimulated later in life may form odontogenic cysts known as odontogenic keratocysts. The vascular supply enters dental papilla during cap stage of development and increases during the bell stage of hard tissue formation. The vasculature enters the dental papilla around sites of future root formation. The pioneer nerve fibres approach the developing tooth germ during the bud/cap stage but do not penetrate the dental papilla until after dentine formation has begun.

Formation of the permanent dentition arises from a proliferation and extension of the dental lamina. The permanent incisor, canine and premolar germs arise from proliferation on the lingual aspect of dental lamina next to their deciduous predecessors. The permanent molars have no deciduous predecessors and develop from backwards extension of the dental lamina which gives off epithelial ingrowths giving rise to the first, second and third permanent molars.

Dentinogenesis

The secretion of dentine matrix begins at approximately 17–18 intra-uterine weeks corresponding to the late bell stage, or crown stage, of tooth development. Odontoblast differentiation begins at future cusp tips, spreading apically down a gradient of differentiation down the cuspal slopes. Dentine formation, or secretion of a dentine matrix, starts immediately following odontoblast differentiation. Odontoblast differentiation can be characterized by a distinct change in cell phenotype and morphology. The ectomesenchymal cells of dental papilla have a high nucleus to cytoplasm ratio, little rough endoplasmic reticulum and few mitochondria and therefore have a low synthetic/secretory activity. As these cells differentiate into odontoblasts, they become cells with a low nucleus to cytoplasm ratio and have increased rough endoplasmic reticulum, Golgi and mitochondria and develop a high synthetic/secretory capacity.

The cells of the inner enamel epithelium are critical to the formation of dentine and odontoblast differentiation through molecular signalling. The basement mediates presentation of these molecules which include the growth factors FGF and BMP. As odontoblasts differentiate and secrete pre-dentine, the basement membrane breaks down and the cells of the inner enamel epithelium become exposed to pre-dentine, which signals ameloblast differentiation. As well as a receiving the chemical/molecular signals, the dental papillar cells must also be competent to respond to that signal for differentiation to occur. Competency is achieved by the cells undergoing a requisite number of cell cycles and after the final cell division and cell alignment at the periphery of the dental papilla, the cell nearest the inner enamel epithelium receives these molecular signals from the enamel organ and differentiates into an odontoblast. The other daughter cell remains undifferentiated and exists within the developed pulp as a sub-odontoblast in the cell-rich layer. Odontoblasts are post-mitotic cells and they undergo no further cell division. Once differentiated, they begin to secrete pre-dentine, which is an unmineralized dentine matrix.

The first formed dentine is **mantle dentine** and is approximately 0.15 mm thick. This mantle dentine matrix is synthesized and secreted from both newly differentiated odontoblasts and existing dental papillar cells (the remainder of the dentine matrix is secreted from odontoblasts alone). Mineralization of mantle dentine is via **matrix vesicles**. After mantle dentine formation, odontoblasts continue to secrete pre-dentine which mineralizes to dentine and this dentine, secreted throughout the remainder of tooth development, is termed **primary dentine**. The odontoblasts always secrete a layer of pre-dentine which mineralizes to dentine and, as they secrete pre-dentine, the cells retreat pulpally. As the cells retreat, they leave a single cytoplasmic process within the matrix which allows the odontoblast to communicate with the deeper layers of matrix. This process also creates the tubular structure of dentine, which runs throughout the tissue. These tubules follow an S-shaped course in coronal dentine, but a straighter course in radicular dentine.

There are **two levels of matrix secretion** from the odontoblast and it is this unique secretory pattern that contributes to the unique structure of dentine. The main secretion of structural components (collagen, proteoglycans) into pre-dentine comes from the cell body of the odontoblast. The pre-dentine matrix is secreted around and between the extending odontoblast process and this leads to formation of tubules, with each tubule containing an odontoblast process. This creates the tubular structure of dentine and this dentine matrix secreted from the odontoblast cell body is termed **intertubular dentine**. A second level of secretion of a dentine matrix, rich in tissue-specific matrix components at the mineralization front, is within each dentinal tubule. This is termed **intratubular dentine** or **peritubular dentine** and is found immediately surrounding the inside of the dentinal tubule and is highly mineralized with little or no collagen. It is thought secretion of peritubular dentine is from the odontoblast process.

Dentine forms rhythmically during development with the odontoblast alternating between periods of pre-dentine secretion and quiescence. As a result, incremental lines can be observed and these correspond to a daily rate of secretion of pre-dentine of 4 μm/day. At the boundary between these daily increments minute changes in collagen fibre orientation can be noted. In addition to these daily incremental lines, a 5 day pattern of secretion can also be observed and these incremental lines run at 90° to the dentinal tubules and highlight the normal rhythmic and linear pattern of dentine secretion. These incremental lines are known as the **lines of Von Ebner** and are approximately 20 μm apart. Once secretion of coronal dentine has been completed, the odontoblast reduces is size and becomes a more quiescent, resting cell with minimal secretory capacity.

Dentine Mineralization

Mineralization of dentine is still a controversial subject. In understanding mineralization several important questions need to be addressed. They are:

- what initiates mineralization?
- where does the mineral come from?
- what controls the rate of mineralization?
- where are mineral crystals deposited?

The odontoblasts are essential in the mineralization process and have specific and key roles in initiating and regulating dentine mineralization. They synthesize and secrete the organic matrix that mineralizes; they control the transport of calcium ions into that matrix; and they determine the presence and distribution of specific matrix components (proteoglycans and glycoproteins) that regulate the process. Two basic mechanisms for mineralization exist, called matrix-vesicle-mediated mineralization and heterogenous nucleation or epitaxy.

Matrix-Vesicle-Mediated Mineralization

The biological mineral, hydroxyapatite, which is the constituent mineral in both dentine and enamel, cannot be precipitated directly as it is too complex and requires a high degree of saturation of calcium and phosphate to occur. To obtain hydroxyapatite, **less stable** simpler calcium phosphate called brushite must be precipitated and this is transformed into hydroxyapatite. There is insufficient calcium or phosphate in serum to precipitate brushite so to form hydroxyapatite mineral where none existed before, there is a need for a mechanism to raise calcium and phosphate concentrations within a localized environment in dentine. The matrix vesicles provide the first mineral seen in mantle dentine. These provide a **controlled micro-environment** to concentrate calcium and phosphate, in the presence of a variety of **enzymes** (including alkaline phosphatase). Mineral crystals develop within the vesicles and eventually burst out and become associated with the organic collagenous matrix of pre-dentine or osteoid. These vesicles 'bud off' from the odontoblast process membrane in dentine formation, forming membrane-bound organelles of approximately 30–200 nm in size. As matrix vesicles are the only crystalline structures present in very early mantle dentine formation they have been credited with having an **initiating role** in mineralization.

Heterogenous Nucleation or Epitaxy

In heterogeneous nucleation mineral crystal growth is induced by a solid-phase material on which a crystal lattice can be formed. Hydroxyapatite crystal growth is best promoted on a material that has similar lattice spacings to the crystal, which is a concept known as epitaxy. This solid-phase material with similar lattice spacings is the organic matrix that is secreted by the cells. In this process, there is a 'seeding' of small quantities of hydroxyapatite crystals into the organic matrix and these then grow at the expense of the calcium and phosphate, which passes around the matrix.

Mineralization of Primary and Secondary (Circumpulpal) Dentine

Calcium ions are transported by the odontoblasts to the mineralization site via active transport through the cell. This **intracellular** route actively controls the level of calcium in the mineralizing area, maintaining calcium concentrations that are not in equilibrium with other body fluids. Calcium is deposited onto the type I collagen matrix and mineral crystal deposition occurs at the **gap zone** within the collagen fibrils. A pool of **chondroitin sulphate** (CS), decorin and biglycan is secreted at **mineralization front** and transported intracellularly through the odontoblast process. Although general levels of proteoglycans at the mineralization site and in mineralized dentine are lower than those found in pre-dentine, the CS-rich proteoglycans are distributed in mineralized connective tissues **interfibrally** and associated with the gap zones of the collagen fibres. It is this CS proteoglycan pool that is associated with guiding mineral deposition as the CS may be involved in transport of calcium and phosphate to the gap zone in the collagen. Other important proteoglycans and glycoproteins are essential in directing the mineralization of dentine and ensuring adequate and sufficient mineralization. One such glycoprotein is **dentine phosphoprotein** (DPP). This highly phosphorylated dentine-specific protein is secreted at the mineralizing front. It is **highly acidic** and has a **high affinity** for calcium and hydroxyapatite surfaces. Changes in the conformation of the protein allow it to bind increasing numbers of calcium ions. In high concentrations, it inhibits crystal formation and so by

controlling the release and level of DPP, the odontoblast controls the initiation of mineralization and rate of deposition. Several other proteins have been shown *in vitro* to be associated with mineralization. The classical bone-associated glycoproteins are also found within the dentine. **Osteopontin** is a phosphorylated protein capable of promoting mineralization and **osteonectin** has been shown to inhibit growth of hydroxyapatite crystals while promoting the binding of calcium and phosphate to collagen.

Other Factors Limiting/Controlling Mineralization

Collagen is found in many other soft connective tissues and in pre-dentine, tissues that are not mineralized. Specific glycoproteins and proteoglycans have been shown to have differing roles in promoting and inhibiting mineralization and crystal growth. Included in these proteins are the dermatan sulphate proteoglycans, which are found in pre-dentine but not in mineralized dentine. It is likely that dermatan sulphate species of proteoglycans assist in inhibiting mineralization; however, other factors also regulate mineralization. **Pyrophosphate** is found in soft tissues and body fluids and actively inhibits mineralization. In hard tissues **pyrophosphatase** can be identified, which degrades any pyrophosphate present, allowing mineralization to occur.

There are several reasons why there are these two distinct mechanisms for dentine mineralization. Matrix vesicles are required for the mineralization of mantle dentine, because not only is there a need to produce mineral where none existed before, but the matrix formed is secreted from newly differentiating odontoblasts with some contribution from the dental papilla cells. Not all the matrix components are present and some nucleation sites are not expressed. There is also the need to form a mineral that can be seeded onto the dentine matrix. After mantle dentine has been synthesized and secreted and odotoblast differentiation is complete, odontoblasts express all the matrix components required for nucleation sites and the initial hydroxyapatite crystal seeds grow at the expense of calcium and phosphate that passes into the matrix through the cell.

Tooth Root Formation

Roots are incomplete at eruption and root development is completed approximately 12 months post eruption for deciduous teeth and 2–3 years post eruption for the permanent dentition. The root is formed primarily of dentine but lined with cementum and for root formation to begin, epithelial tissue is required to map out the shape of the tooth and initiate and mediate root odontoblast differentiation and subsequent dentine secretion. The epithelium responsible for this is known as **Hertwig epithelial root sheath** (HERS) and is formed from a downward growth of the cervical loop. The HERS is bilaminar, consisting of cells from both the inner and outer enamel epithelium and grows as a collar enclosing the future root. The inner cells of HERS do not differentiate into ameloblasts; however, they are responsible for inducing cells on the periphery of the dental papilla, adjacent to the HERS to differentiate into odontoblasts for root dentine secretion. As in the crown, a gradient of root odontoblast differentiation and root dentine secretion can be observed from crown to root apex. The HERS fragments once root dentine secretion begins and exposes the root surface to the ectomesenchymal cells of the dental follicle. This stimulates follicular cells adjacent to the root dentine to differentiate into cementoblasts which are responsible for cementogenesis and secretion of cementum. The HERS fragments lie adjacent to the root as cell clusters and are generally quiescent and functionless. These clusters are known as the **cell rests of Malassez** and, although quiescent, can be stimulated to proliferate during periods of inflammation (e.g. pulpitis) and give rise to dental (radicular) cysts.

Two types of **cementum** are formed: cellular and acellular. As cementoblasts differentiate from the follicular cells they begin to secrete collagen fibrils and non-collagenous proteins (e.g. bone sialoprotein, osteocalcin) along and at right angles to the root surface before migrating away from the developing root. As the cementoblasts migrate, more collagen is deposited. This is **acellular cementum** and is the first formed cementum. The matrix secreted by the cementoblasts subsequently mineralizes and during mineralization the cementoblasts move away from the cementum, and the collagen fibres left along the surface of the root eventually join the forming periodontal ligament fibres. **Cellular cementum** is formed once the majority of the tooth development is complete and once the tooth is present in the occlusion. Cellular cementum is formed around the collagen fibre bundles and the cementoblasts become entrapped within the matrix they produce. These cells trapped within the cementum are termed cementocytes. The origin of **cementoblasts** is thought to be different for acellular and cellular cementum. Current thinking is that cementoblasts responsible for acellular cementum arise from the ectomesenchymal cells of the dental follicle adjacent to the developing root dentine whereas cementoblasts responsible for the synthesis and secretion of cellular cementum migrate from the adjacent area of bone. Interestingly, cellular cementum is not commonly found in teeth with one root, however in premolars and molars it is found only in the part of the root closest to the apex and in interradicular areas between multiple roots. It is also thought that the inner cells of the HERS have very brief secretory phase prior to it fragmenting. This results in the secretion of a thin hyaline layer of tissue containing enamel-like proteins. It is most prominent in the apical area of molars and premolars and less obvious in incisors and deciduous teeth.

Differential proliferation of the HERS in multi-rooted teeth causes the division of the root into two or three roots, as local proliferation causes invaginations of the HERS to give rise to multi-rooted teeth. Ingrowth of the root sheath towards the end of root development is responsible for apical closure of the root.

Epithelial–Mesenchymal Interactions in Tooth Development

The mammalian dentition comprises a series of homologous structures whose difference, based on their position in the jaw, relate to size and shape. In this respect incisors form distally and molars more proximally. Mechanisms therefore exist for patterning different regions of future dentition and this occurs at a molecular level in the ectomesenchyme prior to initiation of tooth development. The generation of a tooth in the developing embryo thus requires coordinated molecular signalling between the first branchial arch ectoderm and the underlying neural-crest-derived ectomesenchyme.

Sequential and reciprocal signalling between the epithelial (enamel organ) and mesenchymal (dental papilla) compartments of the tooth germ regulates the formation of the complex shape of individual teeth. Signalling molecules of different families mediate cell communication during tooth development. The majority of these belong to the transforming growth factor β (TGFβ), FGF, Hedgehog (Shh) and Wnt families. These signals regulate interactions between the enamel organ and dental papilla; however, they may also mediate cell–cell communication within each constituent part of the tooth germ. The genes regulated by these different signals include transcription factors and those encoding for cell-surface receptors on cells in either the enamel organ or dental papilla that regulate the competence of those cells to respond to the next signals. These genes also regulate the ability of the cells to respond to new signals that act reciprocally, which maintains communication between the enamel organ and dental papilla.

The appearance of transient signalling centres in the enamel organ during tooth development is crucial to maintaining these epithelial–mesenchymal interactions and thus allowing tooth development to proceed. The first of these centres appears during the bud stage and then again when the enamel knot(s) appear. They may express many different signalling molecules including Shh, BMPs, FGFs and Wnts and regulate coronal development and the initiation of the secondary enamel knot(s) at the sites of the folding of the inner enamel epithelium leading to cusp formation.

One of the first signalling events in tooth development addresses the question of how a tooth knows to become a tooth. Tissue recombination studies have demonstrated that the oral epithelium controls events that commit the neural crest cells of the ectomesenchyme to become teeth and the BMPs and FGFs regulate this process. It is the epithelium that induces cell competence in the mesenchyme to drive subsequent tooth development. The first epithelial signals induce in the mesenchyme the expression of reciprocal signalling molecules (FGF and BMP4), which act back on the epithelium regulating the formation of the primary epithelial band. Further signals then regulate formation of the bud stage and condensation of the ectomesenchymal cells. These cells of the ectomesenchyme maintain the expression of transcription factors (e.g. Msx1) that had been earlier induced by signalling from the oral epithelium. This upregulates the expression of new genes (such as the transcription factor Runx2 and the signalling molecule FGF3), which then regulates the progression from the bud to cap stage. This transition from bud stage to cap stage is a critical developmental step, marking the onset of the development of the crown. At the same time BMP4 expression in the ectomesenchyme is required for the formation of the enamel knot.

Integral to tooth morphogenesis is the enamel knot, a transient signalling centre formed by epithelial cells of the enamel organ at the future cusp tip. The enamel knot is a transient structure of condensed epithelial cells that do not proliferate (they express the p21 gene associated with the exit from the cell cycle). These cells, however, stimulate proliferation in the flanking epithelium, which grows to surround the mesenchymal dental papilla. The enamel knot is the epithelial origin of the signalling molecules (including BMP-4, Shh, FGF4 and 9, and Wnts). The growth factors BMPs and FGFs induce the expression of several transcription factors in the developing dental papilla, many of which are essential for tooth development to progress. These include the transcription factors Msx1 and Pax9. Reciprocal interactions between the mesenchyme and epithelium maintain the enamel knot and mediate the formation of the four cell layers within the developing enamel organ. Shh is another important signalling molecule as its secretion from the enamel knot influences growth of the cervical loops. It also regulates crown patterning (crown shape) by initiating formation of the secondary enamel knots, which determine the sites where the inner enamel epithelium folds (due to differential cell proliferation) and cusp development starts. This reciprocal epithelial–mesenchymal signalling establishes memory and induces differentiation (Feature box 10.1).

To understand how we get teeth of different shapes in the correct position in the dental arch (patterning of the dentition), two theories have been proposed. The **field model** proposes that local factors responsible for tooth shape reside in the ectomesenchyme in specific regions or fields and tell the ectomesenchyme to form a tooth of a specific shape. A second theory, the **clone theory**, proposes that clones of ectomesenchymal cells are already programmed by the epithelium to become a specific tooth with a specific shape. Evidence exists to support both theories and it is likely that both may influence tooth development. The Odontogenic Homebox Code (field theory) is based on observing restricted expression of certain homeobox genes (such as Barx1, Dlx1/2 and Msx1/2, and known to be important in tooth development) in early developing ectomesenchyme. It has been observed that expression of Msx1 and Msx2 is restricted to areas of ectomesenchyme corresponding to regions where incisor teeth will eventually develop but not regions where multi-cuspid teeth will develop. Conversely, expression of the genes Dlx1 and Dlx2 has been observed in ectomesenchyme corresponding to regions where multi-cuspid teeth, but not single-cusped teeth, form. These areas of expression are broad and overlap but may provide the positional information for development of teeth of specific shape in the correct position in the dental arch (Feature box 10.2).

Amelogenesis

Amelogenesis is the formation of enamel and begins with secretion of a partially mineralized enamel matrix by terminally differentiated **ameloblasts** until a full thickness of tissue is achieved. This provides an organic scaffold for subsequent mineralization; however, this matrix already contains in the region of 30% mineral. This is the secretory phase of amelogenesis. Following this, maturation of secreted enamel matrix is achieved beginning from the amelodentinal junction (ADJ) and proceeding outwards. During this phase there is considerable resorption of the majority of the organic matrix, which is replaced by crystal growth.

The secretory stage of amelogenesis begins immediately after the onset of dentinogenesis at future cusp tips and following ameloblast differentiation. Ameloblasts secrete an organic enamel matrix which is almost instantly partially mineralized. This first formed enamel matrix is composed of organic, protein matrix (20% by volume), inorganic hydroxyapatite (16% by volume) and water (64% by volume). The organic matrix is comprised of two families of enamel proteins: the **amelogenins** and the **non-amelogenins**. The amelogenins are small soluble hydrophobic proteins and have a significant role in the regulation of enamel prism orientation, enamel mineralization and crystal growth. The non-amelogenins are a mixture of proteins including **enamelin**, **tuftelin** and **ameloblastin**. Enamelin is a larger acidic protein encoded by the ENAM gene. Mutations in this gene give rise to the autosomal dominant amelogenesis imperfecta, suggesting a role for the protein in amelogenesis. Tuftelin is an acidic glycoprotein suggested to have a role in enamel mineralization, as has ameloblastin. The inorganic phase of this initial enamel matrix consists of small crystals of hydroxyapatite and further crystal growth is observed during the maturation phase of amelogenesis. As a full thickness of enamel is secreted by the late secretory stage, changes become apparent in the first formed enamel next to ADJ. This consists of proteolysis of the amelogenins with concurrent increase in crystal growth and an increase in mineralization. During the maturation stage there continues to be a selective loss of protein (amelogenin) through proteolysis and resorption, loss of water and further growth of mineral crystals.

The ameloblast differentiates from inner enamel epithelium as the first pre-dentine is secreted. A number of changes to the cell are observed as it terminally differentiates including an increase in cell length, increase in synthetic organelles, polarization of the nuclei to the basal third of the cell and the development of a short, stubby process at the secretory pole of the cell. This process is termed the **Tome's process** and is responsible for the formation of the structural unit of the enamel: the enamel prism or enamel rod. The first formed enamel, however, is structureless and is called **aprismatic enamel**. This is because the distinct Tome's process has not yet developed, thus amorphous secretion from cell body of ameloblast is observed. Enamel structure is based on numerous enamel prisms/rods and each is made by one ameloblast and consists of many Hap crystals. These prisms are perpendicular to the ADJ and define the course of the ameloblast as it moves towards the future enamel surface, secreting enamel matrix as it does so.

Once the Tome's Process develops, two sites of secretion exist. One is from the proximal end of the process/cell body and gives rise to inter-rod or **interprismatic enamel**. The second level of secretion is from the distal end of the process and is responsible for the formation of the enamel rods or **prismatic enamel**. One ameloblast (Tome's process) gives rise to one enamel prism, but interprismatic enamel is formed from adjacent cells. Both interprismatic and prismatic enamel have the same biochemical composition but differ in the orientation of hydroxyapatite crystals. Aprismatic enamel has a more random orientation of crystals at the ADJ. This dual level of secretion from the ameloblast gives enamel its characteristic structure, which at the light microscopic level is a fish-scale/keyhole appearance. The Tome's process is always short and remains on the formative surface of enamel matrix and is not embedded in the matrix like the odontoblast process is in the dentinal tubules. Thus, enamel is not permeable like dentine.

Enamel Mineralization

Enamel mineralization occurs in a tissue-specific micro-environment and the size, morphology and stability of the formed crystals are determined by the degree of supersaturation of calcium and phosphate in the fluid phase and is greatly influenced by the presence of a large number of regulators which are the matrix proteins.

Calcium reaches the matrix through the enamel organ by intercellular and transcellular pathways. Active transport systems, using carrier proteins in cell membranes, may be involved and calcium may also flow up through concentration gradients from blood plasma to enamel matrix. The first formed aprismatic enamel is poorly organized with random crystal sizes and morphology. Initial crystals grow by fusion of nucleation sites but once a prismatic structure takes shape growth is increased by length, not width, and controlled by the amelogenin protein which forms **nanospheres**.

The amelogenin nanospheres control hydroxyapatite crystal growth by acting as spacers between the crystals, providing space for new crystal deposition and inhibiting crystal fusion. There is good correlation between the size of the nanospheres and spacing of the enamel crystallites, suggesting that the width of the nanospheres controls the final thickness of the enamel crystals. In the maturation phase of amelogenesis, the matrix proteins have a reduced role to play as most organic material has been degraded through proteolysis and removed. Matrix proteins are removed long before crystal growth ends and these may accumulate in the extracellular space around the ameloblasts where they may inhibit cell activity and so control or limit the thickness of enamel deposition.

During enamel maturation, the Tome's process is lost so thin-layer structureless aprismatic enamel is found on the tooth surface. The ameloblast cell-surface membrane next to the enamel modulates between a ruffled and smooth surface corresponding to proteolytic degradation and removal of the amelogenin nanospheres and influx of mineral ions. There is a reduction in cell height, loss of synthetic organelles within the cell and an increase in surface area with the presence of the ruffled border. Further regressive changes are observed as the cell enters a protective stage. At this point, once enamel formation is complete, the enamel organ regresses to a thin layer of cuboidal cells, known as the **reduced enamel epithelium**, which fuses with the oral epithelium as the tooth erupts into the oral cavity.

Tooth Morphology

Teeth are comprised of a crown and one or more sets of roots (Table 10.1). Within the permanent dentition there are four basic types:

1) **incisors**, which have a horizontal incisal edge;
2) **canines**, with a single large cusp;
3) **premolars**, with two cusps of varying sizes;
4) **molars**, which have four or five cusps.

The premolars are absent in the deciduous dentition (Table 10.2).

When considering the surfaces of the teeth, six terms may be used. For each tooth, the surface pointing around the arch towards the midline is the **mesial** surface. The surface facing away from the midline is called the **distal** surface. The surface facing towards the tongue is the **lingual** surface but, when considering the upper teeth, it may be termed the **palatal** surface. The tooth surface facing outwards, away from the tongue is termed the **vestibular** surface. When referring to the molar teeth the term **buccal** may be used. The biting surface is termed **incisal** for the incisors and **occlusal** for all other teeth.

Development of the Tooth-Supporting Structures

While the development and formation of the cementum has been discussed earlier in this chapter, formation of the periodontal ligament, alveolar bone and junctional epithelium has not yet been considered.

Periodontal Ligament

It is the cells from the dental follicle that give rise to the periodontal ligament (PDL). Formation of the PDL begins with the differentiation of ligament fibroblasts from cells of the dental follicle. During the initial stages of root formation the follicular cells show increased proliferation and the innermost cells of the follicle near the forming root differentiate into **cementoblasts** and the outermost cells differentiate into **osteoblasts**. The centrally located cells differentiate into fibroblasts. These fibroblasts secrete a collagen matrix producing the periodontal ligament fibres, which get embedded in the developing cementum and alveolar bone. At first, all the developing fibres of the periodontal

Table 10.1 Tooth morphology and anatomical features of the permanent dentition.

Tooth type	Features
Maxillary central incisor	Mesial surface straight and at sharp right angle to incisive edge Disto-incisal angle rounded Crown large in proportion to root and inclined palatally Single tapering root, rounded triangular cross-section
Mandibular central incisor	Single root, flattened mesiodistally, curves distally Incisive edge at right angles to a line bisecting the crown labiolingually Root 12 mm long with marked distal longitudinal groove Smallest tooth in permanent dentition
Maxillary lateral incisor	Mesial-incisal angle acute, disto-incisal angle more rounded Incisive edge marked downward slope to shorter distal surface Crown more rounded, shorter and narrower than central incisor Single tapering root to pointed distally curving apex
Mandibular lateral incisor	Larger than first incisor with fan shaped crown, wider incisive edge Incisive edge twisted distally in a lingual direction (follows dental arch) Mesial surface of crown longer than distal, incisive edge slopes Root 14 mm long
Maxillary canine	Single pointed cusp Distal slope longer than mesial Very long single root, rounded triangular cross-section Disto- and mesiopalatal surfaces of root often grooved
Mandibular canine	Distal profile of crown rounded Crown narrower mesiodistally Only this canine capable of bifurcated root Root tends to curve distally, crown leans distally in relation to root
Maxillary first premolar	Two roots, buccal and palatal, curve distally Two sharply defined cusps with buccal larger than palatal Mesial slope of buccal cusp longer than distal Concave canine fossa on mesial surface Occlusal outline more angular than maxillary second premolar
Mandibular first premolar	Two cusps, joined by central enamel ridge, large pointed buccal cusp Two occlusal fossae, distal larger than mesial Lingual inclination of crown on root Single rounded root, may curve distally
Maxillary second premolar	Two cusps, one palatal, one buccal, shallower and equal in size than first premolar No canine fossa Oval occlusal outline Single root, flattened mesiodistally, longer than first premolar

Table 10.1 (Continued)

Tooth type	Features
Mandibular second premolar	Large crown than first premolar
	Usually three cusps, equal in size, less pointed
	Occlusal outline squarish, central fissure curves around buccal cusp
	Single conical root, curves distally to blunt apex
Maxillary first molar	Cusp of Carabelli on palatal surface in 50–70% of cases, four cusps
	Rhomboidal occlusal outline
	Largest maxillary tooth
	Three well-developed, separated roots, palatal longest, buccal curve distally
Mandibular first molar	Five cusps (3 buccal, 2 lingual), occlusal outline rectangular
	Bulbous, lingually inclined buccal surface with two grooves
	Largest mandibular tooth
	Two roots, mesial longer, flattened mesiodistally, grooved longitudinally
Maxillary second molar	No cusp of Carabelli and rhombic occlusal outline more obvious
	Roots less divergent, buccal roots same length
	Smaller overall than first molar
Mandibular second molar	Rounded square occlusal outline
	Four cusps, separated by pronounced central cruciform fissure pattern
	Buccal surface bulbous, lingually inclined terminating in buccal pit
	Two roots, similar to first molar but closer together and less broad
Maxillary third molar	Triangular occlusal outline (distopalatal cusp can be absent)
	Smallest maxillary tooth, crown 'too big for its roots'
	Largest cusp mesiopalatal
	Three roots, short, underdeveloped, convergent often fused
Mandibular third molar	Crown similar to second molar but smaller, four cusps
	Square/rectangular occlusal outline, corners rounded
	Two roots, short, underdeveloped and often fused

Table 10.2 Calcification and eruption dates for the deciduous dentition.

Tooth	Eruption	Calcification begins	Enamel complete
A	6–10 months	4 months i.u	2 months
B	8–12 months	4½ months i.u	3 months
C	18–20 months	5 months i.u	9 months
D	12–15 months	5 months i.u	6 months
E	24–36 months	6 months i.u	12 months

i.u., interuterine.

ligament run obliquely in a coronal direction from tooth to bone. This changes as the tooth erupts and remodelling of the follicle into a PDL begins at the cemento-enamel junction and proceeds in an apical direction. The part of PDL fibres present in the cementum and alveolar bone are called **Sharpey's fibres**. Some of the multipotent cells of the dental follicle that are capable of producing bone, cementum and the ligament will be preserved as undifferentiated progenitor cells in the mature PDL, primarily in association with the perivasculature, and are known as periodontal ligament stem cells.

The fibre bundles that exit the cementum and alveolar bone and form the periodontal ligament are called principal fibres. Depending on the location of these fibres they can be **dentoalveolar fibres** or **gingival fibres**. The dentoalveolar fibre groups of the PDL are:

- alveolar crest group: near the cervical region,
- horizontal fibre group: near the midroot,
- oblique fibre group: immediately above apical group,
- apical fibre group: near the apical area of the root,
- interradicular group: between two roots.

The gingival fibre group of the PDL are:

- dentogingival group: these fibres are the most numerous, extending from the cervical cementum to the lamina propria of the gingiva,
- alveologingival group: these fibres extend from the alveolar crest to the lamina propria of the gingiva,
- circular of circumferential fibres: continuous around the neck of the tooth,
- trans-septal fibres: these fibres extend from the cervical cementum of one tooth to the cervical cementum of the other.

The Dentogingival group and alveologingival group fibres embed in attached gingiva and free gingiva and also called attached gingival group and free gingival group fibres.

Alveolar Bone

As the tooth root begins to form and cementum is secreted, bone is formed in the adjacent area. Like with other types of bone in the body, the cells responsible are osteoblasts but, in this case, have differentiated from the cells of the dental follicle. As with the formation of primary cementum, collagen fibres are created on the surface nearest the tooth and remain there until attaching to fibres of the developing periodontal ligament. The alveolar bone is found on the alveolar process, a thin piece of bone separating the teeth. It is composed of outer and inner alveolar plates and the individual tooth sockets are separated by interdental septa. The bone lining the tooth socket is the alveolar bone proper whereas the remainder of alveolar process is supporting bone of the mandible or maxilla. The alveolar plate can be known by a number of anatomical terms which are directly related to its function and appearance histologically or radiologically:

- **cribriform plate**, due to the presence of sieve-like holes throughout its structure;
- **bundle bone**, due to the numerous bundles of collagen fibres that pass into it;
- **lamina dura**, a clinical term based on the dense appearance of the alveolar bone in radiographs.

The remaining bone found in the alveolar process is compact and cancellous (spongy) bone.

Junctional Epithelium

The junctional epithelium is a collar-like band of non-keratinized stratified squamous epithelium which extends from the cement–enamel junction to the base of the gingival sulcus. Coronally, it is approximately 15–30 cells thick and apically narrows to one to three cells. Its length is between 0.25 and 1.35 mm. It is initially derived from the reduced enamel epithelium (REE), a thin piece of tissue that is the remnants of the

Table 10.3 Calcification and eruption dates for the permanent dentition.

Tooth	Eruption		Calcification begins		Enamel complete	
1 Maxillary	7–8 years	6–9 years	3–4 months	1 year	4–5 years	5 years
Mandibular	6–7 years		3–4 months		4–5 years	
2 Maxillary	8–9 years		10–12 months		4–5 years	
Mandibular	7–8 years		3–4 months		4–5 years	
3 Maxillary	11–12 years	9–12 years	4–5 months		6–7 years	7 years
Mandibular	9–10 years		4–5 months		6–7 years	
4 Maxillary	10–11 years		1½–1¾ years	2–3 years	5–6 years	6 years
Mandibular	10–12 years		1¾–2 years		5–6 years	
5 Maxillary	10–12 years		2–2¼ years		6–7 years	7 years
Mandibular	11–12 years		2¼–2½ years		6–7 years	
6 Maxillary	6–7 years		At birth		2½–3 years	
Mandibular	6–7 years		At birth		2½–3 years	
7 Maxillary	12–13 years		2½–3 years	3 years	7–8 years	
Mandibular	12–13 years		2½–3 years		7–8 years	
8 Maxillary	18–21 years		7–9 years		12–16 years	
Mandibular	18–21 years		8–10 years		12–16 years	

Root development: primary complete about 12 months after eruption; permanent complete about 3 years after eruption.

enamel organ. At the completion of enamel formation, the enamel organ collapses in on itself (becoming several cell layers thick) and sits covering the crown of the tooth until eruption. The REE is replaced once the tooth erupts and is rapidly lost and replaced by squamous epithelial cells. The transformed REE and oral epithelium fuse and form the dentogingival junction and the junctional epithelium. Final conversion of REE to junctional epithelium may not occur until 3–4 years post eruption (Table 10.3).

11

Craniofacial Development

Abigail S. Tucker

Department of Craniofacial Development and Stem Cell Biology, King's College London, London, UK

Learning Objectives

- To be able to describe the anatomical development and function of the jaws and temporo-mandibular joint.
- To understand the principle of taste and the formation and anatomy of taste buds.
- To describe the development of the skull vault and the role of sutures as growth centres.
- To be able to list examples of craniofacial syndromes and how they are inherited.

Clinical Relevance

An understanding of the cellular and molecular mechanisms controlling craniofacial growth and development is important not only in explaining the fully developed anatomy of the head and neck but also to understand the mechanism by which craniofacial abnormalities such as cleft lip and palate arise.

Introduction

The face and skull together form the craniofacial complex. Classically these two parts are known as the **viscerocranium**, which includes the jaws and support skeleton, and the **neurocranium**, which houses the brain.

In this chapter the anatomy, function and development of key parts of the craniofacial complex will be discussed, followed by sections on syndromes that affect the craniofacial region.

Jaws and Support Skeleton

The lower jaw of mammals comprises the **dentary** bone, which is also known as the **mandible**. The upper jaw is formed from the fusion of the maxilla, lateral and medial nasal processes and the frontonasal process. The maxilla and mandible both derive from the **first pharyngeal** (branchial) arch. The highly reduced tongue skeleton and Reichert's cartilage are derived from the second pharyngeal arch.

Basic Sciences for Dental Students, First Edition. Edited by Simon A. Whawell and Daniel W. Lambert.
© 2018 John Wiley & Sons Ltd. Published 2018 by John Wiley & Sons Ltd.
Companion website: www.wiley.com/go/whawell/basic_sciences_for_dental_students

The skeletal elements of the jaw can be divided into those that form by **endochondrial ossification** or **membranous ossification** (also known as intramembraneous ossification), or remain as **persistent cartilage**. Endochondrial ossification occurs when a bone is formed overlying an initial cartilaginous template. In contrast, membranous ossification occurs when a bone forms *de novo* without the need for a cartilaginous template. Both of these processes occur in the head, with endochondrial ossification found in the cranial base and middle ear, while membranous ossification is responsible for the majority of the jaws and cranial vault. In addition some cartilages are not converted to bone but remain as cartilages throughout the animal's life, such as those associated with the external ear and nose.

During embryonic development the craniofacial region is initially formed by a cartilaginous skeleton, known as the **chondrocranium**. The bones then form during a second wave of development and form the **dermatocranium**.

One of the first cartilages to form is **Meckel's cartilage**, which runs the length of the developing mandible. Meckel's cartilage is of particular interest as it forms the first structure of the lower jaw and in mammals has a number of fates (Figure 11.1). In the most rostral region (rostral means towards the front of the craniofacial region) it remains cartilaginous and holds the two arms of the mandible together in the midline, forming small nodules of cartilage on the dorsal surface of the **symphysis.** Further back in the jaw Meckel's becomes completely surrounded by the dentary bone and is reabsorbed by the action of chondroclasts (cartilage-absorbing cells) and through matrix metalloproteinases (MMPs) that degrade protein components of the extracellular matrix (ECM). There is also some evidence that the cells of Meckel's cartilage in this region can transform into bone cells (osteoblasts) and therefore take part in the final structure of the dentary. Although Meckel's cartilage is no longer visible postnatally, it acts as a scaffold onto which the bone is laid, and is therefore important as a template for the jaw. The most proximal part of Meckel's transforms into bone and forms the first two **ossicles of the middle ear**, the malleus and the incus. These join with the stapes to form the three-ossicle chain found in all mammalian ears. In contrast, all non-mammal land vertebrates have only one middle ear bone, the stapes (also known as the columella) (Feature box 11.1, Figure 11.2).

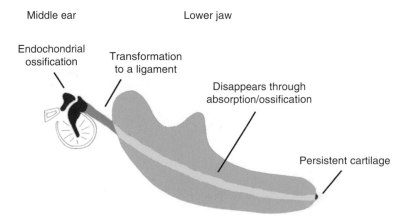

Figure 11.1 Fates of Meckel's cartilage. Meckel's cartilage at the symphysis remains as persistent cartilage (blue). The main body of Meckel's disappears during embryonic development (yellow). The most proximal part undergoes ossification and forms two of the three middle ear bones (red). The part between the lower jaw and middle ear transforms into the sphenomandibular ligament (green). Forming dentary bone in orange.

Feature box 11.1 Comparison of the mammalian and non-mammalian jaw

In all mammals the lower jaw (mandible) is made up of a single bone, the dentary. In all other jawed vertebrates (fish, amphibians, reptiles, birds) the lower jaw is made from a complex of overlapping bones. Presence of a single bone in the lower jaw is therefore one of the defining features of mammals, and is widely used by palaeontologists to classify animals as mammals based on their fossilized skulls. In mammals the dentary bone is therefore often referred to as the mandible. The dentary bone is named as it classically houses the teeth in a range of vertebrates. In mammals the jaws are articulated by a joint between the dentary bone of the lower jaw and the squamosal bone of the upper jaw, known as the temporomandibular joint (TMJ) in humans. In all non-mammalian jawed vertebrates the jaw articulation is found between the quadrate (or palatoquadrate) and articular part of Meckel's cartilage; the TMJ is therefore unique to mammals (see Figure 11.4). In mammals the main body of Meckel's is resorbed while in non-mammals it persists, providing a key structure for the lower jaw. A central question in evolution for the last 200 years has been what happened to the skeletal elements that formed the primary jaw joint in non-mammalian vertebrates? Evidence from comparative anatomy, developmental biology and the fossil record has shown that some of the bones of the jaw in non-mammals became incorporated into the middle ear in mammals during evolution, creating the unique three-ossicle (bone) ear. The presence of three bones in the middle ear and a single bone in the jaw are therefore intricately linked and part of the same evolutionary history (Figure 11.2).

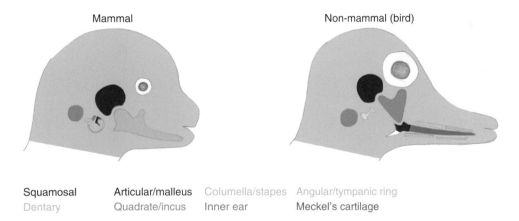

| Squamosal | Articular/malleus | Columella/stapes | Angular/tympanic ring |
| Dentary | Quadrate/incus | Inner ear | Meckel's cartilage |

Figure 11.2 Jaw articulation in mammals and non-mammals. A comparison of the jaw articulation. Mammal on left, bird on right. The homologous skeletal elements are shown in the same colour to illustrate the shift in function, position and size of these elements during evolution.

As the most proximal part of Meckel's cartilage forms part of the middle ear it is important that the jaw and ear become physically separated during embryogenesis, to prevent sound transfer to the ear when eating. This is achieved by the transformation of Meckel's cartilage, in between the dentary and the ear ossicles, into two ligaments, the **sphenomandibular** (also known as the malleomandibular) ligament and the anterior malleolar ligament. The sphenomandibular ligament is involved in jaw joint movement by limiting the distension of the mandible, preventing dislocation. The connected anterior malleolar ligament attaches the **malleus** (the first middle ear ossicle) to the anterior wall of the tympanic cavity and may stabilize the mandible. This transformation of cartilage

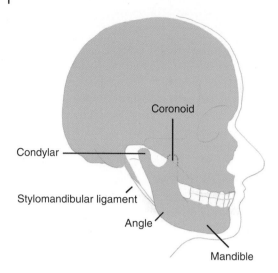

Figure 11.3 Schematic of the human skull showing the processes of the mandible (dentary bone) and its connection to the rest of the skull.

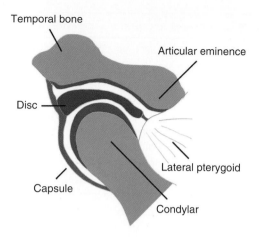

Figure 11.4 Schematic of the TMJ showing the position of the disc at the junction of the upper and lower jaw.

into ligament allows the ear and jaw to function independently. The embryonic history of Meckel's cartilage highlights the complex fate of structures in the craniofacial region.

The Temporomandibular Joint

The human mandible can be divided into the main body, known as the **ramus**, the **alveolar bone**, which forms the sockets for the teeth, and, at the back of the jaw, the articulation with the upper jaw, known as the **temporomandibular joint** or TMJ. The jaw joint is found between the **condylar process** of the mandible and the **glenoid fossa** of the temporal bone in the upper jaw (Figure 11.3). The temporal bone is a compound bone created by fusion of a number of separate bones including the squamosal, petrosal, styloid, mastoid and tympanic ring.

The TMJ is not a typical joint. A disc separates the condylar from the glenoid fossa and slides in and out, forming a gliding joint. This is known as a **ginglymoarthrodial joint** as it is hinged and sliding (Figure 11.4). As the

TMJ is involved in both mastication and speaking it is often thought to be the most frequently used joint in the human body.

When the mouth opens the condylar initially rotates involving the lower synovial space. With further opening the condylar slides forward along the articular eminence. The articular eminence limits the forward movement of the condylar. The movement is also restricted by the temporomandibular ligament and the stylomandibular ligament.

The condylar process of the mandible is a **secondary cartilage**. After the dentary bone is formed a second wave of cartilage initiation occurs located at specific areas, often associated with articulation sites. These later-forming cartilages are known as the secondary cartilages. In all mammals a secondary cartilage caps the back of the dentary, forming the condylar process. The condylar is largely replaced by bone during embryogenesis but remains cartilaginous at the articular surface until adult life. The condylar cartilage has three important roles: it forms the articulation surface for the TMJ, it forms the disc of the TMJ and it acts as a growth centre. Cells at the condylar articulation surface **proliferate** and then **differentiate**, becoming **hypertrophic** before undergoing endochondrial ossification. This allows the

Feature box 11.2 TMJ disorders

Pain associated with the TMJ is common, particularly in females, and is known as TMJ dysfunction (TMD). TMD is characterized by pain and can be associated with restricted movement of the mandible and clicking noises. Approximately 20–30% of the population can be affected by TMD. TMD can have multiple causes and the mechanisms behind the pain are poorly understood. The clicking or popping noise is created when the disc suddenly moves to and from a temporarily displaced position. If the disc fails to move back into position the jaw can become locked in position.

TMJ pain has been suggested to be caused or aggravated by poor occlusion, although the evidence for this is circumspect. Orthodontic treatment to reduce TMD-associated pain is therefore not currently recommended. In contrast, bite plates, also known as occlusal splints, are often recommended by dentists. Such plates are generally worn at night to reduce abnormal muscle activity.

mandible to grow, making space for the permanent dentition. Asymmetrical growth of the condylar leads to asymmetrical mandible growth, creating problems with functional occlusion and with the aesthetic appearance of the face. Endochondrial ossification of the condylar process appears to be stimulated by mechanical signals, with ossification being severely delayed in mice without teeth or on a mash (soft) diet.

During embryonic development the **disc** forms from the top layer of the developing condyle, separating from it to form a space for the synovial capsule above and underneath. This occurs at approximately 12 weeks during human development. Interaction with the forming condyle is vital for correct glenoid fossa formation, and if the glenoid fossa and condylar do not meet successfully the fossa is defective.

Congenital defects associated with the condylar include ankylosis of the disc to the condylar head or to the glenoid fossa, or formation of a small condylar. In addition condylar defects are associated with some craniofacial syndromes, such as Treacher Collins syndrome (mandibulofacial dysostosis) and oculoauriculovertebral (OAV) spectrum (which includes hemifacial microsomia and Goldenhar syndrome). Problems in the TMJ in adult life can lead to TMJ disorders (see Feature box 11.2).

Above and below the condylar on the mandible are the main muscle attachment sites for the jaw-opening and -closing muscles, which attach to the **coronoid** process (superior to the TMJ) and **angle** (inferior to the TMJ) (Figure 11.3). In many animals the inferior process projects out and is known as the angular process rather than angle (see Feature box 11.3). Similar to the condyle, a secondary cartilage is also associated with the anterior border of the coronoid process during embryonic development in humans. As with the condylar cartilage, the coronoid cartilage acts as a growth centre, increasing the size of the coronoid, but is lost before birth. The muscles that attach to the coronoid and angle also influence the shape of these skeletal elements, with large muscle attachments leading to larger processes due to mechanical force. In mice loss of the **tendons** that allow the **muscles** to attach to the developing angular bone leads to a loss of this process, while severing the muscles that attach to the coronoid process in a guinea pig leads to a reduction in the size of this process. The final shape of cranial skeletal elements is therefore determined not just by the initial layout of the bone but also by the presence and persistence of secondary cartilages and by muscle attachment, which together shape the skeletal elements in an integrated way.

Feature box 11.3 Dentary variation across mammals

Above and below the condylar on the mandible are the main muscle attachment sites for the jaw-opening and -closing muscles, which attach to the coronoid process (superior to the TMJ) and angle (inferior to the TMJ) (Figure 11.3). The shape and size of the condylar and angle (also known as the angular process) vary considerably throughout mammals and are closely linked to diet. Most herbivores, for example, have a small coronoid process and therefore a weak muscle attachment and poor jaw closing muscles. Carnivores, in contrast, generally have a large coronoid, accommodating a large muscle attachment and allowing fast closure of the jaws, essential for predation. The shape of the angular process also varies: mammals with an upright stance (head at a 90° angle to the neck), such as humans, have an angle instead of an angular process that sticks out. In contrast, in mammals where the head is in the same plane as the neck (such as the mouse) a large angular process forms as a muscle-attachment site. Intriguingly it is also possible to tell the difference between a marsupial and placental mammal based only on the angle of the angular process. Marsupials have an inwardly inflected angular process in contrast to the placental mammals where the angular process forms in the same plane as the rest of the dentary. It is therefore possible to predict the diet, stance and lifestyle of a mammal simply by studying the shape and size of the proximal region of the mandible.

Cranial and Facial Sutures

To allow space for the **brain** to grow during childhood the brain case is constructed of a network of bones separated by **sutures** (Figure 11.5). Down the middle of the skull runs the sagittal suture, while across the skull at a 90° angle to the sagittal suture runs the coronal suture. The coronal divides the parietal bones from the frontal bones at the front of the head. Where the two sutures meet on top of the head the anterior **fontanelle** forms. Interestingly from studies in the mouse it has been shown that the frontal and parietal bones have a different embryonic origin, despite both being formed by membraneous ossification. The frontal bones are derived from neural crest, while the parietal bones are derived from the mesoderm. Near the base of the skull the lamboidal suture separates the parietal bones from the occipital bone.

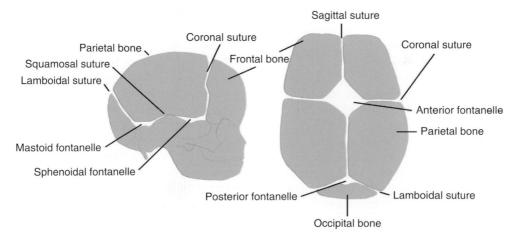

Figure 11.5 Skull vault: sutures. Sagittal (left) and anterior (right) views of the skull of a newborn outlining the sutures and fontanelles that separate the skull bones.

The sutures not only divide up the bones of the skull but also act as **growth centres**, with new bone being laid down at the margins of the sutures. Once the brain has reached its adult size the sutures ossify and the skull bones fuse together and no more expansion of the skull is possible. Fusion of the coronal, sagittal and lamboidal sutures occurs between the ages of 22 and 26, with the squamosal suture fusing in an adult's 30s. If the sutures prematurely fuse together this leads to **craniosynostosis** (see Feature boxes 11.4 and 11.5) and the skull becomes distorted as it grows asymmetrically to try and house the expanding brain.

Feature box 11.4 Genetics

As humans we have 23 paired chromosomes: one set from our mother, the other from our father. Genetic defects can be caused in a number of ways depending on the mutation involved. If the mutation is on the X chromosome it is known as X-linked, while mutations on the non-sex chromosomes are known as autosomal. In some cases a mutation needs to occur in only one copy of a gene for a phenotype to be observed. This is known as a dominant mutation. In other cases a single mutation on a gene can have no obvious effect, the other copy of the gene being able to maintain function. A phenotype in this case is only observed if both copies of the gene have a mutation. This is known as recessive. Mutations can be inherited or occur *de novo* (spontaneously).

Feature box 11.5 Craniosynostosis

In craniosynostosis the sutures fuse prematurely. It is a relatively common craniofacial defect with an incidence of 1 in 2500 live births. Suture fusion can be restricted to one suture or multiple and can be symmetrical or asymmetrical. Fusion of the sutures prevents growth of the brain in that direction, and the other sutures usually compensate by expanding, giving the skull a misshapen appearance. For example, if the coronal suture prematurely fuses the sagittal suture compensates and the skull widens to counter the inability to grow between the frontal and parietal bones. Patients with craniosynostosis need surgery to break open the sutures and to pull the skull bones apart to allow growth. Unfortunately these surgically induced sutures fuse again as the bones eventually meet and repeat operations are required to re-break them to allow further growth.

Craniosynostosis can be non-syndromic or syndromic (i.e. associated with a specific syndrome). The most common syndromic forms, such as Crouzon, Apert and Pfeiffer syndromes, have been shown to be caused by overstimulation of the fibroblast growth factor (FGF) signalling pathway. In these syndromes mutations in FGF receptors lead to too much FGF signalling causing premature bone formation at the sutures. Apert, Crouzon and Pfeiffer syndromes are autosomal dominant, so that a mutation in one copy of the FGF receptor can lead to the syndrome. Although characterized by craniosynostosis these three syndromes vary significantly in other aspects; for example, Apert is associated with mental retardation and limb defects whereas Crouzon syndrome is associated with no mental retardation and normal limbs. Intriguingly, mutations in the same gene can cause different syndromes (Crouzon and Pfeiffer syndrome can both be caused by mutations in Fgfr2), while mutations in different genes can cause the same syndrome (Crouzon syndrome can be caused by mutations in either Fgfr2 or Fgfr3). In addition to premature suture formation, Apert and Crouzon syndromes are associated with a narrow high arched palate and dental crowding. This results in malocclusion and delayed eruption. The maxilla is usually small, complicated by premature fusion of the facial sutures, resulting in a permanent underbite.

Sutures between bones are also found in the face and palate and again are essential for allowing growth as the face grows during infancy and adolescence.

Facial sutures readily respond to changes in their mechanical environment. The facial sutures can remain patent until late into an adult's life (60s–70s). Unlike the cranial sutures, facial sutures do not sit upon a **dura**, which may account for the differences in the timing of closure. In contrast to many of the other facial sutures, the mid-facial suture fuses in the late teens. Palatal expansion is therefore possible in young adults. Facial sutures are exposed to tensile, compressive and shearing stress during masticatory function. Manipulation of bone growth at the facial sutures is possible using **orthodontic treatment**, which can remodel the maxilla.

The Tongue

The tongue is important for mastication, speech and taste. It is formed by a contribution from the first three **pharyngeal arches** (with a possible contribution form the more caudal arches), with muscles derived from the somites. There are eight muscles, four of which are intrinsic and not attached to the bone. These change the shape of the tongue. The remaining four muscles are extrinsic, attached to the bone and change the position of the tongue. Congenital malformations of the tongue include **ankyloglossia**, where the lingual frenulum that tethers the tongue is short, **macroglossia**, where the tongue is very large, and **microglossia**, where the tongue is small, often associated with micrognathia, cleft tongue and bifid tongue.

The tongue contains concentrated taste buds in **taste papillae**, of which mammals have three types: **folliate**, **fungiform** and **circumvallate** (Figure 11.6). In addition the tongue is covered in a lawn of cone-shaped **non-gustatory filiform papillae** that have a mechanical role, cleaning the mouth, spreading saliva and moving food particles.

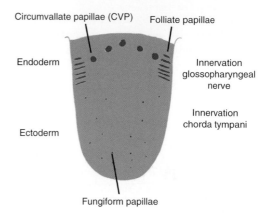

Figure 11.6 Tongue structure. Schematic showing the layout of taste buds, their embryonic origin and their innervation across the tongue.

The fungiform papillae are localized to the anterior of the tongue and house one taste bud per papilla. This part of the tongue is thought to be ectodermal in origin and is innervated by the **chorda tympani** nerve, a branch of the **facial** nerve. In contrast the folliate and circumvallate papillae (CVPs) are larger and house hundreds of taste buds. These arise at the back of the tongue from epithelium that is derived from the endoderm and are innervated by the **glossopharyngeal** nerve. The CVPs are found in a chevron pattern at the back of the tongue. Humans have 4–12 of these CVPs, but the number varies across the Animal Kingdom with mice having only one. Taste buds are aggregates of receptor cells. These cells convert a chemical stimulus into a neuronal input to mediate the sense of taste. Each taste bud comprises a bundle of round 100 cells containing type I, II and III cells. The type I cells are support cells. The type II cells transduce sweet, bitter and umami (savoury) tastes, while the type III cells transduce sour tastes (Figure 11.7). Taste cells are continuously renewed from the surrounding epithelium.

In addition to housing many taste buds, the tongue plays a central role in swallowing. The process of swallowing is known as **deglutition** and can be divided into three stages: oral, pharyngeal and oesophageal.

Oral surface

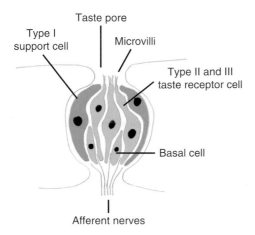

Figure 11.7 Diagram of a taste bud showing the contribution of different receptor cells, basal and support cells to the bud.

The oral stage involves mastication of food, with coordinated action by the tongue and muscles. These include the muscles of mastication (masseter, temporalis, pterygoid) and the buccinator and orbicularis oris muscles, which keep food contained within the oral cavity. Drooling, such as observed in patients with facial palsy, is due to a failure of these muscles to contract. After this voluntary stage the involuntary pharyngeal stage occurs, where chewed food is passed through the oropharynx and into the oesophagus, aided by the relaxation of the cricopharyngeus muscle. During this stage it is important that the oral cavity (oral pharynx) is shut off from the nasal cavity (nasal pharynx) and from the larynx. This is achieved by the contraction of the soft palate and laryngeal muscles. Finally, during the oesophageal stage the food (bolus) moves down the oesophagus, controlled by the peristalsis of the oesophageal muscles. Difficulties with swallowing are known as **dysphagia** and can lead to food aspiration, choking, coughing and regurgitation. Dysplagia is usually caused by another health problem including dementia, oral/oesophageal cancer, gastro-oesophageal reflux disease (GORD), head injury or stroke.

The Palate

The palate can be divided into the **soft palate** at the back of the mouth and the more anterior **hard palate**, with the **primary palate** behind the upper incisors. The palate forms from the palatal shelves, which rise up on either side of the oral cavity and fuse in the middle line to separate the oral cavity from the nasal passages (Figure 11.8). The roof of the soft palate houses some taste buds. The hard palate is lined by ridges that run across the surface of the palate in stripes. These ridges are known as **rugae** and can be used in forensic identification.

Problems during the development of the palate result in a **cleft** palate, which occurs at an incidence of 1 in 700 live births, with an open connection between the oral and nasal cavity known as **velopharyngeal inadequacy** (VPI). Clefts can occur in a number of ways; for example, the palatal shelves can fail to elevate, or they can elevate but fail to meet or they can meet but fail to fuse together (Figure 11.8). In some cases where the shelves fail to elevate this is due to the tongue failing to drop during embryogenesis, which then forms a physical block to the movement of the shelves. If the shelves are too small they may elevate but not grow together, again resulting in a cleft. In order for the shelves to fuse in the midline the epithelium that surrounds the shelves at the point of contact needs to be removed to create a seamless roof above the oral cavity. The epithelial cells in the midline seam appear to do this by a combination of approaches, including cell migration, programmed cell death (apoptosis) and a transformation from an epithelial fate to a mesenchymal cell type (**epithelial–mesenchymal transformation** or EMT). If the cells persist then a submucosal cleft forms. In this case the cleft is often difficult to detect, as the palate can appear intact, but may cause speech problems due to underlying muscle and bone abnormalities.

Cleft palates are routinely operated on soon after birth to allow separation of the

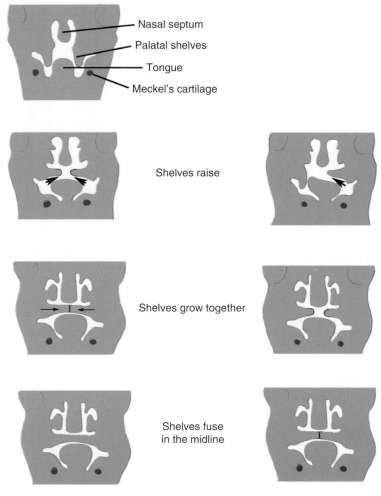

Figure 11.8 Palate development and clefts. Virtual frontal sections through a human embryonic head. Left-hand side: normal palate development. The shelves on either side of the tongue rise up, grow together and then meet in the midline. Once they have met in the midline the epithelial seam is lost to form a continuous palate separating the oral and nasal cavities. Right-hand side: defects associated with palate development. Either one or both of the shelves can fail to rise. The shelves can rise but not grow together or the shelves can meet but the midline epithelial seam remains, leading to a submucosal cleft.

airways as VPI is associated with problems with feeding, ear disease, swallowing and speech. **Submucosal clefts**, however, are often left untreated depending on the individual case.

Cleft palates are often found in combination with **cleft lips**. In the case of cleft lips the facial processes of the upper jaw (maxillary and medial nasal processes) fail to fuse correctly during embryonic development, leaving a cleft. Normal fusion involves coordinated expansion of the processes, with active fusion and programmed cell death

required to break down the epithelial seam. These clefts can be partial, complete, unilateral or bilateral. Cleft lips are repaired soon after birth to close the gap between the processes. Clefts of the lip and palate are often associated with dental defects. Most commonly this involves **hypodontia**, observed in 80% of non-syndromic cleft patients. The most frequently missing teeth are the upper permanent lateral incisors. In addition to missing teeth cleft patients can also have **supernumerary** lateral incisors, observed in 40–73% of patients and associated with the

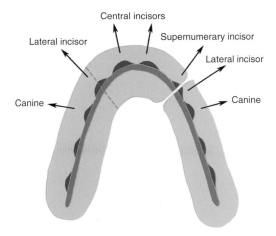

Central incisors

Lateral incisor

Supernumerary incisor

Lateral incisor

Canine

Canine

Figure 11.9 Primary tooth formation in cleft lip patients. Schematic showing the layout of developing tooth germs across the upper jaw with the placode (a thickening of the epithelium) for the lateral incisor forming at the fusion point between the maxillary and medial nasal processes. A cleft in this region splits the tooth placode leading to either loss of the tooth or the formation of supernumerary lateral incisors.

primary dentition. The presence of these extra teeth is due to the fact that the lateral incisor tooth germs appear to be derived from placodes on the maxilla and medial nasal process that normally fuse together when these facial processes fuse. In the case of clefts the dental placodes do not fuse and form separate tooth germs on either side of the cleft site (supernumerary teeth), or fail to form a tooth germ at all (hypodontia) (Figure 11.9).

Craniofacial Syndromes

In addition to the syndromes associated with craniofacial defects already described dentists may come across a number of other syndromes which lead to dental defects that need specialist care (examples can be found in Feature boxes 11.6 and 11.7). In some cases it can be the dentist who is able to first detect

---

Feature box 11.6 Ectodermal dysplasia

Ectodermal dysplasias are a group of closely related conditions, of which more than 150 different syndromes have been identified. These syndromes are united in that they show defects in structures derived from the ectoderm, which include teeth, hair, nails, sweat glands, salivary glands, sebaceous glands and skin. Ectodermal dysplasias occur at an incidence of approximately 7 in 10 000 live births and can be life threatening as infants are often unable to regulate their temperature correctly due to a lack of sweat glands. These ectodermally derived organs all share a common developmental pathway early on in their formation, in that they are derived initially from a thickening of the epithelium, known as a placode, which invaginates into the surrounding mesenchyme to form a bud-like structure. In fact, some endodermally derived organs (such as the tracheal submucosal glands) also go through placode and bud steps during their development, and are also defective in ectodermal dysplasias; therefore ectodermal

dysplasia is in fact not just restricted to the ectoderm. These various organs, such as hair and teeth and glands, not only share similar mechanisms of development but also utilize shared molecular pathways that control these early events. One of these pathways is the ectodysplasin (EDA) signalling pathway, mutations in which cause hypohidrotic ectodermal dysplasia (HED). HED occurs at an incidence of 1 in 100 000 live births. Hypohydrotic refers to the fact that the sweat glands (*hidrotic*) are reduced or absent (*hypo*). In addition to loss of sweat glands, patients have missing or sparce hair, missing or misshapen teeth, missing or reduced sebaceous glands and respiratory tract glands and missing or reduced salivary glands. The mortality is particularly high in the first 2 years of life if the syndrome is undiagnosed, diagnosis being complicated by the fact that lack of teeth and sparce hair are unhelpful diagnostics in babies.

The dental defect can affect both the primary and secondary dentition with teeth forming as simple peg shapes or with flat-tened cusps. The enamel also appears com-promised in patients with HED. In addition, the reduction in output of saliva caused by the defective salivary glands leads to a dry mouth and compromises the formation of the salivary pellicle. This leads to a loss of the buff-ering capacity of the saliva in the mouth and a subsequent higher incidence of oral infec-tions and caries. These factors need to be taken into account when treating the teeth of patients with ectodermal dysplasia.

HED can be caused by mutations in a num-ber of genes associated with the EDA pathway. Mutations in the ligand (ectodysplasin) lead to X-linked HED (XLHED), as the EDA gene is on the X chromosome. The mutation is X-linked recessive. This means that females with one copy of the mutation are phenotypically quite normal, while males with one copy of the mutation express the disorder. Mutations, however, can also be found in the receptor for EDA (EDAR) and intracellular binding compo-nents of the pathway (EDARADD). These

mutations can be autosomal recessive or auto-somal dominant, depending on the nature of the specific mutation. Importantly for this pathway naturally occurring animal models are available for study and therefore we know a lot about how this pathway works and the mechanisms behind the defects. Mice with mutations in Eda, for example, have hair defects, missing and misshapen teeth and reduced branching of their salivary glands. In 2003 experiments on mice with XLHED, where pregnant mothers were injected with a fusion protein of Eda (Eda-Fc), led to an almost com-plete rescue of the ectodermal dysplasia phe-notype. Importantly, postnatal injections of affected mice were still able to rescue the defect in sweat glands. In 2007 similar postna-tal rescue experiments were performed in dogs with mutations in Eda, leading to a rescue of the permanent dentition and gland development in injected animals. This has lead to the first clinical trials of injecting Eda-Fc into patients with XLHED, providing a possible simple treatment for a genetic disorder.

Feature box 11.7 Holoprosencephaly

Holoprosencephaly (HPE) is caused by a mid-line defect in the embryonic forebrain and has an incidence of 1 in 200 spontaneous abor-tions and 1 in 16 000 live births. As such it is the most common defect in the forebrain and mid-face. In the most severe cases, known as alobar holoprosencephaly, the forebrain does not divide into the two cerebral hemispheres and there are severe facial abnormalities, including the merger of the eyefields leading to cyclopia, and the absence of a nose. Slightly less severe is lobar holoprosencephaly in which the brain hemispheres do separate and the facial abnormalities are less extreme. In the mildest form (microform) the brain is unaffected and the only evidence of a midline problem is the formation of a single central incisor in the upper jaw. This is known as soli-tary median maxillary central incisor (SMMCI)

syndrome. A single symmetrical incisor forms in the midline affecting both primary and per-manent dentitions. This is mainly an aesthetic problem and is treated at the permanent den-tition stage by moving the central incisor to one side with the addition of an artificial inci-sor as an implant or a bridge. Despite its mild phenotype, SMMCI has been recognized as a risk factor for HPE in the next generation and as such can be thought of as a potential pre-dictor of HPE. SMMCI and HPE are associated with mutations in the Sonic hedgehog (Shh) signalling pathway. This is an important sig-nalling pathway in embryonic development controlling the patterning of diverse struc-tures such as the limb, spinal cord, brain and tooth. In addition, mutations in the Shh path-way have been linked to the development of cancers, such as basal cell carcinoma.

the problem. For example dental anomalies, including supernumerary and impacted teeth, are associated with **Gardner's syndrome** at an incidence of 30–75%. Gardner's syndrome is a variant of familial adenomatous polyposis (FAP) caused by a mutation in the adenomatous polyposis coli (APC) gene with defects driven by changes in the Wnt signalling pathway. Some 68–82% of patients develop **osteomas**, located in the sinuses and mandible, associated with a similar high incidence of **odontomas**. Of key importance is that Gardner's syndrome patients have a very high susceptibility to developing **colon cancer**. Identification of these at risk patients is therefore possible through an examination of their teeth.

Understanding craniofacial biology is therefore an essential part of a dentist's toolkit.

12

Saliva and Salivary Glands

Gordon B. Proctor

King's College London Dental Institute, London, UK

Learning Objectives

- To be able to describe the anatomy and structure of the salivary glands.
- To understand the formation of saliva and the mechanism of secretion.
- To list the constituents of saliva and their function.
- To describe the role saliva has in the physiology of the mouth.

Clinical Relevance

The oral cavity is bathed in saliva which plays an important role in digestion and mucosal protection. The constituents of saliva and the rate at which it is produced vary and knowledge of salivary physiology is important not only for the normal physiology of the mouth and teeth but also when treating patients that have reduced salivary output (xerostomia). Such patients have significant discomfort and are at increased risk of conditions such as dental caries. Recent research has suggested that saliva may represent an important secretion that could be used for the diagnosis of both oral and systemic disease.

Introduction

Salivary glands are present in a huge range of animal species from insects to humans and fulfil an array of important functions. For example, silk is produced by the silkworm (*Bombyx mori*); female *Anopheles* mosquitoes (e.g. the malaria-transmitting species *Anopheles albimanus*) produce saliva containing anophelin, a thrombin-inhibiting anticoagulant; similar types of anticoagulant are produced by snake venom glands along with a range of neuro- and other toxins; and cave swiftlets (*Collocalia linchi*) make a nest using their saliva (which is used in the much sought-after bird's nest soup). The characteristics of saliva produced by different mammalian species often reflect diet; thus the giraffe produces a thick mucinous saliva that allows it to cope with the thorny acacia shrub that features prominently in their diet while sheep produce large volumes of saliva that stabilizes digestion and fermentation of the cellulose-rich diet in the rumen.

Basic Sciences for Dental Students, First Edition. Edited by Simon A. Whawell and Daniel W. Lambert.
© 2018 John Wiley & Sons Ltd. Published 2018 by John Wiley & Sons Ltd.
Companion website: www.wiley.com/go/whawell/basic_sciences_for_dental_students

'Amylase' is frequently offered as a response when asked to name a component of human saliva and by extension it is often thought that the main function of our saliva is for food digestion. Amylase may provide a small amount of digestion of dietary starch but the main functions of saliva are to enable formation and swallowing of the food bolus and to provide protection of the oral and upper digestive tract. To achieve these broad functions saliva in the mouth is formed from three paired major salivary glands – parotid, submandibular and sublingual – along with an estimated 500–1000 small, minor submucosal salivary glands, and together these provide a film of saliva that coats and protects the oral mucosal and tooth surfaces. The rate of production of saliva increases greatly when are senses are stimulated by tasting, smelling and chewing food and the increased production facilitates swallowing and clearance of food from the mouth. The sensory stimuli result in salivary secretion due to a nerve-mediated reflex since salivary gland secretion is dependent upon nerve-mediated signals. At other times salivary secretion is maintained at a lower, resting rate. The mobile but slow-moving film of saliva in the mouth replenishes/replaces proteins adsorbed to the underlying soft and hard oral surfaces and lubricates and protects these surfaces.

Recent research has suggested that saliva represents an important secretion that could be used for the diagnosis of both oral and systemic disease (see Feature box 12.1).

Salivary Gland Anatomy and Structure

Salivary glands are **exocrine glands**; that is, they secrete onto an oral **mucosal surface**. During embryonic development major salivary glands form as initial proliferating epithelial buds that arise from the oral epithelium and grow into the underlying mesenchyme. A **tree-like ductal structure** devel-

ops through a process of branching morphogenesis and canalization. The development process requires a controlled exchange of molecular signals between epithelial cells and mesenchymal cells. The ductal structure of the major adult salivary glands is well demonstrated by sialography, an imaging technique whereby X-ray contrast medium is injected into the opening of the main excretory duct of the gland on the oral epithelium, either Stenson's (parotid) duct or Wharton's (submandibular) duct (Figure 12.2).

At the ends of fine branches of the major salivary gland ductal tree are glandular **secretory endpieces** referred to as acini (grape-like), which are collections of saliva-secreting epithelial cells. The mechanisms by which **acinar cells** secrete saliva are discussed later but the histological appearance of acinar cells is determined by the types of secretory protein synthesized by the cells and stored in large granules, which can fill the cytoplasm. The content of the storage granules is an indicator of the types of saliva produced, which can be broadly divided into **mucin**-containing and non-mucin-containing salivas. Mucins are the main components of mucus, a protective layer found on most mucosal surfaces in the body, and salivas containing greater amounts of mucin tend to be viscoelastic, which is an important characteristic for retention of saliva on oral mucosal surfaces and maintenance of lubrication and hydration of the surfaces. **Parotid gland acinar cells** produce **watery saliva with little or no mucin** and characteristically stain strongly with the routine histological dyes haematoxylin and eosin (H&E; Figure 12.3a). The submandibular gland contains mixed populations of acinar cells, some of which are mucin-producing and pale-stained with H&E. Most of the acinar cells in sublingual glands are mucin-producing and consequently the saliva secreted is viscous and sticky. Some acinar cells in these glands contain less mucin, possibly because it is not fully formed in the storage granules of cells, and have a 'serous' appearance with H&E staining. Most of the minor salivary glands in

Feature box 12.1   Saliva as a diagnostic fluid

Saliva has a complex composition of cells, bacteria, nucleic acids, proteins, hormones and small molecules (Table 12.1) and these components are potential biomarkers that can be used in monitoring of our health and disease. A **biomarker** can be defined as a characteristic that can be objectively meas ured and evaluated as an indicator of normal biological processes, pathogenic processes or pharmacological responses to a therapeutic intervention.

We are very familiar with the idea of blood tests as an aid to disease diagnosis; these range from counting of red blood cells, determining the presence of autoantibodies to measuring blood electrolytes. The use of blood biomarkers to diagnosis disease in specific organs really depends upon the relationship between blood levels of the component and how they relate to the disease process. For example, the effectiveness of prostatespecific antigen as a biomarker of prostate cancer depends upon how well blood levels of the protein reflect levels and disease

activity in the prostate. The same issues must be evaluated when considering salivary biomarkers. Components of saliva originate from **different sources** (Figure 12.1) and might therefore provide biomarkers of different physiological or pathological processes. The great advantage of saliva over other biomarker fluids is the ease with which it can be collected; no needle and no major invasion of privacy is necessary, making it possible to sample multiple times to monitor disease progression. Currently saliva is used to determine exposure to viruses, for example **HIV** or **hepatitis B** by the presence of antibodies. Levels of steroid hormones such as cortisol, oestrogen and progesterone can be assayed to determine stress and susceptibility to premature childbirth. There has been a large growth in the use of saliva to **test for drugs of abuse**, for example cannabis and methamphetamine. It is likely that a variety of tests will be developed for monitoring the levels of prescribed medications, for example psychoactive drugs, to ensure that treatment is effective.

Saliva is an obvious candidate as a biomarker fluid for monitoring oral diseases such as caries, periodontitis and squamous cell carcinoma, since it is in contact with the tissues involved. Some progress has been made in demonstrating alterations in the salivary content of components thought to be involved in oral disease. For example, matrix metalloproteinase 8 (MMP8) is a collagen-degrading enzyme released by neutrophils and fibroblasts and is elevated in saliva from patients with periodontitis. MMP8 and other proteins elevated in saliva from patients with periodontitis might be used to monitor progression of the disease and response to therapeutic intervention. A group of mRNA molecules have been found to be elevated in saliva from oral cancer patients and may be used in future to monitor patients with pre-malignant oral conditions who have an increased risk of developing cancer; this would help in making decisions about surgical intervention and disease treatment.

Table 12.1   Saliva composition and diagnostics.

Cells (epithelial cells, neutrophils)
Microorganisms (bacteria (10^8–10^9/mL),
    viruses, *Candida*, protozoa)
Microparticles (0.1–1 µm)
Exosomes (<0.1 µm)
Mucin glycoproteins (MUC5B and MUC7)
Proteins (e.g. statherin, proline-rich proteins,
    histatins)
Immunoglobulins (SigA, IgG)
Peptide hormones, cytokines (e.g. interleukin 8)
Peptides
Amino acids
Enzymes (e.g. amylase, carbonic anhydrase 6,
    elastase)
Electrolytes/ions (hypotonic, calcium-saturated)
Lipids
Steroidal hormones (e.g. oestrogen,
    testosterone and cortisol)
Small signalling molecules
DNA
Messenger RNA (cellular and cell free)
MicroRNA

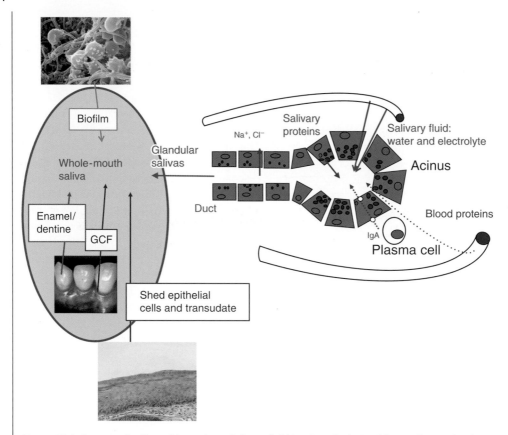

Figure 12.1 Sources of salivary biomarkers. Salivary fluid is primarily derived from salivary gland secretion. Most of the protein content of saliva is due to salivary proteins synthesized and secreted by salivary acinar cells. However, saliva in the mouth also contains epithelial cells shed from the mucosal surfaces, blood cells (neutrophils) from gingivae and oral microorganisms, mainly species of bacteria. Small amounts of blood and tissue fluid proteins enter saliva mainly from the gingivae. GCF, gingival crevicular fluid.

Blood-borne molecules also enter saliva but the amounts present depend upon the type of molecule. **Steroid hormones** freely move into saliva in amounts that reflect the circulating levels of free (not bound to albumin or other blood proteins) hormone. Thus saliva has been used as a fluid for monitoring levels of some steroid hormone. Proteins and other larger molecules from blood tend to enter saliva in very small amounts and the use of saliva to monitor disease-associated blood-borne proteins depends upon the sensitivity of methods used for detecting and quantifying such proteins; as the sensitivity and technology is improving continuously the opportunities are increasing.

the oral submucosae are mucin-producing and the acinar cells stain similarly to those of the sublingual gland (Figure 12.3b). The histological dye combination of periodic acid–Schiff reagent and Alcian blue can be used to stain mucins and demonstrates how fewer acini of the submandibular gland are mucin-producing compared to the sublingual gland (Figures 12.3c and 12.3d).

Following secretion saliva enters the ductal system, moving through the smallest (intercalated) ducts, through striated ducts, interlobular collecting ducts and finally the single main excretory duct of the gland.

(a) (b)

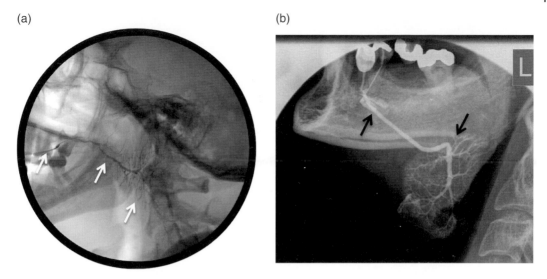

Figure 12.2 Ductal systems and positions of major salivary glands. Injection of radio-opaque contrast medium into the main ducts of salivary glands enables imaging of the ductal systems. (a) Positive image of the contrast medium in the parotid gland. (b) Negative image of the contrast medium in the submandibular gland. The opening of the main parotid duct at the level of the upper molars is clearly seen (arrows).

Myoepithelial cells surround acini and intercalated ducts and provide contractile support to these structures (Figure 12.3e). The process of salivary secretion is dependent upon a rich supply of arterioles surrounding ducts and acini and a rich autonomic innervation with parasympathetic and sympathetic nerves supplying acinar and ductal cells. **Minor salivary glands** lie just beneath the oral mucosal surface in the submucosa and thus have a short ductal system with intercalated like duct cells but fewer recognizable striated duct cells. The interlobular collecting ducts tend to open directly onto the mucosal surface (Figure 12.3b).

How is Saliva Formed by Salivary Glands?

The Salivary Reflex

Afferent mechanisms
Secretion from the parotid, submandibular and sublingual glands is evoked by interaction of tastants with different receptors on **taste buds** located predominantly in the epithelium on the dorsum of the tongue and following activation of **mechanoreceptors** also found on the dorsum of the tongue, on other mucosae and in the periodontal ligament. Minor mucus salivary glands may also increase secretion in response to taste stimulation but perhaps movement and tactile stimulation of the mucosa play a more important role in secretion by labial and palatine minor glands. The submandibular and sublingual glands but not the parotid gland increase secretion in response to different smells associated with food. In addition to taste the sensation of cold or hot in the mouth can evoke a flow of saliva and this is mediated by temperature-sensitive transient receptor potential (TRP) channels, which also respond to pungent stimuli such as chilli (capsaicin). There is no evidence of a **conditioned salivary reflex** in humans, as observed by Pavlov in his experiments on dogs. The watering of the mouth experienced before consumption of food is most likely associated with smell or with muscular compression of the main excretory ducts and expulsion of the saliva.

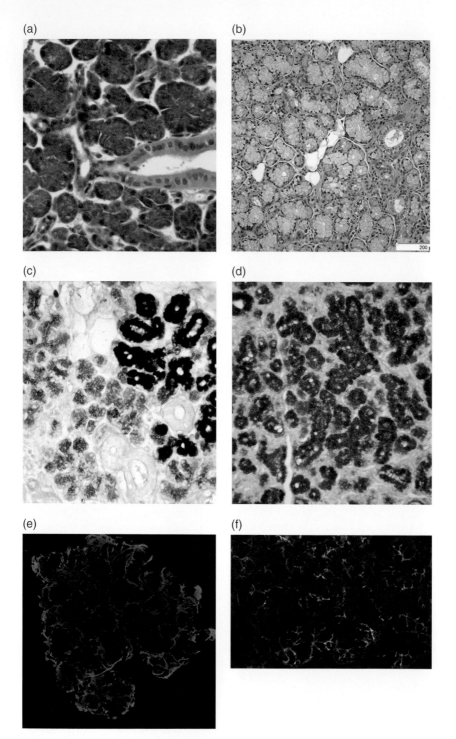

Figure 12.3 Histological appearance of salivary gland cells revealed by microscopy. The acinar cells of salivary glands have an appearance that depends upon the proteins and glycoproteins stored in granules in the cytoplasm. (a) Acinar cells of parotid glands stain darkly with H&E. (b) Minor mucus gland acinar cells contain abundant mucin-containing storage granules that do not stain with H&E. (c) When mucin-containing cells are stained with periodic acid–Schiff (PAS) reagent and Alcian blue, mucins stain dark blue. In this panel the staining reveals that submandibular glands have some mucin-containing and many non-mucin-containing acini. (d) Sublingual gland acinar cells, mostly mucin-containing; all are stained dark blue with Alcian blue. (Note: the images in a–d are taken at different magnifications.) (e) Myoepithelial cells are supporting cells that 'wrap around' the outside of acini and small ducts as revealed by fluorescent staining in this three-dimensional image. (f) The apical membrane of acinar cells is different from the basolateral membrane and contains the membrane-bound water-transporting protein aquaporin 5 as shown by the fluorescent staining in this three-dimensional image.

Central Integration of the Salivary Reflex

Taste receptors in the anterior epithelium of the tongue generate signals in **afferent sensory nerve fibres** of the **facial nerve** (CN VII), which innervate the nucleus of the solitary tract (NST) in the **medulla oblongata**. A similar function is performed by the **glossopharyngeal nerve** (CN IX), which innervates the posterior third of the tongue (Figure 12.4). The integration of the salivary reflex in the central nervous system is not completely understood. Interneurones conduct signals from the NST to the the superior and inferior salivary nuclei which are the salivary centres located in the medulla, and to the sympathetic salivary centres in the upper thoracic segments. **Efferent nerve fibres** from the superior salivary nucleus conduct efferent signals via the chorda lin-

gual nerve to the submandibular ganglion and thence to the submandibular and sublingual glands. The parotid gland is supplied by efferent fibres from the inferior salivary nucleus in the glossopharyngeal nerve (tympanic branch) to the otic ganglion and postganglionic fibres in the auriculotemporal nerve. Sympathetic innervation of the major salivary glands arises from the thoracic spinal cord and the superior cervical ganglion. Minor salivary glands are supplied by parasympathetic nerve fibres in the buccal branch of the mandibular nerve, the lingual nerve and the palatine nerve. Touch and temperature evoke afferent signals in sensory fibres of the **trigeminal nerve** (CN V), which innervate the trigeminal nucleus in the lower pons; interneurones presumably connect the trigeminal nucleus with the salivary centres.

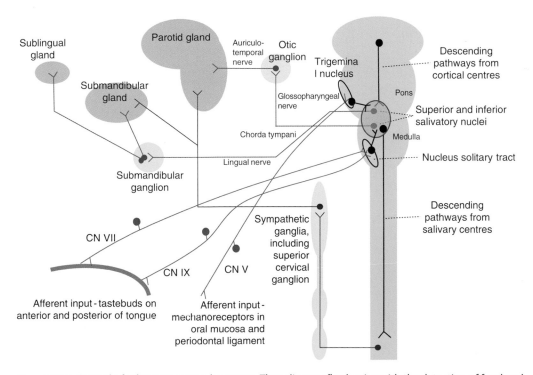

Figure 12.4 Control of salivary secretion by nerves. The salivary reflex begins with the detection of food and tastants such as acid and salt by taste buds and mechanoreceptors on the tongue; in addition the chewing of food is detected by mechanoreceptors in the periodontal ligament around teeth. Signals in afferent sensory nerves (green) are relayed to the salivary centres from where efferent parasympathetic nerves conduct signals to the salivary glands (blue). Sympathetic efferent nerves (red) arise from the thoracic spinal cord. Nerves within the CNS (black) innervate the salivary centres and influence nerve-mediated signals to the salivary glands.

The salivary reflex is profoundly influenced by central nerves from other nuclei in the brain supplying the salivary nuclei in the medulla oblongata. There are various inputs from the frontal cortical areas which can enhance or suppress impulse traffic from the salivary nuclei to salivary glands; this is the cause of reduced salivation and dry mouth experienced during fear and anxiety.

Efferent Autonomic Regulation of Salivary Secretion

Salivary glands receive a rich innervation of **autonomic parasympathetic and sympathetic nerves** which are in contact with many cell types including acinar, ductal, myoepithelial cells and smooth muscle cells of blood vessels. Salivary secretion is dependent upon an intact parasympathetic innervation; if the parasympathetic nerve supply to a salivary gland is cut then secretion of saliva

almost completely stops. The extent of sympathetic innervation of salivary glands varies greatly; the parotid and submandibular glands receive extensive sympathetic innervations while mucus-secreting glands such as the sublingual and minor salivary glands receive a sparse adrenergic innervation that appears to be directed to blood vessels rather than salivary acini and ducts.

Receptor-Mediated Signalling and Secretion in Salivary Glands

Cell Signalling of Fluid Secretion

The main neurotransmitter released from parasympathetic nerves is acetylcholine, which acts on **muscarinic acetylcholine receptors** (mainly subtype M3) on acinar cells (Figure 12.5). The dependence of salivary secretion on acetylcholine signalling is demonstrated in cases of poisoning with the

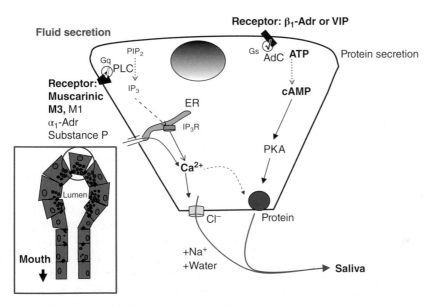

Figure 12.5 Intracellular coupling of salivary secretion in acinar cells. Fluid secretion is dependent mainly upon activation of muscarinic M3 receptors by acetylcholine released from parasympathetic nerves. The intracellular coupling mechanism is characterized by an elevation of calcium released from the endoplasmic reticulum (ER) and activation of chloride release. Protein secretion is mainly activated by release of noradrenaline by sympathetic nerves and activation β_1-adrenoceptors; vasointestinal peptide released from parasympathetic nerves binds to vasointestinal polypeptide (VIP) receptors. Intracellular signalling is characterized by an increase in cyclic AMP (cAMP), which activates protein kinase A leading to exocytosis of protein storage granules and release of protein into saliva. Gq and Gs, G proteins; PLC, phospholipase C; PIP_2, phosphatidylinositol biphosphate; IP_3 – inositol triphosphate; IP_3R, IP_3 receptor; AdC, adenylate cyclase; PKA, protein kinase A.

berry of deadly nightshade (*Atropa bella-donna*), which contains high concentrations of the alkaloid atropine, an antagonist of cholinergic muscarinic receptors; poisoining is characterized by a very dry mouth in addition to the ventricular fibrillation, dizziness and other effects of muscarinic blockade. Acinar cell activation of fluid transport is achieved through increases in **intracellular calcium** concentration and binding of calcium to ion-transporting proteins in cell membranes. Acinar cell muscarinic receptors are G-protein (Gq)-coupled receptors and binding of acetylcholine leads to the activation of the enzyme phospholipase C which generates secretory signals by acting on the substrate phosphatidylinositol 4,5-bisphosphate (PIP_2). This produces an increase in the **intracellular secondary messenger** inositol triphosphate (IP_3).

IP_3 interacts with IP_3 receptors (IP_3Rs) on the endoplasmic reticulum of acinar cells causing release of **stored calcium** from the endoplasmic reticulum into the cytoplasm. Increased cytoplasmic calcium originates in the apical region of acinar cells, where IP_3Rs are concentrated, and is propagated to other parts of the cell through calcium-induced activation of further calcium release via Ryanodine receptors. Cytoplasmic calcium levels are tightly controlled by rapid removal of calcium through the actions of plasma membrane and endoplasmic reticulum calcium pumps which are powered by energy released from the hydrolysis of ATP. Sustained salivary secretion requires influx of extracellular calcium across the plasma membrane of acinar cells in order to maintain raised levels of intracellular calcium and continued activation of cell membrane ion transport proteins referred to as store-operated calcium entry (SOCE). This is a research area where knowledge has greatly increased over the last 10 years.

Cell Signalling of Protein Secretion

Salivary protein secretion by acinar cells occurs by a different mechanism to fluid secretion and the intracellular signals leading to secretion are different; the principal neurotransmitter involved is noradrenaline released from sympathetic nerve endings. **Noradrenaline binds to β_1-adrenoceptors** on acinar cells and increases in G-protein (Gs)-coupled adenylate cyclase activity with the generation of increased levels of intracellular cyclic adenosine monophosphate (cAMP) from adenosine triphosphate (ATP). Parasympathetic nerves also release the peptide neurotransmitter vasointestinal polypeptide (VIP) and binding of VIP to the VIP receptor (VPAC1) on acinar cells can also give rise to substantial salivary protein secretion via release of VIP and Gs-protein-coupled increases in **intracellular cAMP**. Parasympathetic nerve-evoked protein secretion can also be caused by acetylcholine acting through elevated intracellular calcium and activation of protein kinase C.

Salivary Gland Secretory Mechanisms

Salt and Water Secretion by Acinar Cells

The directional movement of salivary fluid and protein into acinar lumina of salivary glands and to the mouth is dependent upon **salivary acinar cell polarity**; that is, the **apical pole** of the cell has a cell membrane which contains different ion transport proteins compared to the opposite (basolateral) pole. The cell polarity is created by close interaction between adjacent cells with the formation of tight junctions and is maintained by interaction of the basal aspect of cells with basal laminae and the connective tissue matrix of the gland. **Tight junctions** are protein complexes formed principally by interaction of transmembrane proteins of adjacent cells. The tight junctions of acinar cells allow the movement of some ions, water and small molecules and are therefore 'leaky' tight junctions. In the ductal system of salivary glands the ductal epithelial cells are similarly polarized but in this case the tight junctions are watertight, indicative of a greater number of tight junctional contacts between cells; similar differences in the leakiness of tight junctions are seen in different parts of the kidney tubular system.

Acinar cells secrete salivary fluid and there is a minimal contribution to overall volume of secretion by the ductal system through which saliva passes to the mouth. Salivary acinar cells are salt-secreting and it is the movement of salt across the acinar epithelium from tissue fluid into acinar lumina that leads to water movement and formation of salivary fluid (Figure 12.6). Movement of salt across acinar cells is possible because of the activity of the **sodium/potassium ATPase** (sodium pump) located in the basolateral membrane of acinar cells which maintains a low intracellular sodium concentration relative to the extracellular tissue fluid. This difference in sodium concentration, the sodium gradient, provides the impetus for movement of ions (principally sodium and chloride). Inhibition of sodium pump activity with the alkaloid ouabain inhibits salivary secretion.

Salivary secretion is also dependent upon a **chloride channel in the apical membrane** of acinar cells; when intracellular calcium is increased during stimulation (see earlier in this chapter) the chloride channel opens and chloride is released into the acinar lumen. Sodium follows the movement of chloride into the acinar lumin by a paracellular (passing between cells) route. The accumulation of **salt** in the acinar lumen leads to **movement of water by osmosis**, most likely by

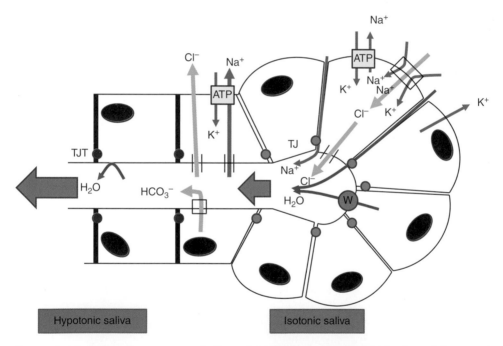

Figure 12.6 Secretion of components of saliva and modification of composition by ducts. Saliva secretion is dependent upon the low intracellular sodium concentration created by the active sodium pump (ATP). Saliva secretion begins with the movement of sodium and chloride into the acinar lumen; water follows due to the osmotic gradient of salt and enters the acinar lumen by moving between cells or through the water channel (W), aquaporin 5, present in the apical membrane. Different ion transport membranes in the acinar cell membranes allow the salt and water movement: a chloride channel in the apical membrane is opened on glandular stimulation; sodium follows, travelling between acinar cells through leaky tight junctions (TJL). Chloride enters acinar cells through a chloride co-transporting protein in the basolateral membrane which utilizes the concentration gradient of low intracellular sodium to drive chloride into the cell. Saliva secreted by acinar cells is isotonic. Ductal cells remove sodium and chloride due to the presence of membrane transporter proteins and the low intracellular sodium concentration created by the sodium pump. The tight junctions (TJ) between ductal cells are not leaky and do not allow the movement of water; also there is no water channel in ductal cells. Ductal cells can secrete bicarbonate (HCO_3^-). Following modification by ducts, saliva becomes hypotonic.

both paracellular and transcellular routes. The movement of water through the acinar cell is possible because of a water channel (aquaporin 5) present in apical membranes of acinar cells (Figure 12.3f). Water therefore is drawn into the acinar lumen and ductal system either by flow through aquaporin channels or around cells and through the tight junctions. The continued movement of salivary fluid is possible because of a co-transporter protein on the basolateral membrane of acinar cells that allows entry of chloride (coupled with movement of sodium along its concentration gradient) into the cell to replace chloride lost across the apical membrane into the acinar lumen.

Salt and Absorption by Ductal Cells

Saliva entering the mouth from major salivary salivary glands is hypotonic, enabling the tasting of salt in food. Saliva secreted by acinar cells is isotonic and as it flows through the ductal system of the major salivary glands salt is removed, principally by **striated duct cells**, and saliva is rendered hypotonic. The degree of hypotonicity is dependent upon salivary flow rate; consequently, stimulated saliva secreted at an increased flow rate has a higher salt concentration. The removal of sodium and chloride by ductal cells is dependent upon creation of a transmembrane gradient for sodium by the sodium/potassium ATPase (sodium pump) located on the basolateral membrane. In fact striated duct cells are particularly enriched in this enzyme and with the abundance of basolaterally located ATP generating mitochondria are well equipped to transport large amounts of salt out of the cell and into the glandular interstitium. Sodium ions are absorbed by ductal cells from the ductal lumen through a sodium channel in the apical membrane and as sodium enters the cell it is removed across the basolateral membrane by the sodium pump. Membrane ion-transporting proteins also remove chloride from saliva in the ducal lumen, across the ductal cell and into the interstitium (Figure 12.6).

Bicarbonate is an important component of saliva since it plays a major role in buffering salivary pH near neutrality and preventing dissolution of tooth mineral, which increases in the presence of acid (see later). Salivary acinar cells can secrete bicarbonate but it appears that ductal cells also play a major role in bicarbonate secretion into saliva. Since the **bicarbonate concentration** of stimulated saliva is many times higher than that of unstimulated saliva ductal bicarbonate secretion is most likely stimulated by autonomic nerves. Other ions transported by salivary gland cells including calcium, phosphate, thiocyanate, iodide and nitrate fulfil important functions (see later). Calcium appears to enter saliva predominantly by being packaged in protein storage granules and released during protein exocytosis (see later). The calcium concentration of glandular saliva does not vary greatly under different stimulation conditions. Phosphate secretion by salivary glands is less well understood but there are phosphate-transporting proteins in membranes of salivary gland cells. Thiocyanate, iodide and nitrate are all actively transported into saliva from the circulation/gland tissue fluid. There are membrane transport proteins in salivary duct cells (called the sodium iodide symport and sialin) that transport these ions into saliva.

Protein Secretion by Salivary Gland Cells

Most salivary gland **protein secretion** is due to **exocytosis of protein storage granules** in acinar cells. When cells are stimulated via autonomic nerves storage granules fuse with the apical membrane of acinar cells and the content of protein is released into saliva. The packaging of proteins into storage granules at high concentrations requires accumulation of calcium ions to shield the high density of negative charges, particularly in the case of granules that store mucins, which are large, highly glycosylated, negatively charged proteins.

Some proteins are secreted into saliva by other mechanisms. Immunogobulin A (IgA; in its dimeric form with bound J chain) is secreted by plasma cells present in the interstitium of salivary glands and enters saliva as SIgA. The mechanism of salivary secretion requires IgA to bind to a receptor (epithelial polymeric immunoglobulin receptor, pIgR) on the basolateral membrane of salivary acinar and ductal cells and the receptor transports the IgA across the cell and into the lumen of the acinus to be released as SIgA, a complex of the secreted IgA and Secretory component, the cleaved product of pIgR.

The Composition and Functions of Saliva

Saliva performs a number of important functions that are essential for the maintenance of oral health. The properties and effectiveness of saliva are dependent upon its composition which is largely determined by secretions from the major and minor salivary glands and components derived from the surfaces in the mouth: the mucosal surfaces, tooth surfaces and gingival crevices.

Saliva clears substances from the mouth, buffers pH, maintains tooth mineralization, facilitates wound healing, neutralizes some harmful dietary components, regulates the oral microbiota, provides lubrication, prevents dessication and provides a barrier for the oral mucosa. Most of these functions depend upon the interaction of the components of saliva with oral surfaces and the latter are very varied, being composed of soft epithelial tissue surfaces with varying degrees of keratinization and roughness along with the tooth surfaces which are hard and composed of tooth mineral.

The rate at which saliva is delivered to the mouth shows a wide variation between subjects. The properties and composition of mixed saliva in the mouth differ depending upon whether secretion is stimulated, by tasting, smelling and chewing food, or unstimulated (Table 12.2). **Unstimulated** is used to describe a state when no exogenous stimulus is present but in physiological terms

Table 12.2 Rate of salivary flow from different glands.

	Resting		Stimulated	
	mL/min	%	mL/min	%
Whole-mouth saliva	0.35	100	2.0	100
Parotid glands	0.1	28	1.05	53
Submandibular and sublingual glands	0.24	68	0.92	46
Minor glands	<0.05	4	<0.1	1

there is always some endogenous stimulation in the conscious subject. **Parotid saliva** makes a greater contribution upon stimulation, resulting in a saliva that is less viscous since parotid gland acinar cells do not secrete mucins.

Oral Clearance and the Salivary Fluid Film

The volume of saliva in the mouth varies between subjects (0.5–2.1 mL) with a mean of 1.1 mL just prior to swallowing. Following a swallow the volume is 0.4–1.4 mL with a mean of 0.8 mL and much of this residual salivary volume is present as a film on all of the mucosal and hard tissue surfaces of the mouth. The thickness of the **film of saliva** has been estimated by measuring the wetness of filter paper strips applied to different surfaces; the anterior tongue has a layer of approximately 50–70 μm and the buccal surface 40–50 μm, while the anterior hard palate has a layer of only approximately 10 μm (Figure 12.7). Teeth have a much thinner layer of fluid saliva on the enamel surface. The rate of secretion of saliva into the mouth and the **movement of the saliva fluid film** over oral surfaces determines how quickly substances are cleared from the mouth through swallowing. This is of great importance to oral health since clearance of sucrose, acid and bacteria is required to prevent excessive tooth demineralization.

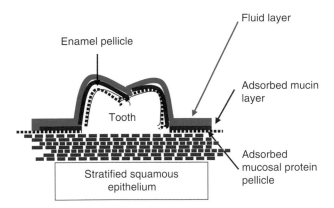

Figure 12.7 Saliva on surfaces of the mouth. Saliva forms a fluid layer or film over all of the surfaces of the mouth and the film thickness depends upon the surface. The enamel surfaces of teeth have a thin fluid film of less than 5 μm while the anterior tongue has a film thickness of approximately 70 μm. Underneath the fluid layer are protein pellicles, adsorbed (bound) layers of salivary proteins and mucin which have a thickness of approximately 50 nm. All of these layers are important in providing salivary function in the mouth. The adsorption of the lubricating/hydrating mucin layer is dependent upon adsorption of other salivary proteins to the surfaces of epithelial cells and teeth. The layer is protective and renewable.

Subjects with chronically dry mouth, for example due to the side effects of medications or the salivary gland autoimmune disease Sjögren's syndrome, are particularly susceptible to bacterial or non-bacterial tooth demineralization due to slow salivary clearance (see Feature box 12.2).

The Acquired Protein Pellicle

In addition to the fluid layer, oral surfaces have a thin adherent layer of protein, a pellicle. The protein pellicle on enamel and mucosal surfaces is mostly composed of salivary proteins. It has been shown that the protein pellicle on enamel surfaces is also contributed by proteins derived from the gingival margins (Figure 12.7). The **acquired enamel pellicle** provides a lubricating layer that reduces wear and attrition of surfaces and has been shown to reduce acid-induced enamel demineralization providing further protection in addition to that provided by stimulated saliva; thus tooth surfaces with thicker pellicles are less susceptible to enamel loss compared to those with thin pellicles. Although the enamel pellicle is reduced by tooth brushing and can be almost completely removed by tooth polishing, it rapidly reforms in minutes due to the strongly interacting calcium-binding proteins present in saliva.

Functions of Salivary Proteins

There are over 2000 proteins present in saliva and these are mostly derived from salivary glands, oral mucosal surfaces and gingival margins. The total amount of protein in saliva is approximately 2–4 mg/mL and most of this total is due to a smaller number of abundant proteins, the most abundant of which are amylase, mucins, proline-rich proteins, histatins, cystatins and statherins. **Mucins**, particularly the large salivary mucin (MG1 or MUC5B) make saliva a **viscoelastic**, sticky fluid and are important in the formation of the film and pellicle (see previous section). On oral mucosal surfaces, like other mucosal surfaces in the body, there is a mucin-rich layer that is protective, providing lubrication (reducing abrasion) and presenting a barrier to microorganisms. The protective properties of the mucin layer are enhanced by the presence of **other innate defence factors**: SIgA, lactoferrin, lysozyme and a range of smaller

---

Feature box 12.2 The dry mouth

Saliva is crucial for maintaining oral health and it is therefore not surprising that those individuals who have a long-lasting significant reduction or absence of saliva suffer from oral disease and discomfort and difficulty in undertaking everyday tasks, such as the normal eating and tasting of food. **Dry mouth (xerostomia)** is more prevalent in older age groups, most likely because it is a frequent side effect of many prescribed medications and older subjects tend to be more medicated; the more medications taken the more likely it will be experienced. Some medications that cause dry mouth have a mechanism of action which can be directly linked to the **xerogenic** (dry-mouth inducing) effect. For example, **anti-cholinergic** medications are prescribed for subjects with irritable bladders (urinary incontinence) since the blockade of muscarinic (M3) receptors suppresses bladder contractions which tend to be abnormal in sufferers. However, since the same type of receptor is important in nerve-evoked secretion by salivary glands blockade leads to a reduction of stimulation and consequently a dry mouth. Other drugs used in the treatment of depression, for example **tricylic antidepressants** and noradrenaline/serotonin-reuptake inhibitors, appear to activate α2-adrenergic receptors in the central nervous system and have a negative impact on impulses in the salivary centres of the medulla leading to reduced salivary gland stimulation and dry mouth. However, there are many drugs linked with the complaint of dry mouth for which we do not have an obvious mechanism of action that might interfere with signalling of salivation. The most severe forms of long-lasting, irreversible dry mouth are seen in patients treated with external **irradiation of the head and neck** for squamous cell carcinoma and sufferers of the autoimmune disease **Sjögren's syndrome**. In patients receiving irradiation for head and neck cancer the salivary glands receive over 50 rads of irradiation and this results in an irreversible loss of secretory function probably due to the destruction of stem and progenitor cells in salivary glands and therefore reduced replenishment of salivary gland acinar cells. In patients with Sjögren's syndrome salivary secretion is greatly reduced. This is due partly to destruction of salivary gland secretory cells as a result of the autoimmune disease but also because of the chronic inflammation and the effects of cytokines interrupting normal secretory signalling in salivary glands. This is a research area requiring further study.

The effectiveness of therapeutic intervention for chronic dry mouth depends on the cause. Stimulation of secretion with sugar-free chewing gum may help in treating medication-induced dryness. For more severe dryness pharmacological stimulation with **pilocarpine** or **cevimeline** (cholinergic agonists described as parasympathomimetics) may be helpful, although unpleasant side effects can occur. Saliva substitutes (artificial saliva) can be prescribed but most of the commercially available substitutes do not adequately replace saliva and so patients frequently resort to drinking water, which is also an inadequate replacement for saliva. Further research is required on the development of **saliva substitutes** that will be accepted by patients.

---

cationic antimicrobial proteins including histatins from salivary glands and defensins from epithelial cells. The acquired enamel protein pellicle is enriched in (phosphorylated) proteins that interact with hydroxyapatite: acidic proline-rich proteins, statherins, histatins and cystatin. These proteins act together as inhibitors of spontaneous precipitation of calcium phosphate ($CaPO_4$) salts and prevent secondary crystal growth by adsorbing on the enamel. **Statherin** has also been shown to bind to calcium in saliva and enables saliva to be a body fluid saturated with calcium and phosphate.

The proteins of the acquired enamel pellicle and the mucosal pellicle are important in determining the microorganisms that colonize these surfaces and hence the commensal flora of the mouth, now also referred to as the the the **oral microbiome**. The early colonizing streptococcal species possess adhesins which interact with salivary protein motifs on surfaces and many of these bacteria have been shown to survive on mucin-containing layers by utilizing the mucin as a nutritional source. There are also salivary proteins, most notably **salivary agglutinin**, but also statherin, mucin and some basic proline-rich proteins, that aggregate microorganisms in saliva and enable clearance from the mouth.

To 'lick your wounds' is an often-used phrase and it is well known that wounds in the oral mucosa heal more rapidly than wounds in the epidermis. Saliva does contain growth factors, such as epidermal growth factor (EGF), that enhance epithelial cell proliferation but more recently it has been realized that a group of proteins called **histatins** is able to enhance epithelial cell migration and facilitate wound closure. Histatins tend to be degraded by oral bacteria but synthetic, resistant forms of histatins are currently being explored in treating wounds.

Certain salivary proteins, the proline-rich proteins, have been found to interact with dietary components that have an astringent (dryness-inducing) property and this may represent a protective mechanism since many of such substances can potentially have a negative impact on digestion.

Functions of Ionic Components of Saliva

Saliva is maintained approximately at neutrality (pH 6.5–7.4), achieved by a **bicarbonate pH-buffering system**. Bicarbonate is present at higher concentrations in stimulated salivas from the parotid and submandibular glands (20–30 mM) compared to unstimulated salivas from these glands (1 mM). Stimulated saliva is therefore able to neutralize dietary acid and acid generated from bacterial metabolism of dietary sugars. Bicarbonate and protons react to form water and carbon dioxide that is lost to the atmosphere since the solubility of carbon dioxide remains relatively constant. The reaction of carbon dioxide with water and the bicarbonate buffering reaction are catalysed by **carbonic anhydrase 6** secreted into saliva by salivary glands and it may be that this is particularly important in buffering on tooth and mucosal surfaces in the mouth. Bicarbonate also facilitates solubilization of mucins in saliva either by its buffering effects or by interacting with calcium.

The total calcium concentration of saliva is approximately 2 mM. Saliva is described as being **supersaturated** with calcium; that is, given the pH of saliva the calcium concentration is higher than would be expected for an equivalent water-based solution buffered at the same pH. Supersaturation is achieved by the presence of calcium-interacting proteins, most notably statherin, secreted by salivary glands. Protein-bound calcium provides a reservoir for maintaining free calcium levels in saliva. The effect of high calcium and phosphate concentrations in saliva are that they limit demineralization of tooth enamel and facilitate remineralization, particularly sub-surface remineralization.

Thiocyanate, iodide and nitrate are actively transported into saliva and appear to fulfil an antimicrobial or bacteriostatic function. Thiocyanate (SCN^-) and iodide are oxidized to antimicrobial hypothiocyanate ($OSCN^-$) and hypoiodide by the enzyme salivary peroxidase in the presence of bacterially derived hydrogen peroxide and this has the effect of limiting bacterial growth at sites of plaque formation. Nitrate is reduced to nitrite by bacteria which colonize anaerobic sites on the anterior tongue and nitrite has been shown to limit growth of oral bacteria. The generation of nitrite by oral bacteria has recently be shown to also play a role in moderating systemic blood pressure and vasodilation of small vessels through the relaxation of endothelial cells. Nitrite is actively absorbed through the stomach mucosa upon swallowing and transported into the bloodstream. In fact, a nitrate cycle is operating in the body, since dietary nitrate is actively absorbed in the stomach, transported in the bloodstream and actively absorbed by salivary glands to be transported into saliva; thus high-nitrate-containing foods such as beetroot have been shown to have a beneficial effect in lowering blood pressure. It is increasingly apparent that saliva plays an important role in moderating taste and food preferences. Unstimulated saliva has a low salt concentration relative to other body fluids, allowing detection of lower levels of dietary salt by receptors in taste buds.

13

Introduction to Dental Materials

Paul V. Hatton and Cheryl A. Miller

School of Clinical Dentistry, University of Sheffield, Sheffield, UK

Learning Objectives

- To understand the nature of chemical bonding.
- To be able to describe the microstructure of metals, alloys, ceramics, glasses, polymers and composites.
- To be able to describe the physical and mechanical properties of commonly used dental materials.
- To be aware of the legal, regulatory, safety and biocompatibility issues in relation to dental materials.

Clinical Relevance

It is essential for dentists restoring teeth to have a thorough understanding of the physical and chemical properties of these materials including their appearance, compatibility with each other with sound tooth structure and ability to withstand the challenging environment of the mouth over time. This information will not only inform their choice of material but prepare them for future developments in a very active research field.

Introduction

The healthy human tooth is a complex structure that performs a number of important functions related to the ingestion of food and communication. The role of teeth in eating is primarily mechanical and includes biting and mastication. In addition to this important function, teeth have an important role in speech where specific sounds require contact between soft tissues, such as the tongue, and teeth. Finally, healthy teeth are associated with the human smile as well as other facial expressions, and there is a strong psychosocial relationship between the appearance of teeth and a sense of well-being in an individual. These important functions are not, however, the only determinants of the properties of an ideal dental restorative material. The oral environment represents a

---

Basic Sciences for Dental Students, First Edition. Edited by Simon A. Whawell and Daniel W. Lambert.
© 2018 John Wiley & Sons Ltd. Published 2018 by John Wiley & Sons Ltd.
Companion website: www.wiley.com/go/whawell/basic_sciences_for_dental_students

very challenging environment for a synthetic material. It is moist due to the flow of saliva, subject to temperature fluctuations and the pH may fall to below 4.0 following ingestion of certain substances such as carbonated drinks. Moreover, the mechanical forces generated in the mouth when biting may far exceed 500 Newtons. Finally, the mouth and tooth surfaces are colonized by a large number of microorganisms that have the potential to damage synthetic materials, for example by releasing the acidic products of microbial metabolism.

When teeth are damaged by trauma or disease, they become increasingly unable to perform the important functions identified above. It is also very likely that the patient will experience discomfort or even considerable pain. Untreated, dental problems rarely resolve, and it is far more likely that teeth will continue to deteriorate and progress to a more serious problem such as the development of an abscess. It is vital then that the modern dentist has available a range of effective dental materials and related technologies to treat trauma, disease or congenital abnormalities when presented. The ideal dental restorative material must restore function including aesthetics, and provide a durable repair that will continue to perform for many years in a demanding environment.

The subject of dental materials science is concerned primarily with the synthetic materials used to repair or replace tooth tissue. It also, however, encompasses those materials used elsewhere in the repair of other oral tissues, and materials used to assist the dental team in their treatments (Feature box 13.1). The subject also interfaces with other emerging technologies, most importantly the development of new advanced manufacturing methods and related advances in the field of 'digital dentistry'. Finally, dentists and allied healthcare professionals have to also understand that there are legal and regulatory requirements that impact directly on their use of dental materials, and these have important implications for both purchasing and clinical selection.

To summarize, the oral cavity is an exceptionally demanding and hostile environment for any synthetic substance, yet dental materials make an enormous contribution to the successful treatment of many millions of patients each year. The reasons for this success are complex and multifaceted, and include the manufacture of good-quality materials by industry, an effective regulatory environment (at least in the developed world) and ongoing innovation to improve performance. However, it is the dentist and their team that make the most important

---

Feature box 13.1 Dental implants

Dental implants, which are also sometimes referred to as endosseous implants, are medical devices that are placed directly into the jaw or skull bones to support a prosthesis, for example a crown, bridge or denture or in some cases a facial prosthesis. Although ceramics such as alumina and zirconia have been used to produce dental implants, mainly due to their superior aesthetics, titanium implants are by far the market leader accounting for the majority of implants placed.

Titanium is a highly reactive metal and will react within millisecond to form an oxide layer when exposed to air. It is this layer that permits the implant to osseointegrate (bone growth within extremely close proximity to the implant without fibrous tissue).

A significant amount of research has been aimed at enhancing osseointegration; mostly this involves increasing the surface area of the titania (titanium dioxide) layer by the introduction of pores or roughness. For example, Nobel Biocare's TiUnit® surface is produced by electrochemical treatment whereas Straumann's SLA® implant surface is the result of sand blasting with large grit before acid etching with hydrochloric and sulphuric acids.

contribution through their excellent knowledge of the materials they are handling, knowledge that underpins the safe and effective use of dental materials. It may be argued that 'dental materials' is therefore the most important subject related to basic science in the undergraduate curriculum. Knowledge of materials science helps to explain the properties of materials, and therefore the structure–property relationships in dental materials systems that underpin the successful and durable repair of tooth tissue in a challenging environment. Knowledge of materials science will also prepare the dentist for lifelong learning throughout their career, which is essential given the inevitable changes in materials and health technologies that will impact on the clinic in the decades to come.

The Structure of Matter

All materials are built from atoms and understanding how these atoms form a solid (atomic structure) is key to understanding the physical and chemical properties of the material. Moreover, atomic level substitution or manipulation can dramatically change the properties of a material. Therefore to truly comprehend and appreciate the properties of materials, the atomic structure and thus atomic bonding must first be understood.

There are many types of bonds which can be grouped into two categories: primary and secondary. Primary bonds are **covalent**, **ionic** and **metallic bonds** and secondary bonds, which are weaker, include **van der Waals'** and **hydrogen bonds**.

Covalent Bonds

Covalent bonds are the strongest bonds and are formed when electrons are shared between elements, resulting in strong compounds. These directional bonds enable the constituent elements to attain the stable inert gas structure. Diamond, the hardest-known naturally occurring material on Earth, is created from covalent bonds between carbon atoms arranged in a 3D structure.

Ionic Bonds

Ionic bonds are non-directional and formed from the donation and acceptance of electrons between elements, giving rise to compounds. For example, to become stable, an atom such as sodium loses an electron and chlorine gains an electron. Hence if sodium and chlorine are able to interact the compound sodium chloride, $NaCl$, is formed from the electrostatic attraction and hence there are ionic bonds between positively charged Na^+ ions and negatively charged Cl^- ions.

Metallic Bonds

Not surprisingly metallic bonds are found only in metals. Metallic bonding is non-directional and is where the electropositive metal atoms give up their valence electrons. The negatively charged ions form a sea of free electrons around the positively charged ions. These free electrons are more or less able to freely move through the solid which gives metals their high electrical and thermal conductivities.

Van der Waals' Bonds

Van der Waals' forces are a result of electrostatic attraction or repulsion between molecular entities other than those due to bond formation or to the electrostatic interaction of ions or of ionic groups. Van der Waals' forces arise from three types of interaction: dipole–dipole, dipole–induced dipole and London (instantaneous induced dipole–induced dipole) forces.

Hydrogen Bonds

Hydrogen bonds are permanent dipole–dipole interactions and are the bonds between hydrogen atoms and atoms of the most electronegative elements such as nitrogen, oxygen and fluorine.

The Nature of Materials and Examples in Dentistry

Metals and Alloys

Metal and metallic alloys are used widely in dentistry. Dental amalgam, an alloy of metals such as silver, tin, copper and mercury, is widely used as a filling material; crowns are constructed from alloys of gold, platinum or palladium; orthodontic braces are generally made from steel alloys and dental implants from titanium.

Metals are solid (the exception being mercury) materials (elements, compounds or alloys) that are usually hard, opaque, lustrous and good conductors of heat and electricity. Metals are generally malleable, and hence can be cold worked (mechanically shaped by hammering, pressing rolling or drawing through a die at ambient temperature without breaking or cracking). They can also be cast (heated until molten and poured) and produced by amalgamation.

Microstructure of Metals

When a metal is cooled, it solidifies by a process called **crystallization**, which can be either **homogeneous**, resulting in single-crystal metals, or, more commonly, **heterogeneous nucleation**. In the latter, an impurity in the metal acts as a nucleus from which the crystals will grow in the form of spherulites or dendrites. The crystal will continue to grow until the grains impinge on each other at the grain boundaries and all the material has solidified. In many circumstances, a finer-grained material is preferable; this can be achieved by rapid cooling or the use of grain-refining agents that increase the number of nucleation sites.

The atoms of metallic structures within the grains are close-packed and arranged in regular 3D lattices. Generally the atoms are in perfect crystal structures, but occasionally an irregular defect occurs, knows as a dislocation. Under very high stress a dislocation will move through the lattice until it reaches a grain boundary.

When force is applied at ambient temperature to deform a metal it is know as **cold working**, which is often in the form of drawing or rolling. The ability to cold work a metal is directly related to its plasticity, the extent to which the material can be deformed without fracture. When the applied force is tensile, the maximum degree of extension gives a measure of the metal's ductility. This is often characterized by the metal's ability to be drawn into a wire. When a metal is hammered or rolled into a sheet (i.e. deformation under compressive stress) we exploit the material's **malleability**.

Alloys

Alloys are a mixture of two or more metals or a metal and a non-metal, produced by melting the components together. Upon cooling the alloy can form one of three solid phases: a solid solution, a mixture or an intermetallic compound.

A **solid solution** is a homogeneous mixture of the constituents at the atomic level to form a mixed crystal lattice. There are two types of solid solution: substitutional and interstitial. In substitutional solid solutions the atoms of one starting crystal replace those of the other. These may occur when the atoms have similar valencies, sizes and crystal structure, for example an alloy of gold and copper. If, however, there is a large difference in atomic size of the components, the smaller atoms are able to occupy positions normally vacant in the lattice of the larger atoms. This is known as an interstitial solid solution, an example being carbon in iron, forming 'carbon steel'.

Solid solution alloys can also be a combination of substitutional and interstitial solutions. Stainless steel is an excellent example as the carbon atoms fit into the lattice interstices and some of the iron atoms are replaced with nickel and chromium atoms.

The constituents may be soluble over the complete range of compositions or over a specific finite range. Solid solution alloys are useful as their properties can be tailored for specific applications by altering the relative amounts of each constituent and/or the temperature at which the liquid is solidified.

An alloy **mixture** is when two or more substances are combined but each component retains its original chemical characteristics.

Intermetallic Compounds

When a metallic solution solidifies, alloys of two or more metals that have a limited mutual solubility may form new phases at certain ratios. These new phases are known as intermetallics or intermetallic compounds and have crystal structures different from their constituent metals. The phases exist in distinct local environments and often are of well-defined, fixed stoichiometries. Dental amalgam may contain the intermetallic phases of silver or copper and tin in the form of Ag_3Sn and Cu_3Sn.

Ceramic and Glasses

Ceramics
Ceramics are inorganic, non-metallic compounds that are usually crystalline in nature, although occasionally the term ceramic is used to encompass inorganic amorphous materials (i.e. glasses). This section refers only to crystalline ceramic materials; amorphous materials are described in the following section.

Ceramics are brittle, hard materials with high melting points. Therefore they are weak in tension, but have very high compressive strengths. They have an ordered 3D structure and are both covalently and ionically bonded compounds of typically metal ions and non-metal ions, such as those of carbon, nitrogen, oxygen, phosphorous or sulphur.

In contrast with metals and most glass production that is achieved via melting, ceramic articles are produced from powders in several stages:

1) powder synthesis,
2) preconsolidation processing (milling/grading/additives),
3) compaction or shape forming (to produce what is known as a 'green body'),

4) drying,
5) densification (sintering).

Dry pressing, isostatic pressing, plastic forming, extrusion, injection moulding, slip casting and tape casting are all methods used in ceramic processing to produce the **green body** ready for drying and sintering.

Ceramics are used widely in dentistry, for example porcelain is used for crowns, bridges and veneers; and alumia and zirconia for cores.

Glasses
Glasses are hard, brittle, non-crystalline solids that have no long-range order, although they do possess short-range order. To understand the fundamentals of glass formation, it is necessary to consider the changes in volume with respect to temperature of a liquid (Figure 13.1). Starting at high temperature (a), cooling the liquid (line a–b) results in a gradual decrease in the volume (with the exception of hydrogen-bonded liquids) until the melting point (T_m) is reached. Below this point crystallization may occur, but only if there are sufficient nuclei present and a high-enough crystal growth rate. During crystallization there is a significant decrease in volume (along the line b–c) as the atoms/molecules become ordered. Upon further cooling the material becomes more dense (c–d) until crystallization is complete.

If crystallization does not occur just below T_m, the liquid passes into a supercooled state. The volume continues to decrease gradually with temperature, due to rearrangement of the atoms/molecules in the liquid. As viscosity increases, the atoms in the liquid become less and less mobile until they cannot rearrange themselves fast enough to reach the equilibrium volume characteristic of that temperature. The glass state line then departs from the supercooled liquid line (a–b–e) as the atoms are essentially 'frozen' in position and into a fixed configuration. The glass transformation range is the range of temperatures near where the volume/temperature relation departs from the supercooled liquid line (a–b–e) and follows the glass line.

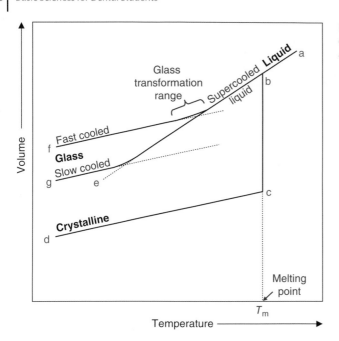

Figure 13.1 The volume/temperature diagram for a glass-forming liquid. Letters are referred to in the text.

The glass line is often fairly straight with a gradient similar to that of the crystallization line (c–d). The material is in the glassy state at point f when fast cooled and point g when cooled more slowly.

The disordered nature of a glass is best explained with reference to silica (SiO_2) that can exist in several crystalline forms and as an amorphous material. The crystalline forms of SiO_2 are based on SiO_4 tetrahedra joined at their corners. Vitreous silica also contains SiO_4 tetrahedra joined at their corners, but the relative orientations of the neighbouring tetrahedra that are variable in the glassy state but constant in the crystalline material. This difference is shown schematically in Figure 13.2, which is a two-dimensional representation of silica. Both crystalline and glassy forms are composed of SiO_3 triangles joined at the corners; the glass has disorder due to changes in Si–O–Si angles (bond angles) and a slight change in bond length (see Figure 13.3).

Two factors govern the ability of a substance to form a glass: its chemical composition and the rate of cooling from the melt. These factors determine whether or not crystal nucleation and growth will occur during cooling and hence whether glass will form. Glass melting is not the only way of producing a glass; other methods include the sol–gel route and vapour deposition. An example of a glass used in dentistry is 45S5 Bioglass® which is used in periodontology under the commercial name of PerioGlas® and as NovaMin® as a component in toothpaste (see Feature box 13.2 for more details).

Glass-Ceramics

Crystallization must be avoided to form a glass. However, glass-ceramics may be produced when nucleation and growth are controlled. Crystallization is achieved by subjecting a suitable glass to a specific heat-treatment schedule. This results in the nucleation and growth of one or more crystal phases within a glassy matrix. The degree of crystallinity can be controlled depending on the specific application, and is usually in the range of 90–99% with the remaining percentage as residual glass.

A significant advantage of glass-ceramics over other materials is their ability to be formed into complex shapes by traditional glass-forming techniques such as casting, blowing, pressing and rolling. Compared

Figure 13.2 Schematic two-dimensional representation of the structure of silica SiO$_2$ in its (a) crystalline and (b) vitreous forms.

(a)   (b)

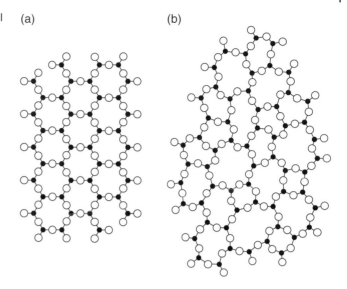

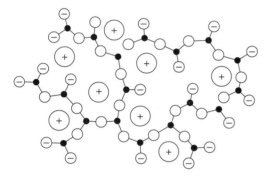

Figure 13.3 Schematic two-dimensional representation of the structure of mixed-oxide glass.

with engineering ceramics such as alumina or silicon carbide, glass-ceramics can be produced at significantly lower temperatures.

Another advantage of glass-ceramics is their strength and toughness compared with their parent glasses and other conventional ceramics such as porcelain. High mechanical strength can be attributed to factors including the lack of pores (compared with conventional ceramics and their resistance to abrasion and therefore the formation of surface flaws (compared to glasses).

Feature box 13.2 45S5 Bioglass

The first glasses found to have the ability to bond to living bone contained SiO$_2$, Na$_2$O, CaO and P$_2$O$_5$ in specific proportions. The most well-known and researched of all the bioactive glasses is 45S5 Bioglass®, which was developed by Hench and coworkers in the late 1960s. It has a molar composition of 46.1SiO$_2$· 24.4Na$_2$O·26.9CaO·2.6P$_2$O$_5$. Among bioactive glass, the use of 45S5 Bioglass is prevalent as it is both osteoconductive (encouraging the growth of new bone on its surface) and osteoinductive (a process in which immature cells are stimulated to differentiate into (pre) osteoblasts that ultimately begin new bone formation). Substituted compositions based on 45S5 Bioglass® have been developed with one of the more promising for bone augmentation being strontium-substituted bioactive glasses that are capable of more potent bone tissue regeneration via selective cell stimulation. The main application of 45S5 Bioglass in dentistry is as a synthetic bone-graft material to augment periodontal defects, commercially know as NovaBone's PerioGlas®. However, more recently 45S5 Bioglass (commercially registered as NovaMin®) has been added to toothpaste (Sensodyne® Repair and Protect, GlaxoSmithKline, UK) to reduce hypersensitivity via the formation of a hydroxyapatite-like layer that occludes dentine tubules.

Feature box 13.3 Lithium disilicates

Modern dentistry demands materials that provide outstanding aesthetics, high strength and efficient fabrication. Lithium disilicate ($Li_2Si_2O_5$) glass-ceramics are ideal for the production of monolithic single-tooth restorations, which can be cemented or adhesively bonded. Ivoclar Vivadent Inc. hold the patents on lithium disilicates and produce a number of variations. The glass-ceramics can be pressed from a pre-manufactured ingot (IPS e.max Press) or milled from pre-manufactured blocks (IPS e.max CAD). Therefore lithium disilicate restorations can be produced by digital fabrication.

Essentially lithium disilicates are composed of silica, lithium dioxide, phosphorous pentoxide, alumina, potassium oxide and other components. These are mixed and melted to produce a glass, which is poured into a mould of blocks or ingots. The blocks then undergo slightly different heat-treatment cycles depending on the final product or shaping method to be used. Pressable lithium disilicate (IPS e.max Press) is produced implementing a traditional sequential nucleation and crystal

growth heat-treatment schedule. This results in a crystalline content of around 70%, where the lithium disilicate crystals are needle-like in shape (3–6 μm long) and embedded in a glass matrix. The machinable materials (IPS e.max CAD) again utilize a nucleation and crystal growth regime, but each step is done separately, as the block has to be machined in its softer 'nucleated' state (or 'blue block' according to Ivoclar), where the article consists of 40% platelet-shaped lithium metasilicate crystallites (0.5 μm). The machined article then undergoes the crystal growth heat treatment, resulting in lithium disilicate crystals of around 1.5 μm and a crystallinity of 70%.

The colour of lithium disilicate glass-ceramics is influenced by the inclusion of polyvalent ions, dissolved and homogeneously distributed throughout the glass matrix. The translucency/opacity of the materials is controlled by the difference in refractive index between the glassy matrix and the crystals. The bigger the difference, the more light is scattered, which produces an opaque material, and vice versa.

Also propagating cracks travel through a homogeneous phase in glasses, whereas in glass-ceramics these cracks may be deflected, slowed down or even stopped by the phase boundaries. Lithium disilicate ($Li_2Si_2O_5$) glass-ceramics are an example of glass-ceramics used in restorative dentistry (refer to Feature box 13.3 for further details).

Polymers

Polymers are large molecules consisting of many repeating subunits (monomers), and they are most commonly generated by the relatively rapid assembly of these subunits in the reaction termed polymerization. Polymers are widely employed in a variety of dentistry applications, and indeed are encountered in many forms in everyday life. Nature too uses polymers as structural

materials, with collagen recognized as a self-assembling polymer that is the most important structural protein in living systems, including mammals. While the vast majority of natural and synthetic polymers are organic (i.e. carbon-based), a number of important systems are inorganic. The most important of the latter is arguably polydimethylsiloxane (PDMS), also known as silicone rubber.

With respect to organic polymers, the most important of these is a range of materials based on methacrylate resins. Two examples of methacrylate monomers are provided in Figure 13.4. Methacrylate refers to monomers (and therefore polymers) derived from methacrylic acid, one the most simple being methyl methacrylate $CH_2 = C(CH_3)COOCH_3$. **Poly(methyl methacrylate)** or **PMMA** is used extensively in

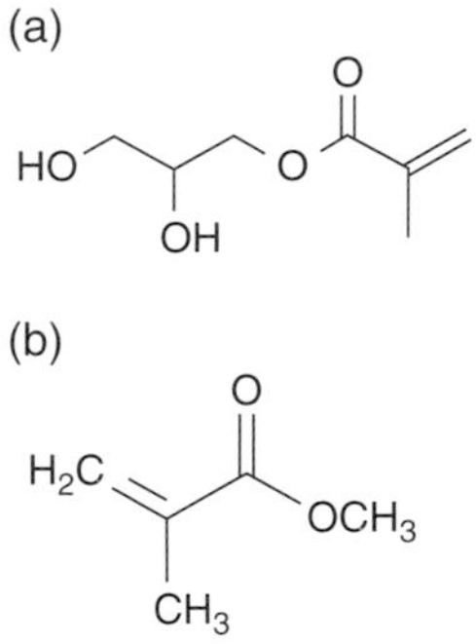

(a)

(b)

Figure 13.4 Examples of different monomers that are used to create polymeric materials used in dentistry (a) glycerol methacrylate and (b) methyl methcrylate

the manufacture of several devices in dentistry including removable dentures. It is used for several reasons including its toughness and its relatively good biocompatibility. It is readily processable and easily shaped in the dental technology laboratory, it is cheap, it may be coloured to resemble gingiva or teeth, and it is also very durable in the oral environment. In addition to PMMA, other methacrylate systems are used extensively in the preparation of aesthetic resin composites and are discussed in more detail in the next section.

Composites

In simple terms, a composite might be any material formed from a combination of two or more different substances. In materials science the composite is formed from at least two of the different classes of materials summarized above. The combination of substances gives rise to a material with properties that are usually very different to the parent materials, and there are many examples of engineering composites with special properties that are utilized for very demanding applications in construction, aviation or other sectors where conditions are extremely challenging. We have argued that the oral cavity is perhaps one of the most inhospitable environments for a material to function, so it is not surprising that high-performance composite materials are employed widely in dentistry (Feature box 13.4). The situation is a little confused because, while composites is a general term for a wide range of materials formed by mixing different parent materials, in dentistry the term 'composite' is most commonly applied to a very specific class of restorative materials. To avoid confusion here, these restorative dental materials are referred to as 'resin composites' in this chapter.

Feature box 13.4 Nanostructure composites

Nanoparticle-reinforced polymer composites have attracted great interest due to claimed advantages over traditional microparticle-reinforced composites. Predicted improvements are primarily attributed to high specific surface area, resulting in strong interfacial forces between the nanoparticle and the matrix. Properties of the nanocomposites and microcomposites have been investigated using advanced microscopy techniques and found to have a bimodal distribution of small (200–500 nm) and large (1–4 μm) irregular filler particles with sharp edges protruding from the surface, a non-uniform packing density and heterogeneous mechanical properties, all associated with high friction and wear. The failure mechanisms were dominated by large particle removal with scratching and indentation. On the other hand, the nanocomposite had a more homogeneous distribution of nanoparticles (40–70 nm) that had a spherical shape, a more uniform packing density, and more homogeneous mechanical properties resulting in lower friction and wear. The failure mechanism was dominated by a more uniform removal of nanoparticles from the polymer matrix. The tribology and mechanical performance of nanoparticle-reinforced composites reported here, combined with their good aesthetics, suggested that they have the potential to become superior direct restorative dental materials.

Dental resin composites are a large family of direct aesthetic restorative materials that are most commonly formed by polymerization of a methacrylate monomer in combination with an inorganic particulate filler, for example quartz. Resin composites are not the only composite materials used in dentistry; other important examples including glass ionomer cements (GICs) and more complex hybrid systems such as resin-modified glass ionomer cements (RM-GICs)

Physical and Mechanical Properties

When a dental practitioner chooses a material to use in the mouth, many factors have to be considered. Moreover, in dentistry many of the materials used are supplied as two or more components that are mixed together prior to use. Therefore the dental team need to consider properties of the unmixed compounds before use (e.g. storage conditions, shelf life), of the components during mixing and setting (e.g. heat generation, setting time, viscosity) and of the set material (e.g. strength, toughness, solubility).

Mechanical Properties

The mechanical properties of a material are used to indicate how the material or component will respond in use. In other words, they indicate how the material will perform in response to applied forces. In dentistry a material or product usually has a minimum value that it must achieve. This is to ensure it can function as required in the mouth. For example, a material must not fracture or deform under biting forces or changes in temperature.

Stress and Strain

The stress and strain of a material can be measured using a classic tensile testing machine. The ends of a specimen are clamped

and a force is applied, under which, in the case of tensile force, the specimen will deform, its cross-section will become smaller and its length greater. The stress and strain values can then be calculated:

$$\text{stress}\,(\sigma) = \text{force/original cross-sectional area}$$

and

$$\text{strain}\,(\varepsilon) = \text{change in length/original length}$$

The units of stress are pascals (Pa), which are Newtons per square metre ($N \cdot m^{-2}$), and strain does not have units as it is a ratio of lengths.

When stress is plotted against strain, as shown in Figure 13.5, other important mechanical properties can be measured, including a type of elastic modulus, Young's modulus, as well as the yield and ultimate stress, and the resilience and toughness.

The yield stress (σ_y), sometimes called the elastic limit, is the point where the material starts to deform permanently under a load. Until the yield stress is reached the material

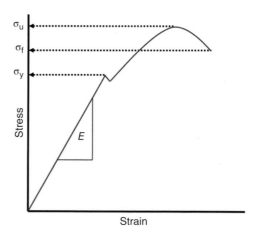

Figure 13.5 Stress/strain curve of a ductile material showing the elastic (Young's) modulus (*E*) given by the gradient of the linear region. Also shown are yield stress (σ_y), ultimate strength (σ_u) and fracture stress (σ_f). The area under the curve in the linear, elastic region is the resilience and that under the whole curve is the material's toughness.

will revert back to its original shape once the load is removed. However, once the yield stress is exceeded, permanent deformation (plastic deformation) will exist even when the applied stress is removed.

The ultimate strength (σ_u) is the maximum of the curve and the maximum stress a material can withstand, whereas the fracture stress (σ_f) is the point at which the material breaks. In ductile materials this is a lower value than the ultimate stress. The area under the elastic region of the curve provides the resilience of the material whereas the total area beneath the whole curve gives a value of toughness. Resilience can be described as the amount of energy that can be absorbed elastically (without deformation) and toughness is the amount of energy that a material can absorb to the point of fracture when subjected to strain. As both properties are a measure of energy, the units of resilience and toughness are joules (J).

Young's Modulus
The Young's modulus (E; the most commonly used form of elastic modulus) of a material is simply the ratio of linear stress to linear strain, and is equal to the gradient of the stress/strain curve in the elastic region. The elastic modulus is a measurement of the stiffness, with Système International (SI) units of Pa (pascals), often given practically as megapascals (MPa) or gigapascals (GPa).

Fracture Toughness
Fracture toughness (K_c), expressed in $MPa \cdot m^{\frac{1}{2}}$, is the property of a material which describes the resistance of a material containing a crack to brittle fracture. In design, usually the yield strength is considered with an appropriate margin, but the fracture toughness also needs to be seriously considered to prevent brittle fractures, which are rapid and often catastrophic.

Impact strength is the capacity of a material to withstand a sudden application of load. The SI unit is joules because impact strength is expressed in terms of the energy required to fracture a sample.

Fatigue
In dental use many products are subjected to fluctuating, often cyclic, loads over a period of time. Although these loads are too small to cause catastrophic failure, the accumulation of stress, especially around a stress riser (defect, pore, point), can cause a crack to propagate through the material until failure occurs. Fatigue properties are either given as fatigue life (the number of cycles to failure) or fatigue limit, also known as fatigue strength (cyclic stress required to cause failure for a set number of cycles). In testing of fatigue (and in service) careful consideration needs to be given to shape, surface finish and homogeneity as these can all significantly affect the results achieved.

Hardness
Hardness is the ability to withstand surface indentation when a compressive force is applied. Hardness is often measured by indentation techniques such as Knoop, Vickers, Brinell or Rockwell, which differ in the geometry of the indenter. The hardness of the material is directly proportional to the size of the indentation and is given as a number. This number is commonly referred to as the hardness number, is larger for soft materials and smaller for hard ones. The hardness of a material can also be measured with a scratch test; therefore hardness gives an indication of a material's resistance to wear (abrasion).

Rheology
Rheology is the study of the flow of matter. The study of the rheological characteristics of a liquid or paste generally involves the examination of viscosity, which is a measurement of a liquid's resistance to deformation under stress. An example of a liquid with low viscosity is water, whereas syrup has a high viscosity.

Newtonian fluids have a single coefficient of viscosity for a specific temperature. Although this viscosity changes with temperature, it does not change with the strain rate.

However, most liquids are non-Newtonian; that is, their viscosity changes with strain rate. For example, tomato ketchup is a non-Newtonian fluid, which displays shear-thinning (pseudoplastic) behaviour; its viscosity is reduced (it becomes more fluid) by applying a stress, for example in the form of shaking or squeezing. Some non-Newtonian materials show the opposite behaviour, with viscosity going up with stress; these are known as shear-thickening (dilatant) liquids. An example is cornflour and water.

Viscosity is a crucial property of the working and setting times of many dental materials that are produced by the combination of two or more components. The blending induces a chemical reaction which causes the mixture to set from a fluid to a ridged solid. The **ease of handling** is determined by the initial viscosity whereas the **working time** terminates when the viscosity is so high that manipulation or moulding becomes impossible.

Viscoelastic materials deform with both viscous and elastic characteristics under stress and therefore display time-dependent strain.

Thermal Properties

Thermal Conductivity

Thermal conductivity is the ability of a material to conduct heat. Materials with a high thermal conductivity conduct heat faster than materials with low thermal conductivity; therefore, the latter are often used as thermal insulators.

Heat transfer by conduction takes place when a temperature gradient exists in a material and is directional from hotter (high molecular energy) to colder (low molecular energy); that is, energy is transferred from the more energetic to the less energetic molecules when neighbouring molecules collide. Thermal conductivity is therefore the rate of heat flow (Watts per metre, $W \cdot m^{-1}$) per unit of temperature gradient under steady state conditions, hence the units of thermal conductivity are $W \cdot m^{-1} \cdot {}^{\circ}C^{-1}$ and it is an equilibrium property.

Thermal Diffusivity

Most thermal changes in the mouth are transient, so we also have to consider thermal diffusivity, which is related to thermal conductivity by the following equation:

$$D = \lambda / (\rho \cdot Cp)$$

Where D is thermal diffusivity, λ is thermal conductivity, ρ is density and Cp is heat capacity.

The relationship between thermal diffusivity and thermal conductivity demonstrates that when transient heat is applied to a tooth or dental material a proportion will be expended, raising the temperature of the tooth/materials, whereas the remainder will be conducted to the pulp. To limit the amount of heat transferred to the patient's tissues, materials with low thermal diffusivities are generally preferred.

Thermal Expansion

When heated most materials expand. The expansion is due to the increase amplitude of atomic/molecular vibrations due to the absorption of heat energy. For solids, the measure of thermal expansion is often stated as linear coefficient of thermal expansion, which is the fractional length change per degree of temperature change. In dentistry it is crucial to minimize thermal expansion mismatches between restorative materials and tooth tissue and between neighbouring materials, for example cores/substructures and crowns.

Exothermic Reactions

It is quite common in dentistry to use materials that are formed by the combination of two or more substances that are mixed together and set *in situ*. Unfortunately, this setting reaction is often exothermic in nature: heat is generated and transferred to the surrounding tooth tissue. Therefore care should be taken with large restorations, especially those in close proximity to the pulp cavity.

Durability

The mouth is an extremely aggressive environment; pH levels can range from around 1.5 (gastric acid) to 10.5 (milk of magnesia and some toothpastes) and temperatures from around 0 to 70 °C; this is combined with mechanical (chewing) and abrasion (brushing) forces. The durability of natural tooth tissue and restorative materials relies on the ability to withstand this environment, and relates to the physical and chemical properties of the materials.

Ideally materials used on the oral environment should not dissolve, erode or corrode. The extent to which a material dissolves in a fluid is measured by it solubility. Classically erosion is a process by which material is removed and transported away, therefore it has both chemical and mechanical components. However, in dentistry the term is commonly used to describe the destruction of enamel and dentine by acid attack, which can be compounded by mechanical forces such as brushing. Corrosion is the deterioration of a material, usually a metal, in its environment. It is an electrochemical process and basically can be considered as destructive oxidation.

These three types of degradation can lead to the leaching of constituents into the oral environment. Therefore it is essential that not only must dental materials not have adverse reactions to the body, but any leached constituents must also be safe both locally and systemically.

Colour and Aesthetics

Colour and related aesthetic properties such as translucency are among the most important functional properties of a restorative dental material. Natural tooth tissue is typically found in a range of shades, and a key objective in aesthetic dentistry is to match the appearance of a restoration so closely to the patient's teeth that it is not easily detectable. An example of a dental shade guide for tooth tissue is given in Figure 13.6.

The science of healthy tooth colour is relatively complex, as it is related to enamel shade, surface roughness, lighting and the environment (e.g. the presence of an adjacent restoration), all combined with the subjective interpretation of the observer. In simple terms, the colour is determined by the different interactions of light with tooth tissue. Light can pass through the tooth (transmission), it may be reflected at the surface or it may be scattered within the tooth structure itself. The off-white, ivory colour of a typical healthy tooth results from the absorption of light that occurs as part of this interaction. Tooth tissue may of course be discoloured, either by external staining by coloured foods, such as tea and red wine, or internal staining that occurred during tooth formation (e.g. tetracycline staining). The staining of the tooth surface is termed extrinsic staining and may be relatively easily removed with an abrasive toothpaste or peroxide-based bleaching agent. Intrinsic staining is more challenging, but can be reduced through internal bleaching or use of composite or ceramic veneers. Tooth colour and the wider subject of aesthetics are important subjects in dentistry, and a key consideration for any dentist planning to restore or repair tooth tissue.

Adhesion

Adhesion is the state or act of attachment of two different materials or substances together so that they may not easily be separated, obviously an important subject in

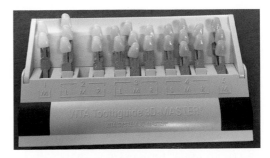

Figure 13.6 Shade guide for assessment of tooth colour and selection of appropriate dental material.

dental materials science where restorations need to permanently remain in place. The forces that are responsible for adhesion in dentistry may include chemical bonding and physical forces ranging from molecular interaction up to the micrometre and millimetre scale. It is such a vast and complex field that 'adhesive dentistry' is considered to be a specific subject within the profession, and there are thousands of published papers including review articles on different aspects of adhesion. In considering the literature, it is generally important to focus on the most recent articles as the field of adhesive dentistry has evolved rapidly in the past decade. The earliest attempts to anchor restorative materials to prepared tooth surfaces were generally unsuccessful because they did not remove the smear layer of denatured tooth, and early direct restorative materials such as amalgam relied upon mechanical retention to remain in place. One early breakthrough in the 1950s was the discovery of acid etching of enamel, but it was not until the 1980s that stronger chemical bonds could be achieved with dentine via removal of the smear layer by acid etching, facilitating the wider use of more aesthetic composite materials.

Safety, Biocompatibility and Adverse Reactions

Dental materials science frequently focuses on the relationship between the chemistry of a material and its functional properties, particularly those properties related to clinical performance. There is, however, another important subject where it is essential that dental students (and dentists) have good knowledge, and that is related to the safe use of a material. The term 'safe' is rather more complex than it first appears when used in this context, as in reality no dental material is absolutely safe for reasons that will be explained. The safety and biocompatibility of dental materials is a vast subject and in reality dental materials are as safe as reasonably practicable due to a series of risk management processes that start with the manufacturer and end with the correct use by the dental team. This section contains a brief overview of the key elements related to safety and the legal requirements that govern the sale and use of dental materials in Europe.

Adverse Reactions to Dental Materials

Many dental materials contain substances that are potentially hazardous to health, and even relatively benign materials may become harmful in specific situations. In 1995, work showed the presence of over 130 common allergens in dental materials. Since then the field has undoubtedly increased in complexity, and it is almost certain that new potential hazards will have been introduced. Monomers, acids, photoinitiators, glass or ceramic powders including nanoscale materials, and certain metals and metal ions found in dental materials are all capable of either direct toxicity or of eliciting an inflammatory or allergic reaction in a sensitized individual. Examples of potentially hazardous substances found in dental materials include methacrylate monomers, mercury, aldehydes, nanoparticles and some forms of ceramic debris. These substances become safe when integral to the dental material as a result of correct handing in accordance with manufacturer's instructions and clinical competency.

Given the number of potential hazardous materials and the volume of dental interventions carried out per year, it might be expected that the incidence rate of adverse reactions to dental materials would be relatively high. However, all scientific studies to date show quite the opposite. Adverse reactions to dental materials are very rare, especially among patient groups. One study estimated that the likelihood of an adverse reaction to a dental material in a patient was less than 1 in 100 000, and determined that occupational exposure was a greater risk (although still very low). If dental materials contain hazardous substances, why are do few adverse reactions occur? The reasons are complex, but may be summarized as follows.

- **Materials chemistry**: in almost all cases the final form of a material in the mouth is its least hazardous form. For example, monomers used in dental composite resins or denture base may be toxic and carry an additional risk of allergy, but when used correctly in the patient they perform their functions in the form of a polymer or composite. Likewise the mobility of mercury is reduced substantially in a dental amalgam restoration, while it is very unlikely that a patient would ever inhale hazardous ceramic dusts from a dental ceramic.

- **Regulatory environment**: most countries have regulations in place to govern the use of materials in medicine and dentistry, and in European member states we observe national laws that are based on European directives in this area (e.g. Medical Devices Directive 93/42/EEC). For the purpose of complying with European law, almost all dental materials are classified as 'medical devices'. The legal definition of a medical device is relatively complex, but essentially it covers all materials that are used in or on the body for the purposes of treating a disease or injury; that is, for a 'medical purpose' (no distinction is made between medical and dental in the regulations). This legislation places obligations upon the manufacturers of dental materials to ensure that their products are as safe as can reasonably be expected and that they are fit for their intended purpose. The regulations also require post-market surveillance for all medical devices on the market to detect any serious adverse events.

- **Dental materials industry**: partly in response to the regulatory environment, and partly because of the need to maintain a good reputation among purchasers and clinicians, the mainstream dental materials industry makes its own important contri-

bution to device safety. This is achieved through a number of mechanisms including the use of a high-quality, traceable raw materials, the adoption of good manufacturing practices (GMP) and other innovations such as improved packaging to reduce the risk of physical contact with the contents.

- **Correct handling**: in all interventions, as long as the dental team handles the material correctly in accordance with the manufacturer's instructions the patient should never come into prolonged contact with hazardous components in such a way as to cause injury or an adverse event. Only in cases of true allergy might a patient suffer an adverse reaction, although these are generally type IV hypersensitivity and are not life-threatening.

While cases of toxicity and adverse reaction to dental materials are very rare, the dentist is still required to remain vigilant, being in the best position as they are to observe an unusual tissue response. Note, though, that general dental practitioners are not professionally qualified to diagnose an allergic reaction to a dental material, and where such an event is suspected the patient would typically be referred to a specialist or to their GP. Examples of suspected or diagnosed toxic and allergic reactions to dental materials illustrate that, while rare, adverse events are still possible with dental materials.

Legal and Regulatory Requirements

As noted, all developed countries have some form of regulation in place to govern the sale and clinical use of dental materials, and in Europe these are based on the Medical Devices Directives. These require all materials to meet a set of essential standards, and approved materials are awarded a CE mark to indicate compliance and permit sale throughout the European free market. Most importantly for the practising dentist, these regulations make it illegal to use a dental material (or any medical device) that does not carry a genuine CE mark on its packaging. Further details on the award of a CE mark are provided in Feature box 13.5. It is important to understand how the CE mark is awarded, and why a dentist should not use materials obtained from an unusual source or supplier where there is a real risk that a counterfeit material has been supplied. While there has not yet been a report of a

counterfeit material causing harm, they are known to exist and dentistry needs to learn lessons from related cases such as the PIP breast implant scandal.

Biocompatibility Testing

One feature of the European regulatory framework described here (and indeed a feature of all advanced international regulatory

---

Feature box 13.5 The award of a CE mark to a medical device

All dental materials are classified as 'medical devices' for regulatory purposes. To be placed on the market for sale in the European free trade area, a dental material must first be awarded a CE mark to demonstrate that it conforms to the Medical Devices Directives. Each member state in the European Union has an individual with the authority to award a CE mark, and in the UK this is the Secretary of State for Health. He or she delegates this authority to the Medicines & Healthcare Products Regulatory Agency (or MHRA), an executive agency of the Department of Health. The MHRA is responsible for the regulation of medicines, medical devices, some forms of equipment and even clinical software used in healthcare including dentistry. It can also lead on the investigation of serious adverse events and other harmful incidents, and may prosecute individuals or companies who are found to have breached the Medical Devices Directives. For the purposes of these regulations, medical devices are placed into one of three categories based on an estimation of risk. Low-risk devices that are intended for transient use and are not blood-contacting are class I, while the highest-risk devices where failure could result in serious injury or death are placed in class III. Dental materials are typically class II medical devices, a large category divided into classes II(a) and (b). Established dental materials such as dental amalgam that were used extensively before

the imposition of regulations in 1999 were automatically awarded a CE mark, but new dental materials introduced since then have to undergo biocompatibility testing as part of the process leading to the award of a CE mark.

To be awarded a CE mark, all dental materials have to be manufactured according to defined standards to maintain quality and reduce the risk of injury to healthcare professionals and patients. To submit a new dental material for approval, manufacturers work with private companies who have been licensed by the MHRA to act in the capacity of a Notified Body (e.g. BSI Ltd). Notified bodies check documentation and manufacturing facilities to advise companies, and prepare a case for submission to the MHRA for the award of a CE mark. It is important to note that the award of a CE mark demonstrates compliance with European regulations, and this is essentially a risk-management process. Risk management can never guarantee that a product is safe and efficacious; indeed, the use of medical devices including dental materials still carries a risk to the patient. Ultimately it is the responsibility of the clinician to ensure that they use a material correctly, in accordance with the manufacturer's instructions and for the intended purpose. Use of a medical device for a different clinical purpose is termed 'off label' and in these situations the clinician assumes an even greater degree of personal responsibility.

systems) is the requirement for new dental materials to undergo biological evaluation to investigate their biocompatibility. Biocompatibility is a relatively complex term that is more than a simple description of non-toxicity, with the most widely accepted definition provided by David Williams being 'the ability of a material to perform with an appropriate host response in a specific application' (from the *Williams Dictionary of Biomaterials*, 1999). The definition for the first time recognized that simply because a material was safe and effective in one clinical application did not mean that it would be so in another. In addition to compliance with national or European regulations, biocompatibility data may be generated as part of a scientific study and/or contribute to a manufacturer's marketing or promotional material. Students and clinicians therefore need to be familiar with this subject.

Biocompatibility testing may be broken down into three simple categories: *in vitro* testing, *in vivo* testing and clinical evaluation and clinical trial.

- ***In vitro* testing**: this describes the evaluation of a material 'in glass', using molecules or more often cultured cells to gain an insight into safety and performance with a view to predicting clinical behaviour. While attractive for a number of reasons including cost effectiveness, these data are of limited value compared to the other tests. The main limitation is that cultured cells are a poor representation of the complex physiology of the whole human body, in particular our homeostatic and detoxification mechanisms. It has been used, however, to successfully screen materials as well as in the investigation of specific cell–material interactions.
- ***In vivo* testing**: this describes the use of animals in research, in this case to predict the response of tissues to materials or their extracts. While it is certainly superior to *in vitro* testing as a predictor of human

tissue reaction and clinical performance, it still suffers limitations. Animals are not identical to humans in terms of anatomy and physiology, and the patient population is more diverse (in terms of age, habits, expectations and pre-existing conditions) than any animal model. This is also a more controversial subject than *in vitro* testing, with several groups opposed to the use of animals in research. Despite the limitations, *in vivo* testing has contributed substantially to our knowledge of materials safety and performance, and it may also form an essential part of the requirements for the regulatory approval of a material.

- **Clinical evaluation and clinical trial**: while technically these are usage tests rather than a means to investigate biocompatibility, the breadth of the Williams definition means that biocompatibilty data will most likely be generated. Clinical trials data is obviously superior to *in vitro* and *in vivo* testing, but are not always as good a representation of performance in practice as might be assumed. The reasons are complex, but include (1) the dentist or dentists involved in a clinical trial may have specialist knowledge of the intervention and the material being used, (2) the patients may have been selected carefully and (3) other extrinsic factors including time available for surgery and availability of follow-up care may be different to that available in general practice. Clinical trials data are very valuable, but are not an infallible prediction of long-term clinical performance when the material is placed on the market.

To summarize, widespread biocompatibility testing is part of the story that explains the relatively good performance and excellent safety record for modern dental materials. Combined with the regulatory framework and good manufacturing practices of the major suppliers, these form a risk-management strategy that have made dental materials some of the safest medical devices on the market today. It must be emphasized though that these practices only reduce risk; dental materials do contain harmful substances and it is the duty of the dentist to use them correctly to ensure patients are not harmed. Moreover, the dentist and their team are in the best position to observe a problem with a material, and no amount of pre-clinical testing will compensate for clinical vigilance.

Conclusions

This chapter summarizes both the underpinning science and practical application of materials in dentistry. It is far from comprehensive, but introduces the reader to subjects that should form the basis for more detailed study as part of a programme for professional dental educational at all levels.

The oral cavity is clearly a hostile environment for any dental material or device, and it is necessary for students and dentists to understand the complex relationships between basic materials science, functional properties and clinical performance. This need is increasingly recognized by the main national and international guidelines on dental education, and most modern curricula also now include consideration of wider related issues including biocompatibility, safe use, and the legal and regulatory requirements for the correct selection of dental materials in the clinic. The pace and scale of innovation in dentistry and dental materials continues to escalate, and continual professional development and lifelong learning are now essential for all clinical and related staff in order to continue to deliver the highest standards of care.

Index

Basic Sciences for Dental Students, First Edition. Edited by Simon A. Whawell and Daniel W. Lambert.
© 2018 John Wiley & Sons Ltd. Published 2018 by John Wiley & Sons Ltd.
Companion website: www.wiley.com/go/whawell/basic_sciences_for_dental_students